OUR ELDERS SPEAK

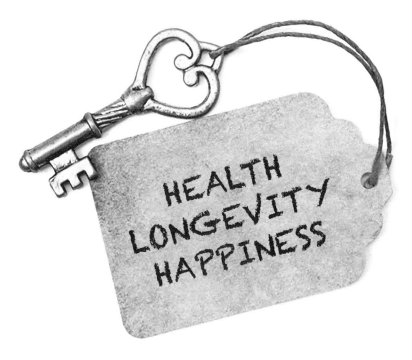

HEALTH
LONGEVITY
HAPPINESS

discover *the*
real keys *to*
vibrant health
longevity *and*
happiness

YOUR MOST IMPORTANT HEALTH QUESTIONS ANSWERED

Panel Discussion with
FRED BISCI, Ph.D.
BRIAN CLEMENT, Ph.D., L.N.
RABBI GABRIEL COUSENS, M.D.
VIKTORAS KULVINSKAS

*Representing over 200 combined years of experience helping
hundreds of thousands of people around the globe
restore and retain vibrant health.*

OUR ELDERS SPEAK
Published by Awareness Press

Printed in the United States of America
First Edition Print 2015

ISBN 978-0-9968080-0-2

Awareness Press
8580 Southwest 21st Court, Ft. Lauderdale, FL 33324

For anyone past, present, or future that wants to live life to its fullest potential, this book is written for you.

"Brilliantly presented! The 112 key questions and answers in a forum format with four elders representing 200 years in the healthcare field makes difficult concepts easy to understand. 'Our Elders Speak' is the ultimate 'go to' manual for health and longevity."

- Edwin Riley, Ph.D. author, teacher, expert on stress reduction
www.stressreduction.com

"These 4 health teachers have changed my health walk and my life. I know the information they share in this book will open your eyes and help you understand what true health is all about."

- Paul Nison Raw Food Author & Chef
www.healthwatchman.com

OUR ELDERS SPEAK

With over 200 years of combined experience as holistic health practitioners and leaders and experts in the Living Foods Movement, Our Elders—Fred Bisci, Ph.D., Brian Clement, Ph.D., L.N., Rabbi Gabriel Cousens, M.D. and Viktoras Kulvinskas—have been teaching a healthy therapeutic diet and lifestyle to thousands of people around the world. They started this movement, this awareness all the way back as far as the 1950s and 1960s with Ann Wigmore. Over the years, Our Elders have refined their teachings—eliminating and adding based on their clinical findings and personal experience—to come up with a very strong and powerful formula for a vibrant healthy lifestyle. Through continuous research and passionate teachings, Our Elders have helped many people restore and retain vibrant health.

Our Elders original message has become diluted and caused confusion. Many inspired people with good intentions became self-proclaimed "experts" offering opinions based on a narrow focus or financial gain as opposed to years of clinical research or personal long-term experience. Unsubstantiated information spread via the Internet.

As a result, not only are the Elders seeing people in their clinics who are sick from a myriad of diseases and conditions, but they are also seeing people who are sick because they failed miserably in their alleged "healing" diets. These people were eating what they presumed was good and healthy, only to find themselves worse off than when they started.

Let us get back to what really works and listen to the valuable lifesaving information Our Elders share with us. They answer over 100 questions in this panel discussion and help you discover the keys to vibrant health, longevity and happiness.

Let's listen closely as *Our Elders Speak!*

"I think that if we can coordinate this information and put it together into one book, a lot of people will start to reconsider whether what they're doing is going to lead to optimal health."
– Fred Bisci

"My hope is that we can help you improve your life and your health and the health of all of humanity." – Brian Clement

"This book will provide an experienced foundation for people to cultivate a deeper understanding." – Gabriel Cousens

"We as a group, have over 200 years of history in the live food clinical, research, personal experimentation and counseling, while observing for decades the results of our guidance."
– Viktoras Kulvinskas

TABLE OF CONTENTS

WHO ARE OUR ELDERS FROM THE HEALTH AND LIVING FOODS MOVEMENT?

FRED BISCI, Ph.D.

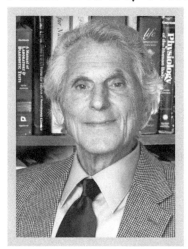

Fred Bisci, born 1929, has lived on 100% raw plant foods for over 50 years. Fred is also a lifestyle/longevity coach, food scientist, detox/fasting expert, and clinical nutritionist. He has counseled and successfully helped tens of thousands of people with this lifestyle approach in nutrition and well-being as well as those with numerous degenerative illnesses and ailments. Fred Bisci's clinical experience and knowledge has repeatedly demonstrated that making a commitment to lifestyle changes is the key to optimal health.

Fred Bisci's history includes hosting his own television show *Eat Your Way to Health*, which had the largest viewing audience in New York City and won the famed Nova Award for best health series. He is author of the book, *Your Healthy Journey (Discovering Your Body's Full Potential)* and has been interviewed and quoted in numerous books and health periodicals. Fred has also appeared on radio and TV shows focusing on health, longevity, exercise and quality of life. Throughout the world, he has conducted seminars and spoken at universities, professional organizations, and business groups on how to lead a long, healthy life.

He has successfully worked with amateur, professional and Olympic athletes, weight lifters, boxers, basketball, baseball and football players, marathon runners, tri-athletes, wrestlers and actors. Fred himself has been a tenacious athlete completing eighteen marathons, two ultra-marathons, was a power-style weight lifter and still leads an athletic life. Fred is dedicated to his family and has been happily married since 1975. He has two daughters, grandchildren and is a constant friend of all types of animals.

Fred's overall mission is to educate people on the failings of modern-day diets. He instead offers a natural, simple, commonsense approach to health, nutrition and longevity. He is a firm believer in this approach and has achieved clinical results by showing people a well-grounded experience to the healing power, peak performance and remedial capabilities of the human body.
www.YOURHEALTHYJOURNEY.org

BRIAN CLEMENT, Ph.D., L.N.

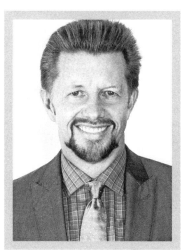

Brian Clement, Ph.D., L.N. has spearheaded the international progressive health movement for more than three and one-half decades. He is the Director of the renowned Hippocrates Health Institute, West Palm Beach, Florida (U.S.A.), the world's foremost complementary residential health center. Over the last half century he and his team have pioneered clinical research and training in disease prevention using hundreds of thousands of participants who provided volumes of data, giving Clement a privileged insight into the lifestyle required to prevent disease, enhance longevity, and maintain vitality. Their findings have provided the basis for Hippocrates progressive, state-of-the-art treatments and programs for health maintenance and recovery——their Life Transformation Program.

Brian Clement has written 20 plus books focused on health, spirituality and natural healing. Among them are *Living Foods for Optimum Health, Longevity, LifeForce*, which Dr. Colin Campbell calls "One of the most important books ever written on nutrition. *Supplements Exposed*, published in 2010, reveals the pharmaceutical fraud rampant in the sales, production, and distribution of worthless and harmful vitamin pills. Additionally, he has authored three volumes for the scientific community *Food is Medicine*. One of his most popular books is his *7 Keys to Lifelong Sexual Vitality* being touted as an important guide to the biology of love. His recent offering, *Dairy Deception* spotlights the hazards of milk, eggs and their offspring.

Brian Clement is a devoted husband and a caring father of four, who along with his wife, Anna Maria Gahns-Clement Ph.D., L.N., co-directs the Hippocrates Health Institute. In addition to his research studies, Clement conducts conferences worldwide on attaining health and creating longevity, giving humanity a roadmap for redirecting, enriching and extending their lives.

A licensed nutritionist, Brian Clement is a graduate of the University of Science, Arts, and Technology where he earned his Ph.D.
www.HIPPOCRATESINST.org

RABBI GABRIEL COUSENS, M.D.

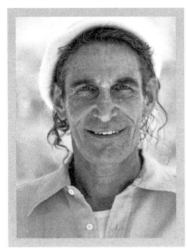

Rabbi Gabriel Cousens, M.D., M.D.(H.), N.D.(h.c.), D.D., Dip. Ayurveda, Dip. American Board of Integrative Holistic Medicine, Founder and Director of the holistic, organic, veganic, eco-spiritual rejuvenation center - Tree of Life Center US (DrCousens.com), Founder and Director of Cousens School of Holistic Wellness (CSHW.org), Founder of the Essene Order of Light and the Modern Essene Way (TreeofLifeFoundation.org), and Founder and Director of Tree of Life Foundation (501c3) (TreeofLifeFoundation.org).

Gabriel Cousens is the author of nine internationally acclaimed books including *Conscious Eating, Spiritual Nutrition, and There Is a Cure for Diabetes*. His forthcoming book, *Conscious Parenting*, provides lucid guidance for parenting a holistic vegan household. Known worldwide as a spiritual teacher and the leading expert in raw, live, plant-source nutrition, Dr. Cousens functions as a holistic physician, psychiatrist, family therapist, and cutting edge researcher on healing diabetes naturally. The *New York Times* calls him, "the fasting guru and detoxification expert". He holds an M.D. from Columbia Medical School, a doctorate in homeopathy, and diplomas in Ayurveda, clinical acupuncture, and holistic medicine. His multi-cultural background as an ordained rabbi, an acknowledged yogi, a four-year Native American Sundancer and Eagle Dancer, and a twelve-year Spirit Dancer, adds insight to his "whole-person enlightenment" teachings. Rabbi Cousens is the founder and rabbi of Congregation Etz Chaim in Patagonia, Arizona. He is joyfully married to Shanti Golds Cousens and is the father of two adult children and grandfather of three granddaughters.

As an acknowledged liberated master he found that the cuisine that best supports the flow of the spiritual kundalini energy is a 95-100% live-food cuisine, for becoming a superconductor of the Divine. This understanding led to his first book, *Spiritual Nutrition and the Rainbow Diet*, which brought the public discussion of spirituality into the live-food movement. His revolutionary work in reversing diabetes naturally is described in the 2nd edition of *There Is a Cure for Diabetes*.

By 1983 Dr. Cousens was eating 99-100% live foods. He found a major improvement not only in support for spiritual life but also in his general physical strength and flexibility as byproducts. At the age of 21, as captain of an undefeated football team, a National Football Hall of Fame member, and All New England middle linebacker and guard, he could do 70 push-ups. At the age of 60, he could do 601 consecutive push-ups. Now at the age of 72, in addition, he can do 33 consecutive pull-ups, versus 10 at the age of 21. Additionally, he is considerably more flexible. At 21 he could not even sit cross-legged; at age 72 he can sit for 2 hours in full lotus.

Additionally, Dr. Cousens' Tree Of Life Foundation Humanitarian Projects are a vehicle for preventing and healing diabetes naturally throughout the world. For his work in Mexico and with immigrant farm workers in Arizona, he received the Cesar Chavez Award in 2013. Dr. Cousens has taught extensively in approximately forty countries on six continents, including Cameroon, Ghana, Nigeria, Ethiopia, United States, England, Canada, Mexico, Nicaragua, Costa Rica, Panama, Peru, Brazil, Argentina, Uruguay, Turkey, Greece, Morocco, Lebanon, Egypt, Israel, South Africa, Australia, New Zealand, Italy, Spain, France, Amsterdam, Denmark, Sweden, Switzerland, Czech Republic, Germany, Poland, Croatia, India, Bali, Thailand, Hong Kong, and Papua New Guinea. His global intent and ongoing service is to spread the awareness of organic, live-food veganism throughout the world for the elevation of planetary consciousness. People have come to programs offered by the Tree of Life Foundation, in Arizona, from 117 countries to receive spiritual teachings and shaktipat, to learn about live food preparation and lifestyle, to study organic, veganic farming, for spiritual fasting, for general detoxification, and to enjoy the healing power and joy of eco-spiritual, organic, vegan live-food vacations. *www.DRCOUSENS.com*

VIKTORAS KULVINSKAS

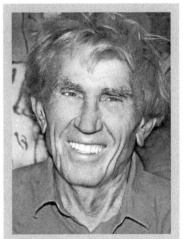

Viktoras Kulvinskas is a Lithuanian World War II survivor who went on to become a college mathematics & computer systems instructor. He was also a computer consultant on notable projects like the Apollo Mission, and worked with M.I.T., Smithsonian and Harvard.

However, Viktor reports he was eating poorly, smoking 3 packs of cigarettes a day and was quite ill and believed he was dying of an autoimmune collapse. Providentially, he became aware of Ann Wigmore and her story of reversing her own cancer with natural methods. After spending time in her program at her healing farm (and recovering), the two began collaboration and eventually founded The Hippocrates Health Institute, with complete dedication to Therapeutic Enzymatic Nutrition for Degenerative Diseases—especially cardiovascular, diabetes and cancer.

The Hippocrates Live Food program has helped millions around the world regain their health through living holistic lifestyles. He is the originator of the popular 7-day instant salad sunflower and buckwheat greens as well as the ever-growing realm of raw seed & nut cheeses.

Viktoras also co-founded with actor/activist and comedian Dick Gregory, The Morbid Obesity and Addiction Center. As Director of Research with the use of enzymatic supplementation he achieved weight loss results for their clients of anywhere from 1 to 2 1/2 lbs per day per person.

He brought the priceless enzyme research of Dr. Howell MD to the awareness of the world, and wrote the introduction to Dr. Howell's book, *Food Enzymes for Health and Longevity*. This propelled the course of alternative medicine, the supplement industry and gave people the power to maintain and regain their health naturally.

Viktoras popularized re-oxygenate, re-enzymize, re-alkalize, re-mineralize, and re-bacterialize the biological terrain for Youthing. He has developed 60 superfood and enzyme supplements.

Viktoras has also authored several books, including the best-seller (manual) *Survival in the 21st Century*. The book documents the successful treatment of cancer, leukemia, obesity, arthritis, diabetes, menstruation, colds, pain and more by using science with anecdotal clients.

Viktoras is a Bishop of The Essene Order.

His other interests and projects include ongoing research in soil-less indoor gardening, probiotic kitchen cuisine and an Essene Biogenic low cost diet.

The father (or now, grandfather) of raw foods continues to lecture, and give consultations worldwide as well as offer retreats in Costa Rica where he resides most of the year.

We hope you will investigate Viktor's personal story and his research, and benefit from his many years of fruitful experience in raw foods, supplementing and holistic living. *www.VIKTORAS.com*

MESSAGE FROM OUR ELDERS

"My message is very simple. I want to give people the maximum opportunity and the tools it will take to develop a happy, healthy and productive life." – Brian Clement

"…an 80% live food cuisine helps one become a superconductor for the Divine. A 95-100% live food cuisine empowers one to be an even more powerful superconductor for the Divine…" – Gabriel Cousens

"My message is to change your lifestyle, avoid processed food and let natural law have dominion in your life…"
– Fred Bisci

"My message is simple—love yourself and love others as yourself…"
– Viktoras Kulvinskas

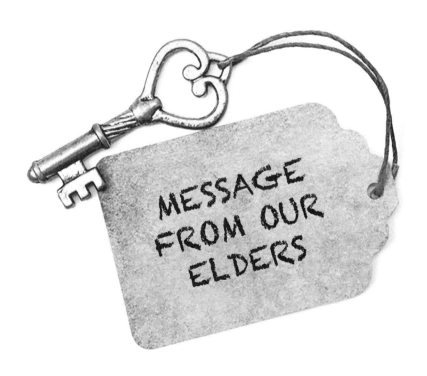

1. WHAT IS YOUR MESSAGE?

BRIAN CLEMENT

My message is very simple. I want to give people the maximum opportunity and the tools it will take to develop a happy, healthy and productive life. If each and every one of us were to find our passion and fulfill it, the destiny of humanity would be radically different than the collision course that we're on today, at the beginning of the 21st century.

As director of the Hippocrates Health Institute—now nearly 60 years in helping people to help themselves—we have seen tens of thousands of people take responsibility for their lives, turn around catastrophic disease, and successfully fight the premature aging process. But to me, the most important gain from all of this is not the health, but the vitality and vigor that are achieved when you find your core purpose. These self-healers go on to become productive members of the human race, contributing positively and constructively toward sustaining not only the planet that we live on, but also the health of fellow humans.

GABRIEL COUSENS

My particular message is a question and a statement. Why we are interested in live foods? The primary reason that I began on the live food path and my primary teaching is that, while one can't eat their way to God, an 80% live food cuisine helps one become a superconductor for the Divine. A 95-100% live food cuisine empowers one to be an even more powerful superconductor for the Divine so that they can best support the ultimate purpose of life—to know God.

FRED BISCI

The health of Americans has come to an impasse. More and more people are developing disease. Many diseases that were unheard of when I was young are now out of control. We are being told that we are healthier and living longer. In one respect this is true. Fewer people are dying in infancy. Surgical intervention, medical technology and improvements in medical science are prolonging lives. Yet, people are sicker than ever before. Our health care system is failing us. We have been programmed to believe that the pharmaceutical companies and the medical industry have our best interest at heart, but we must not forget that health care is a business whose profit motive can't be discounted. We have been,

"Most of the diseases that medical doctors are treating people for are preventable."
– Fred Bisci

and are being fed incorrect information on how to care for ourselves so that we might live healthy lives, slow down our aging process and live a high quality life into very advanced years. Most of the diseases that medical doctors are treating people for are preventable.

My message is to change your lifestyle, avoid processed food and let natural law have dominion in your life the way God intended. This is basically simple. Eat a plant-based diet, drink pure water, get plenty of fresh air and get adequate rest and sleep. Get spiritually grounded, have respect for God in all ways, treat others with unconditional love, kindness and generosity. Eat as many raw foods as you possibly can, respect your body clock and circadian rhythms, do not do anything in excess and be fully aware that we are living on a toxic planet and in a toxic environment. Because of this, we should continue this lifestyle for the rest of our lives, along with ongoing periodic detoxification of our digestive system, our lymph system and all of our organs.

VIKTORAS KULVINSKAS

My message is simple—love yourself and love others as yourself; Jesus, Buddha, Gandhi and hundreds of other teachers have repeated the same message. If you understand the meaning of love, then everything else becomes secondary, for within the word love is contained all that is required for becoming healthy, happy and holy.

I use the foundation of the Bhavagad Gita and herbalogical studies, as well as social, nutritional and clinical experience, to lay the foundation. The Bhavagad Gita discusses three lifestyle choices that are commonly found within the human mass. Most common is the tamasic, which is a simple lifestyle of labor, usually followed with cooked and overcooked foods. Such individuals are not suited for deep intellectual or spiritual work due to limited alkalinity, oxygen levels and enzymatic levels to drive the neurological system.

Rajasic is the second way. The diet is primarily tamasic. However, they are energized by rajasic, highly stimulating foods, such as animal protein, which is rich in uric acids and has stimulating properties and is structurally and chemically almost identical to caffeine. They often indulge in coffee and strong teas, as well as psychotropic and other stimulant behaviors, including living in a world of fear associated with the slaughter of animals. As a result, they are usually in a defensive mode with a drug influence of adrenaline as well as thyroid and disorganized pituitary glandular function. Often, these individuals achieve powerful roles in business and politics but they create chaos and unsustainable lifestyles. They are war-like instead of using diplomacy and negotiation where everyone wins. They want to win the resources, take over a country and enslave others. They are very insecure and continuously trying to accumulate more and more. For balance they are involved in psychotropic medications or alcohol to balance their over-stimulated, fear driven system.

The third way is sattvic. Such individuals are peaceful. They live on nutrition that is available in their location that is created and received the way it is given by the source, found in the trees, in the bush, in the fields, in the grasslands. The food is already perfect and consumed in its raw state for highest alkalinity and perfect solar vibration. It ends up providing high electro-voltage potential for advancement of physical, mental and spiritual development within the context of emotional poise. They are very sustainable and they often achieve high levels of happiness and holiness.

Jesus, the great master, studied under such tutelage in India during the "missing" years of life. His historic message is found in several resources; the Dead Sea and the manuscripts of the Essenes ministry that are found in the Vatican Library and Hapsburg Library as well as the channeling of Edgar Cayce's book, Jesus the Essene.

Besides acknowledging the three lifestyle choices of the Bhagavad Gita, the Essenes had a fourth stage, called biogenic, which optimizes the human potential to the maximum. The biogenic realized in this incarnation their Dharmic potential and the reason for being on planet Earth—no matter at what stage of incarnation the individual might have pursued, making their contribution and moving on into higher vibrational realms. Their nutritional intake is not only raw, but also living—that is, germinated, soaked and sprouted. Even baby greens, such as wheatgrass, were already being grown within that Essene ministry 2,000 years ago.

The Essenes were also involved in the usage of the living food that is found in all forms of microbial cultures. The largest biomass on planet Earth, over 85 to 95% of it, is microbial and they are our strongest allies. The Essenes fasted frequently, one day a week, as well as long 40-day fasts. They were noted for extreme health, highly respected by the Roman Empire for their learning and their extreme cleanliness and wisdom as well as channeling the future. They were also farmers that had a sustainable community in a place where nothing grew before they came, it was the desert. They worked with the laws of nature. They were also great healers, with daily practices to empower the mind and organize it, utilizing the emotional component to empower manifestation.

In my message I have five stages of nutritional and lifestyle development. Stage one is a variation of the tamasic, which is sustainable and leads to reproductive low incidence of disease. A good example of this would have been Western cultures 100 years ago and further back. The food is organic and chemical free, and degenerative diseases appear very late in life. Most individuals also engage in different levels of rajasic type of indulgences with animal protein. The lifestyle is not sustainable from the historic millennium point of view, since it leads to the need of continuous increased grazing lands and territories as their population size increases. The followers of this lifestyle will never be completely healthy, happy or holy due to diminished electro voltage and connection to the source. They can be improved and made more sustainable through the right choice of supplements such as enzymes, which they are lacking, mild herbal laxatives at bedtime, as well as blue-green algae for improved mental and physical development, and, lastly some form of probiotics.

Stage two; veganism as orchestrated by PCRM.org, Physicians Committee for Responsible Medicine. We have seen that by diminishing dead animal consumption, degenerative disease patterns also diminish. Based on science and the clinical experiences of thousands of medical doctors, they concluded that, not only is a properly chosen vegan diet adequate, but anything contrary to veganism is also contrary to good health practices. Individuals who follow this diet enjoy health that is an improvement over stage one. However, eventually, as we've seen at Hippocrates Health Institute, a significant clientele level is of those who practice cooked veganism and hygienists coming in for therapeutic raw food—the Essene way lifestyle.

Stage three would be considered sattvic. The motivation for it is well attested by not only the results we have experienced at the Hippocrates Health Institute, but at all the centers around the world. The value of raw foods, liquid diets, green juices and wheatgrass can't be overstated.

The Science Section of the May 23, 2002 issue of the New York Times featured an article based on the findings of clinical studies conducted by Harvard Medical School, which were duplicated by two other universities years later. The article stated that 100% of people on a Standard American Diet are in a state of inflammatory condition. This is due to the body being saturated with incompletely metabolized proteins, called twisted proteins, which lay the foundation for cancer and heart disorders and over 25 other degenerative diseases. These incompletely metabolized proteins tie up the immune system function and prevent the immune system from doing daily repair work and regeneration; thus, aging and degenerative diseases develop, and, according to Harvard Medical School, most degenerative diseases are due to these twisted proteins.

"The raw foods way—when practiced within a lifestyle habit of exercise, spiritual practice, mindfulness, emotional tranquility, kindness, love and self-realization through meditation—will lead to extremely long lives of health, happiness and holiness." – Viktoras Kulvinskas

The clinical research found in Science News, that I document in my book, Survival in the 21st Century, shows that the incompletely metabolized proteins are the key reducers of oxygen absorption and transport within the blood stream, leading to cardiovascular problems and the appearance of cancer conditions. You can Band-Aid yourself by consuming high volumes of enzymes, and get exceptional results in offsetting and delaying the development of degenerative diseases. However, there is a limit to how much the enzymes can help you. Eventually the toxemia, which is associated with heat-treated products and animal protein will lead to expiration no matter how many supplements you take and how much alternative health care you undergo. The raw foods way—when practiced within a lifestyle habit of exercise, spiritual practice, mindfulness, emotional tranquility, kindness, love and self-realization through meditation—will lead to extremely long lives of health, happiness and holiness. You will experience slow aging and eventually ascension.

The fourth stage is Essenes biogenic youthing lifestyles. In the book of Jubilee found in Survival, one of the ancient manuscripts states, "A time will come when the children will once again study the laws and follow the commandments and there will be no more disease, sadness, and all shall live in cooperation and happiness for thousands of years within childlike bodies." Thus, all the aging patterns have completely been reversed. The foods that are found within this way, as practiced and integrated into the Hippocrates Health Institute lifestyles, consist at least 80% of germinated seeds, some sea vegetables and fermented foods, as well as moderate use of soaked seeds and nuts.

This lifestyle provides the genetic material to reverse genetic damage that might be within any individual and optimizes the DNA code. Every mineral, as an element, is essential. This lifestyles include a weekly juice program, emphasis on some form of daily exercise, development of the attributes of global responsibility, kindness, caring and understanding fully of the loving way through meditation and spiritual practices, having enough rest reflective of the kind of activities in which one indulges, and living in a more sustainable and purer environment. If one decides to live in cities, it is important to use air filtration and all kinds of other quantum tools to minimize the exposure to, and the damage associated with, radiation, electromagnetic fields and the negative vibes of the tamasic-rajasic world.

Jesus never taught reincarnation because he taught the way of living long enough so that there won't be need for it. With this lifestyle, you will have the time to express your Dharma, your reason for being here on the planet, and become a self-realized being in one single incarnation. On this lifestyle you can feed thousands of times more individuals than on any other lifestyle. By removing the muco-phlegm along the gastrointestinal tract, blood vessels and lymphatic vessels within the human organism, one can live on a very low density of nutrients similar to mother's breast milk. Mother's milk, a nutrient that is very low calorie, low protein, and low fat, is provided by nature for the period of the most rapid growth and development.

In 1973, an entire issue of *National Geographic Magazine* was dedicated to longevity. It featured a lengthy study that found that the Huns, Georgians and Ecuadorians in Vilcabamba had the longest lifespans. Their dietary consumption was less than 1500 calories per day, 35 grams, at most of protein daily, as well as about 1/6 of the fat levels that we normally consume in the rest of the world. Dr. Oolong and Dr. Huxley, in a study of a tribe in Papua New Guinea, found that members of this tribe lived on even lower parameters. These people exhibited health, happiness and holiness, and, after extensive examination, were found to be getting over 30 grams of protein from the fixation of nitrogen from the air by the microbial cultures found in a healthy gastrointestinal tract of a vegan. The documentations for these studies are shown in *Survival in the 21st Century*.

The fifth stage is physical immortality. A tremendous amount of research has been done by great biologists such as Dr. Child and Dr. Julian Huxley of University of Chicago. Child, a Nobel Prize recipient, showed that, through the combination of consumption of the optimum nutritional programs for the particular species and fasting periodically, longevity was observed for well over 17 generations showing no signs of aging. Furthermore, Nobel Prize recipient Alexis Carrel, author of *Man the Unknown*, did research with tissues showing that it's possible to go through thousands and thousands of reproductions of cells without any sign of degeneration, provided optimum nutrition was given and toxins were eliminated through wash-like fasting.

Hayflick limit is a gold standard in longevity and life extension research stating that all reproductive cells have a limit of no more than a hundred reproductions before the death gene kicks in and they commit suicide. This concept was shown, by both Child and Huxley, to be erroneous, since cells are really immortal. What we call death is a major stress for most individuals, due to the misleading information. Life and consciousness for every individual is a continuum, going through many different forms, and continuing to re-manifest on physical planes until one learns the lessons and ascends to the next level of vibrational and dimensional potential. The most primary lesson to be learned, that is expressed very clearly, is that we are created in the image of the Creator. Thus, we all have all the attributes of the Creator. We lose this identity through our physical, sensual addictions and becoming addicted to all kind of security issues not realizing that we are gods and goddesses.

Through all these stages, one of the most important parts of my message is the need for meditation in order to discover your true identity. So that you, through clarity and an understanding of your incarnations, will lead to manifestation by becoming aligned to the love resources which can be amplified through the process of prayers and other ritualistic practices that are part of the teachings of the ancient masters.

Unless one identifies with this, in the Buddhist tradition for the majority of people, life is one of misery and suffering. But, if one follows the way, the map is made clear, through meditation, for how to overcome this pain and suffering and discover your true Dharma and self actualization within a path of joy, service and expressing is your divine mission.

2. HOW AND WHY DID YOUR MESSAGE GET LOST?

BRIAN CLEMENT

I'm not sure how our message got lost. I think that there are lots of voices in the room speaking and sometimes economics and access supersede solid, historical, scientifically supported data. Sadly, our world today is governed by money and mass media.

"I'm not sure how our message got lost. I think that there are lots of voices in the room speaking and sometimes economics and access supersede solid, historical scientifically supported data."
– Brian Clement

Slowly but surely, people come to their senses after they have tried shortcuts and half-baked theories. We stand ready to welcome these people when they're ready to take total and full responsibility for their lives.

VIKTORAS KULVINSKAS

In the late 60s, over 50 years ago, I started my own process of discovery, after leaving a successful career in computers and theoretical mathematics as a college teacher. We pioneered the living foods field along with many of the other great leaders on whose shoulders one had to stand in order to get a further view of the future, namely Professor Edmond Szekely of the Essene Order and Professor Ehret of the *Mucusless Diet Healing System*. It took one generation, and we saw the appearance of www.pcrm.org, where veganism was well established. I put in 20 years of teaching the message, and you have to be patient. Then it took another generation, where even Doctor Oz, on the Oprah show, declared, not that an apple a day will keep the doctor away, but, truly green smoothies will keep you alkalized and disease free. The research community is rich with thousands and thousands of papers now showing the therapeutic merit of the flagship nutrient of the living foods scene, "enzymes." The vital chemical is not only enzymes, but also the research associated with chlorophyll - the green factor. These are the two magic bullets.

So I don't think my message has been lost. Hippocrates Health Institute, when we started, had only one or two guests. Now, we have in the hundreds weekly and this is where high profile individuals are indulging in drinking wheatgrass juice. The most popular movement in dietary habits amongst the Hollywood set is raw foodism. The restaurant chains are spreading like wildfire throughout the world in every country. *Wellness Revolution, The Next Trillion* written by a Harvard college professor in the field of economics, points to the direction that the new biggest trend to step into this millennium, into this decade, is the healthcare revolution through complementary, alternative and, especially, the holistic approach. This is where the big money is going to be happening, with over 80% of the world population sick with incurable diseases.

So, when you see an issue of *French Vogue Magazine* with Gisele Bundchen, (my friend and neighbor) on the cover, with an excellent article in which she raves about raw foods, the knowledge spreads. When Wimbledon Champion Venus Williams was forced to retire due to degenerative conditions in 2012, she did the Hippocrates program for eight months, then came back as a top tennis competitor. In light of these two striking examples, how can one even think of raising a question about how the message got lost? The message is growing at an exponential rate.

Karynraw.com who has inspired all these raw food restaurants in the USA does detox classes every month, with hundreds of participants. Their statistics show that when people come in from the mainstream S.A.D. (Standard American Diet) and the fast foods, almost a 100% of them become vegan. Is that considered a lost message? Only 4% stay on raw foods. Those are understandable statistics. What we see is this message is being taken deeply into the hearts of America, because there is no other way out. Cleanse and detoxify with raw foods for healing. The Hippocrates message that we have orchestrated is an evaluation of what is considered a successful raw foodist lifestyle; that being 80% raw will keep you extremely healthy, with high life expectations and performance.

Over 80% of people in the USA are addicted to caffeine, sugar, alcohol, street drugs, pharmaceutical drugs, work, pornography and gambling. A study, which was done of 170 nations, found that the United States was around 150th in terms of happiness. Costa Rica, interestingly enough, was third. Being unhappy means you're not comfortable with yourself and you look for all kinds addictive behaviors to distract the mind from being aware of your own unhappiness. On this path, you look for comfort food and we are seeing this in an epidemic proportion.

This state of affairs provides a big opportunity for the live food community to set up detox centers to help individuals in a fashion similar to Alcoholic Anonymous. Create centers with structured programs where individuals can follow a 12-step program to break the habit of indulging in these so-called comfort foods. You can be part of this revolution by creating your center of activity; be of service to the world. Give with love, kindness and personal life experience by being immersed and reflecting the movement.

GABRIEL COUSENS

The message has not been lost. People who are interested in spiritual life understand the message and understand the confusion that people involved in live foods from a materialistic perspective have created. They find the message that I'm giving about live food to be a breath of fresh air and feel very supported by it. In other words, the message is expanding.

My message, which was more or less revealed in my first book, *Spiritual Nutrition and the Rainbow Diet*, in 1986, actually upgraded the popular primary motivations of health and energy in the live food movement. It allowed people to understand that, if thoughtfully designed, a live food cuisine could help support life's ultimate purpose. I do not believe the message has been lost. I believe it has become the background in a variety of live food circles.

At the same time, I'm aware that there are many people who continue to see live foods from a strictly materialistic viewpoint—about "body beautiful"—about strength, power, and energy. I also think that's okay, because they are not ready to see it from a higher life purpose level. When they are ready, they will be able to fall back on the support that's been established. Live food is the most powerful cuisine to support spiritual life.

FRED BISCI

I think this message got lost because there is so much vested interest that obscures the truth. Processed food giants came in, and, the tastier the processed food became, the more addictive it became. Then advertising and television compounded the confusion. If you look at television now, there are all kinds of things they're trying to sell you, from pharmaceuticals, to drugs, to neutraceuticals. They're trying to convince you that you need all these processed foods to be healthy. People get into this trap where they don't feel good and they don't realize how to eliminate the cause of their disease.

The main reason that this message got lost is greed. Unethical people found a way to pervert the truth and program people into believing that the Standard American Diet was acceptable. Fruits and vegetables are no longer organically grown generally as they were years ago. Animal proteins have been perverted by chemicals, hormones and antibiotics. Most foods are altered chemically for profit and shelf life. Junk food production is at an all-time high, and fast food has become a way of life and an addiction. Professionals and lay people who try to tell the truth are attacked, discredited and ridiculed. Many people are programmed to believe that the truth is really quackery. The truth must come out again so that it becomes less confusing and part of mainstream information. This still remains a big challenge.

Another part of the problem is that there is a lot of confusion about which way to follow the truth. This problem exists in the raw food and vegan community today. No two people are in the same place at the same time. Leave out all the processed food, eliminate or reduce the animal protein. If you have a problem and don't know what to do, get some professional advice.

3. WHY DO YOU THINK THIS BOOK IS SO CRUCIAL?

GABRIEL COUSENS

This book is crucial because the overall consciousness of the planet is struggling to awaken. The materialistic consciousness of the planet, in which everything is reduced to how much money one can make and how many years one can live, has also affected the live food movement. My experience with the live food Elders is that we all, through our life experience, see a larger vision. It is a vision beyond preoccupation with physical health. It is a vision of holistic health, and of sincerely contributing to the evolution of the planet. These live food Elders have maintained that lifestyle and understanding over the years, and our statements are based, not on a few years of experience and reading a few books, but on 40 years or more of real life success and experience. Consequently, we're able to share a quality and depth that keeps people focused on life's purpose and what holistic living is about—a vision expanding beyond a materialistic fixation on vegan live food.

FRED BISCI

Well, it's because the state of health in this country—the healthcare system—is approaching the disaster stage. Many people are now getting sick with lifestyle-related diseases. The human body has the ability to remedy them once you leave out the processed food.

When people come to see me, I put them on a plant-based diet with fruit and lots of vegetables, green juices and sometimes the supplemental juices like wheatgrass and they start to recover their health.

This book is crucial because people have to be made aware that they already have all the tools they need to be healthy; it's really very simple.

This book is the fruition of approximately 200 combined years of scientific study, clinical and personal experience, and devotion. Because of what is happening in the world today with health care, diet and lifestyle, books like this are crucial. There is a lot of good information on the Internet, but there is a lot information that is hype, or simply not true. I truly hope this book will bring some clarity to the situation.

VIKTORAS KULVINSKAS

The book Our Elders Speak is very critical and important at this time in history and comes in perfect time, during the initiation of exponential growth within the raw living food movement to the point where it is becoming the dominant philosophy for eating. There are many newbies and opportunists that have surfaced and will continue to do so, becoming instant "experts" in riding this tidal wave to their own financial benefits, instead of looking at the long term implications on health, happiness, holism, harmony and sustainability.

The principles that are spelled out in this book are the results of not only thousands of years of inspired history initiated by the Essenes and the Vedas...but also naturalist anthropology, which brings to the surface the important principles that can simply become lost. Especially when one is looking for a short-term gain that could be easily accomplished on any of the sugar laden fruitarian approaches or many other directives that are initiated by shallow "experts" who are surfacing on the Internet.

This book has been created by 4 respected leaders in the field who are riding on the shoulders of many prominent men and women who have articulated in history, the past truths by their lifestyle choices. We as a group, have over 200 years of history in the live food clinical, research, personal experimentation and counseling, while observing for decades the results of our guidance. We are the true leaders and the ones that will provide the foundation for the future of planet earth and assuring the thriving survival into the 23rd century and beyond. We are looking generations ahead...remembering, re-birthing and re-creating the perfect genetic evolution that can be accomplished once again...manifesting the highest quality of life through inner and outer harmony, love and service to one another. We are one and all is love. That is our theme and belief. Let us join our hearts together and create the paradisiacal future together!!

BRIAN CLEMENT

I think the Elder's Project in book form is timely and quite important at this stage, since the Internet is spreading lots of information that is not quite substantiated, or derived from a long history of clinical research and practice with people. People are, at this point, obviously taking the opportunity to speak about their opinions, and quite often these opinions come from a very narrow focus and lack of depth and experience.

As we put together the Elders Conference and the Elders Publication, we now can present to you, over 200 years of work with hundreds and hundreds of thousands of individuals globally in clinical settings placing them on plant-based diets.

We speak from compassion first, second from history and substantial professional experience, and third with respect for each of you that are listening and reading. My hope is that we can help you improve your life and your health and the health of all of humanity. I'm going to now answer the questions.

THE SHOCKING TRUTH ABOUT THE STATE OF OUR HEALTH

"The youth of today have a higher risk of developing a degenerative disease than their parents. We're living in a generation where the life expectancy of our children is shorter than those of our parents." - Viktoras Kulvinskas

"In the decades that I've done this work, what I used to see take 70, 80, and 90 years for people to contract, like catastrophic cancers, now takes 20 and 30 years." - Brian Clement

"A person can healthfully consume between 15 and 25 grams of fructose daily, but the average American takes in 81 grams of fructose daily." - Gabriel Cousens

"Mainly, this is a society of excesses. We're overdoing so many things and our stress levels are soaring" - Fred Bisci

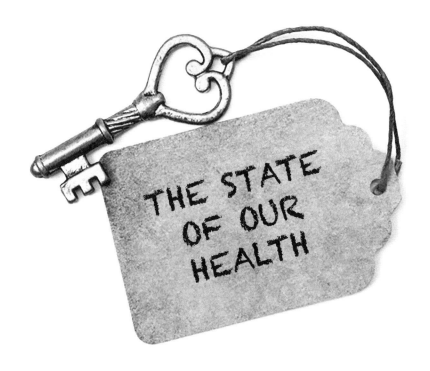

4. WHAT IS THE CURRENT STATE OF OUR HEALTH—SHOULD WE BE WORRIED?

BRIAN CLEMENT

In the more than four decades that I've practiced healthcare, I've seen a radical and rapid decline in health. Currently, I'm presenting a PowerPoint that I put together with a map of just the United States. It shows from 1980 forward how obesity has slowly but surely gobbled up the entire 50 states and it's not stopping. Now, many states have more than 30% of the population who are obese or morbidly obese. That one fact alone should give us pause—so that we, in fact, start to consider what will happen as we gain weight and attract every known disease.

Our children are now afflicted by fast-food mentality due to their parent's addiction to the consumption of these "foods" as trained consumers.

You look at just autism alone. From the early 1980s, statistically, it was 1 out of 10,000. At the beginning of the 21st century, it is 1 out of 50 that contract autism. This one fact is staggering alone. You look at the rise in diabetes and cancer, and the constant and consistent 48% to 50% statistic of people who develop heart attacks and strokes. This also is staggering.

So, why we think it's critical today, and why we should be concerned, is that we are in a rapid decline in our health, and rates of diseases are rising.

VIKTORAS KULVINSKAS

About 30% of the individuals who come to Hippocrates are under 35 years of age. They're suffering from cancer, cardiovascular diseases, MS, rheumatism and many abnormalities. Autism is spreading like wildfire. It is no wonder that the ongoing statistic is that we're living, for the first time, in a generation where the parents are going to outlive their children.

Morbid obesity is spreading, which is an indication of enzymatic deficiency, and an exaggerated enzymatic deficiency in lipase—the enzyme which is supposed to break down and process fat. The consumption of high volumes of food places a severe demand on the body's enzymatic reserves, not only in regards to fats and the storage of fat, but also, the inability to metabolize protein. It was confirmed, according to a 2002 Harvard Nutritional Studies, that states we are indeed in an epidemic of twisted protein. Undigested protein circulates throughout the blood stream, creating complete *stagnation of oxygen transport*, an inflammatory condition and the inability of the immune system to process these proteins.

This is what lays the foundation for every degenerative disease, according to Harvard Medical School. In spite of the genetic degenerations that we see within individuals, if you move into a living food program, you will be in a position to optimize your body and live as long as another individual who has a very strong genetic disposition. You can continuously rebuild your genetic information and every cellular reproduction by providing optimum nutrition internally with an alkaline, enzymatic, high mineral spectrum, green oriented nutritional program. There is no limitation placed on you in terms of creating the highest human potential for yourself.

FRED BISCI

It is not good. Disease and sickness is rampant. Most of the time we are sick because of what we are eating. Should we be worried? No, I don't like the word worried because I don't believe in worrying, but I believe that the state of health has deteriorated to the point where we definitely should be concerned enough to take control of our lives and make changes. I think people should be made aware of all these factors. The truth is we have information now to turn the situation around.

People are getting sicker and sicker from eating processed food. The food giants are taking good, healthy food and turning it into junk devoid of a lot of the nutrients that we need. As time goes on, people consume these foods more and more because these foods are addicting. Processed food is a modern day curse. The public schools in New York City are like war zones. Some of the children are uncontrollable and unteachable because of what they are eating. Most of the school lunches are unfit for human consumption.

The lower GI tract is extremely important; everybody thinks that's where the real problems are. That has not been my experience. I believe that the upper GI and the lymph system are where most of our

"We are a sick country and getting sicker. If you want to become healthy and stay that way you must eat whole food plant-based diet." – Fred Bisci

diseases begin because that's where most of the cellular inflammation begins. The real problem is that the waste products cause fermentation and bacteria proliferation in an anaerobic environment. Your upper GI tract is actually like a second brain. It has that much influence on your cellular metabolism.

Most of the cellular inflammation begins in the upper GI tract, where there are 15 to 20 feet of the small intestine. Everybody has some sludge in there; it's like the cells are suffocating. The lower GI tract you can clean out with enemas, colonics, colon cleansers, etc. The upper GI tract - when you clean that out with probiotics and a healthy plant-based diet, you reduce the inflammation and the body can actually breathe on a cellular level. A plant-based diet can help alleviate and prevent these problems.

I think we have to definitely be concerned, and we have to unify so we can influence and help people educate themselves and make changes for themselves. Then we have a chance to influence and change the system. A lot of the big food giants are buying up the organic farms and, little by little, the laws are being changed here so we've got to be on top of our game. I'm at the point right now where I really don't trust too many people, to be perfectly honest with you.

The public is being deceived and brainwashed by abstract scientific vernacular, which is very impressive and misleading. Much of this is a distortion of the truth. I used to be naive and I used to be a very trusting guy, but now, I really don't put much stock in double-blind studies. As far as I'm concerned, most of them are a joke. A lot of the peer reviews and the scientific information that comes out now is really slanted information that's easily manipulated.

We have to get away from this reductionist mentality and realize that we need a whole-food, plant-based diet, devoid of processed food. The truth? We are a sick country and getting sicker. If you want to become healthy and stay that way, you must eat a whole-food, plant-based diet.

GABRIEL COUSENS

I am not at all worried about my current state of health, as I seem to be getting stronger, younger, and more flexible with each year. I have begun to question the whole concept of social expectations of aging. At the age of 70, I feel more flexible, more fluid, more pain free, and more joyful than I was at the age of 20.

Should the world be worried about its state of health? With each progressing generation we see an increased chronic degeneration of health that is accelerated by degenerate, inflammatory lifestyles. Although we are technically living longer, we are not living healthier. If we define health as in all parameters - physical, emotional, mental, and spiritual - we are not achieving our purpose in life. The worldwide pandemic of type 2 diabetes is a symptom of this problem.

Our concern should be—are we really living the life we were meant to live in terms of our overall evolution? We should be worried that we are not achieving the purpose of life. We should be worried that we are inflamed and degenerating at totally unnecessary rates. Although we are living longer, due to general scientific and cultural support, the question remains: Live longer for what? In asking the right questions about life's purpose, our purpose, and life's meaning, the tremendous vital force we derive from live food may be used to support us in reaching our life purpose and knowing God.

5. WHAT ARE THE MOST DETRIMENTAL CONTRIBUTORS TO POOR HEALTH AND DISEASE?

FRED BISCI

Well, lifestyle of course: processed food, a bad diet, too much animal protein. You can be a very healthy person without any animal protein, if you have the discipline to go into a vegan diet. For people who cannot follow a vegan life style, the animal protein should be clean and in moderation. Not eating animal protein works best for me, but that does not apply for everybody.

I believe the main cause of our diseases—in the way we're eating and living in this country today—is that the body becomes inundated with processed food. It becomes like sludge on the cellular level. There are 70,000 chemicals, that we're aware of, that could be in our food leading to cellular inflammation, problems affecting our organs, and absolutely causing cancer and other diseases to boot.

To fully answer this question would require a separate book in itself, so I am not even getting into cell phones, technology, GMOs and the hundreds of other factors that are affecting us outside of our diet. We have been programmed to believe many things that are not true, in many areas that control our lives. We must educate ourselves and take control of our own lives. Knowledge is power; become empowered. The real science of our existence is amazing. Abstract science is a creation of half-truths.

VIKTORAS KULVINSKAS

There are no singular causes, everything is important. Your attitude, your exercise, your diet, how much you rest—are you living in a very polluted and/or cigarette second hand smoke environment? Next to a nuclear power plant or an airport? From the dietary point of view, the most important thing is to eliminate all dairy products, including organic milk. Anything that is heat treated and/or pasteurized is going to stick to your lungs and lymphatic system, create periodic colds or flu, accelerate the development of malignancies and cardiovascular issues within your system.

Dairy reduces your brainpower, as oxygen levels are greatly interfered with, while also creating an array of digestive disorders. There is no need for dairy products. For more information on this, you can go to www.notmilk.com, as well as take a look at all the research data that I pioneered 40 years ago in my book, *Survival in the 21st Century*.

My advice is, stop all processed foods and go organic and non-GMO, cut down on the size of your meals, chew and exercise your face—you'll look younger. Eat more raw foods that will require more chewing. Consider frequenting organic, vegan restaurants and trying out the wonderful free raw food recipes on the Internet. Minimize the use of your blender; instead use the food processor to chop food up partially, instead of reducing it to a creamy consistency.

Meditate and get happy! That means exercise. Exercise will get you out of the emotional crazies, which drives you to reach for comfort foods. Upgrade your associations. Stop hanging out with those who talk about pills, medicine, and disease. Hang out with those who are progressively talking about optimistic, solution oriented expansion and high vibrations. Eventually, you will be strong enough to handle the negative individuals. There is nothing wrong with going to them and bringing light. We all need to share the light, yet if you can hang out with individuals that talk about darkness and carrying a low vibration, you will also start experiencing the darkness. Support the individuals who have been there for you, creating the way for freedom and becoming healthy, happy and holy.

Dehydration is rampant; increase your water intake. There is only one form of clean water, and that is distilled water. American Water Distiller Company sells a stainless steel distiller for $100 that produces four gallons per day.

Go to retreat centers for detoxification. If you're an alcoholic, go to a detox center. If you're a food addict, you would benefit from some raw foodist retreat place to be with other like-minded individuals. Don't get involved in self-judgment; most people are not successful on their first attempt, and, chances are, you won't be either. You have many emotional addictions, filled with social inculcation by parents, ministry, politicians, teachers—and so many lies. To break from this matrix, it takes time, patience and non-judgment. Don't judge yourself, and love yourself unconditionally.

Keep going back for reinforcements, set up your own support group, and go to Potluck suppers and dinners and meal programs, gatherings of teachers. Just keep on associating with uplifting people, because you become whom you hang out with. That also includes the low-vibe, dead-energy crowd. You'll become like death itself. Cooked, dead food will move you into a less-vibrant and diminished aliveness.

GABRIEL COUSENS

The most detrimental contributor is an inflammatory and degenerative lifestyle, which includes eating junk food, white flour, white sugar, and animal products that are higher up on the food chain (therefore filling people with up to 30 times more toxins, such as radiation, pesticides, herbicides, and GMOs).

The higher we eat on the food chain, the more radiation we take in, the more pesticides and herbicides we take in, and the more death and cruelty we create in the animal kingdom, creating misery, death and cruelty— that misery, death, cruelty and pain also goes into us, contributing to our own degeneration.

In general, the world is living an inflammatory lifestyle that accelerates the aging process. It is living at a level of superficiality that leads to poor physical, emotional, mental, and spiritual health. Without an emphasis on the basics of life—clean, organic live food, clean air, clean water, sufficient exercise, sufficient sleep, meaningful spiritual life, and spiritual joy—we tend to inflame and degenerate. The most detrimental contributor to this state is a lack of love for ourselves and for those people around us. To heal, one has to truly love oneself and love one's life enough to want to heal.

"To heal, one has to truly love oneself and love one's life enough to want to heal." - Gabriel Cousens

BRIAN CLEMENT

Number one is attitude. If we have an attitude that's dismissive, one that is matter-of-fact, what happens is that we wander aimlessly without values and virtue, and when we do this, we disregard our own need and we disregard our own fulfillment. This allows us to be magnets for disorder. And, as we start to eat the wrong foods, lack the necessary movement and exercise, become unconcerned about the water that we drink, the air that we breathe, the clothing that we wear, and the supplements that we take, we become very ill. It's a downward spiral.

So, number one is the mind. And when the mind is clear, focused and understands our purpose, we then tend to eat proper plant-based foods in their organic state, drink water that's not riddled with the chemicals that are found worldwide, make sure that we're breathing the freshest, cleanest air, use filtration systems in cities, wear natural fibers—the list goes on.

6. ARE THERE ANY HIDDEN FACTORS THAT MAY CONTRIBUTE TO POOR HEALTH AND DISEASE?

BRIAN CLEMENT

Well, I think with the invisible factors, as we call them, such as the air we breathe, we are picking up not only chemicals, but also heavy metals particulate. This, in and of itself, contributes to the major diseases such as cancer, cardiovascular disease, asthma, etc.

Globally, they've tested the drinking water for the majority of the population on the planet today and found that, in every case when tested, pharmaceutical drugs are found in that water. Sadly, even sophisticated and expensive water filtration systems fail to remove these, since they are such small particles, subatomic particles sometimes.

We have to be particularly interested in finding water filtration systems, maybe the type we use here at Hippocrates that extracts water from the air. When you're living in humid enough climates you need about 35% humidity on an average to extract water from the air. In this way, we supersede the groundwater and do not have to worry about the pharmaceuticals.

"The clothing that we wear is directly implicated with disease." - Brian Clement

The clothing that we wear is directly implicated with disease. In a book that my wife and I published called *Killer Clothes* we address this particular issue.

The supplements we take. Several years ago, my book, *Supplements Exposed*, explained how more than 90% of the supplements on the market today are dangerous for you to consume and, in the vast majority of cases, are made from petrochemicals, coal tar, turpentine, etc. There are many things that are hidden and that we assume are healthy, that are the exact opposite.

GABRIEL COUSENS

Truly, a lack of purpose; a lack of character development; and a lack of focus on putting God at the center of one's life, are all important factors in looking at longevity. The question we still have to ask is—longevity for what?

FRED BISCI

I don't think anybody is aware of all of them. There are so many things going on in our society that are taking place behind the scenes with food giants and with the pharmaceutical companies. As far as I'm concerned, you don't have to be aware of all the unapparent factors, because we are aware of the apparent factors. We are aware of what it takes to create optimal health for our bodies. We know we have tremendous information now, and we know exactly what to do to improve our situation.

Mainly, this is a society of excesses. We're overdoing so many things and our stress levels are soaring. Many people are internalizing stress, which manifests in different types of disease. My message for the last 50 years is "what you leave out." Once you become aware of what becomes necessary to create superb health, it is not necessary to know the thousands of negative factors that contribute to poor health. The most important factors are to avoid processed food and eat as much raw live food as possible, detox your body, think positively and follow a healthy life style. Medical science has its place, but we must learn how to make the best choices.

VIKTORAS KULVINSKAS

The most obvious are lack of moderation and lousy health practices. To be on a raw food program and to eat huge meals, you will be guaranteed to create some kind of degeneration. I've seen so many hygienists, as well as followers of the 80/20 path, creating a blender mix of food; paw paws, cherries, mangoes, bananas etc.—a full container and having that as a meal. Those actions are going to convert you into a distillery where fermentation sits in. I watched some of the top students of the 80/20 get thinning hairlines, skin conditions, require 10-12 hours for sleeping and have one to two migraine attacks every month. This is not a healthy practice.

Overeating is rampant. If you want to be healthy, you're best served eating between two and three cups at most per meal. This is the size of two fist balls, which is roughly what the capacity of your stomach is. Adapt this protocol, and you'll be able to digest your meal in two to three hours.

There is also the issue of oxygen—many of you are living in an oxygen-deprived environment. The standards for red blood cell count and hemoglobin have been reduced to reflect the diminished averages. By the standards of 100 years ago, everybody in this country is anemic. So how do you get around that? Green chlorophyll foods with every meal. Secondly, the practice of pranayama and cardiovascular exercise, especially with breath retention. The 1027 (in other words 10 followed by 27 zeros) number of chemical reactions that occur every second in your body are all dependent upon oxygen. That's serious multi-tasking within your body to maintain life! And every one of these reactions involves enzymes and oxygen.

Chewing your food well is very important. Even when it is blended or processed, you should spend a great deal of time chewing. Most people think they're very healthy by eating organic old foods. What is old food? It is your vegetables and fruits. You want young food. What is young food? The sunflower greens that I pioneered are an excellent example. Now it's everywhere, along with all microgreens and all the different sprouts. These are foods that will get you young. These will give you a high vitality and energy, as well as being the cheapest foods because you can grow them at home. The importance of minerals is often overlooked—so you'll benefit from consuming sea vegetables on a daily basis. The key factor for health, longevity and low incidents of child fatality is found in cultures that consume fermented foods on a daily basis.

7. WHAT ARE THE MOST COMMON DISEASES YOU SEE IN YOUR CLINICS?

GABRIEL COUSENS

The most common disease I see, in general, is chronic diabetes degenerative syndrome, which is a sugar-related process that also accelerates heart disease, high blood pressure, poorer mental function, senility, cancer, arthritis, general weakness, and degenerative health in all parameters. The other sorts of diseases that I see are more environmentally created diseases, such as exposure to pesticides, herbicides and radiation and also diseases related to poor emotional and mental hygiene. Equally common is chronic fatigue and chronic fibromyalgia.

VIKTORAS KULVINSKAS

Addiction to doctors is on top of that list. It's the leading cause of aging, degeneration and death. Use your doctors for diagnostic help and also for taking care of accidents. Use Google and God as your resources for discovering what the truth is and use these four Elders as the guidepost to truth. The truth is very individualized.

Morbid obesity would be next. I basically worked with Dick Gregory for several years running the nutritional development and research within the Gregory's Morbid Obesity and Substance Abuse Center in Fort Walton and the Bahamas. Our clients were 400-1000 plus pounds. America is starting to look like the three ring circuses of 100 years ago, where the obese were part of the freak show. Now the fat are totally common, while slim healthy individual are more rare. Excess consumption of fats leads to all forms of cardiovascular, circulatory and diabetic diseases. It is widespread, and the most common form is the high addiction to heat treated animal proteins. Pasteurized dairy products are also leading to the precipitation of incompletely metabolized calcium in the joints. That is what's developing all the arthritic conditions we see. Over 85% of arthritis and cardiovascular degeneration is due to consumption of pasteurized dairy products. It also lays the foundation for osteoporosis.

Countries that have the highest consumption of pasteurized dairy products also have the highest incidents of osteoporosis. We have seen degeneration of our children, as 40% are suffering from old age diseases.

Autism is growing exponentially due to vaccinations and terrible childhood foods, all of which are putting stress on our enzymatic reserves and the proper functioning of the immune system. When you introduce poisons into your body by way of vaccines or drugs, you should realize that none of them have a nutritional foundation. You're stressing your immune system, which is strictly driven by enzymes. Alkalinity is the energizing force, but all the mechanics are enzymatic. The wide prevalence of allergies, where one is allergic to the environment and certain foods, is based on an enzyme deficiency. This included myself. Until I got into using enzymatic supplements, I was not able to digest a major segment of raw foods. One should incorporate the consumption of superfoods, with an emphasis on enzymes, probiotics and green food supplements like blue-green algae and spirulina.

BRIAN CLEMENT

Hippocrates Health Institute was founded by Ann Wigmore, who reversed colon cancer after being told by the Harvard Medical Doctors in the early 1950s that she had only months to live. Obviously from that point forward, our name, reputation and history has attracted many people with cancers.

At this point in history, when people are diagnosed with cancer, they should begin immediately to take charge and responsibility for their lifestyles. To date, that is uncommon, although it does occur. We've been historically working with stage 3 and stage 4 cancers, and watching the power of raw and living food and the other tools that we use here at the Hippocrates Health Institute in helping tens of thousands battle cancer. With that said, I can't think of any disorder and any disease that we do not work with. The other inspiring part of this story is that in the recent decade and a half, we have far more healthy people coming for prevention and life extension.

The Hippocrates Health Institute guests are more like your local community. We have people come from around the globe, and they settle with us for weeks, participating in the program - some are very healthy and some have illness. Every known disease to man is at the Institute and we do clinical research on a daily basis. Our medical team uses blood profiles, bio-frequency, medicine units, electromagnetic therapy, cold laser therapy - the list goes on and on and on. We conduct many of these technologies throughout their stay. When one graduates from Hippocrates Health Institute—since we're an educational Institute - for the rest of their life, as part of our gift to them, we counsel them via the mail.

Our medical team gets back blood test reports, medical histories, and throughout that individual's life, we observe them and help them and support them. During this process, we collect data for empirical evidence of their self-healing. We are systematically working with universities, as well as collecting our own in-house data to be published at some later time.

FRED BISCI

In my office, I see many people with a variety of diseases. I see people that have cancer, heart disease, lupus, arthritis, diabetes, dementia—you name it, I see it. I've had a lot of exposure to people trying to change their day-to-day health without going to the ultimate best diet. Of course, I wish everybody would be willing to go to the ultimate best diet, and if they did it correctly and they followed directions and did not succumb to all the confusion and all the hype, then of course their lives would all be a lot easier. Your body is the healer. A whole food, plant-based live food diet devoid of processed food, is miraculous. Your body knows how to heal you, but you must give it the freedom to work its wonders.

"Your body knows how to heal you, but you must give it the freedom to work its wonders." - Fred Bisci

The public comes to me with all of the chronic, and sometimes even acute diseases. Lifestyle change certainly is not a panacea, but most people can be helped, and some dramatically. I have found all chronic disease to be remedial. Most acute disease can be helped. I have seen some unbelievable things happen. Be aware of people who make irresponsible claims. There are many out there.

8. WHAT ARE THE MOST SHOCKING FACTS ABOUT THE STATE OF OUR HEALTH TODAY?

GABRIEL COUSENS

I am shocked at how little people really love and respect themselves. The amount of disturbance connected with eating itself, whether it's obesity—in which we see 48% of people with diabetes being obese and 82% being overweight—or just the reverse of that where people suffer from a variety of eating disorders that all reflect an imbalance between themselves and their own hearts. There is never enough food to feed a hungry soul, and the epidemic of worldwide obesity is evidence of this.

The amount of sugar that people take in their cuisine is another negative statistic. A person can healthfully consume between 15 and 25 grams of fructose daily, but the average American takes in 81 grams of fructose daily.

Third is the lack of hydration. We start about 70 to 75% water and, with age, if we don't pay attention to hydration, we may get as low as 55 to 60% water, and that really undermines our health and contributes to the potential of brain shrinkage with age.

A fourth fact is that millions of people are sleep deprived. Lack of sleep is associated dramatically with lack of health. Sleep deprivation results in 40 times more depression, considerably more endocrine imbalances and blood sugar imbalances, poor regeneration of the neurological nervous system and a weaker immune system. Sleep is a major deficiency today.

Another fact is that most people aren't getting any, or very little exercise. This also weakens our state of health and undermines basic brain health.

BRIAN CLEMENT

In the decades that I've done this work, what I used to see take 70, 80, and 90 years for people to contract, like catastrophic cancers, now takes 20 and 30 years.

The obesity level among our youth has risen and this is yes, diet, and yes, media - where the average western child now watches television or is in front of a computer screen 7 hours a day. Just a couple of generations ago, children were out playing 12 months a year.

The total freedom of corporate interest to spew poisons into the environment is linked to the detection of these poisons in disease globally. A current book that I've published, *Killer Fish*, displays some of this research. *The Hundred Year Lie*, by Randall Fitzgerald, another publication, and Dr. Epstein's book on Toxic Beauty in the cosmetic industry, both provide invaluable information. I would highly suggest that people look at environmental factors.

"...babies born as we speak will commonly die sooner than their parents." - Brian Clement

The lack of adequate exercise is a problem. Current statistics are that less than 5% of the western population exercises adequately. We know exactly what this means from the great work of people like Dr. Kenneth Cooper, who has spent more than a half of a century researching the health benefits of exercise.

I think that what is apparent today is that the youth are surrendering what one and two generations ago people worked hard to develop—respect for women, respect for the environment, respect for their bodies. We see, in great part, the youngest people among us today are discarding things that are very valuable, and social consciousness is waning. There are exceptions and I'm always inspired by some people, because the truth inevitably comes out in those exceptions. Those few people that remain conscious and develop consciousness and rise above even the last generation, I believe will eventually have their voice heard. Just like our voices will be heard when speaking today.

For anyone who's observing today, it's clear that mental illness is starting to become prevalent. Statistically, as we speak, the number one medicines now prescribed globally are antidepressants. My observation is that 8 out of 10 people placed on these drugs seem not to really require psychiatric medicine. Changes in lifestyle and life direction should change the disorder.

I think it is extremely important for people to realize that, statistically; babies born as we speak will commonly die 5 years sooner than their parents. Now, in all of the history of biological science, this is the first time this has ever been observed. When we found out how they developed those statistics, we went one step further and asked, "What will that look like in 25 years if we use the same mathematical formula?" Sadly we discovered that 25 years from the time you're hearing or reading this, children born then will probably die 12 to 15 years sooner than their parents. It's an alarming statistic.

I think that governments of the world are pretty much controlled now by corporate interest, and no matter what side you're on, the end result is that whoever has the most money puts their woman or man in and manipulates them to vote according to their desires, which then degrade the environment and consequently, your health.

We do know now, factually, from a former Food and Drug Administration Director, that the major food industries have full-time scientists developing addictive substances that they put into common foods, so that people constantly and consistently purchase them.

It's extremely important for people to recognize that attitude is the only way that we're going to cause change. What's frightening to me is that so many people have doomsday and negative attitudes. They're looking for the end of the world, rather than the beginning of a new life. They want to be put out of their own pain by believing in demise. I think that the handful of people listening today, the optimists, the realists, will turn the tide. As in human history before, it's been one woman or one man who stands up with values and virtues and speaks truth that leads us out of darkness.

FRED BISCI

I think the most shocking of all is that there really is an answer that's not complicated. Most people are not aware of it. It's not coming in our education. We should have an educational system that's teaching children about how to eat correctly, how to avoid processed foods, how to eat a variety of fruits and vegetables and small amounts of the other foods, how to take care of yourself, how important exercise really is and healthy ways to deal with anxiety and stress and some of the major problems in our society. The truth is really being kept from people because you don't see too much of this in the news media. It's getting better now; more and more people are coming out with more positive suggestions. People are just unaware. To me, it's shocking that some people have any clue that the food they're eating could have an influence on their health.

Also a lot of people don't realize that the major cause of disease is their lifestyle. It's what they're doing, lack of exercise and not getting enough air. People need to maintain healthy thoughts and be spiritually grounded, in addition to leaving out processed foods.

Most of the research is coming from pharmaceutical companies, and is not looking at trying to find ways for people to get healthier. Most double blind studies are a joke. According to most double blind studies, I should have been dead for years. Disease is a business in this country. It's not only big business—it's a billion dollar business. The food giants are taking good food and making junk out of it and making people sick. They're adding fat, sugar and all these different things that will addict us. When you eat processed foods, the salt, fat, sugar, preservatives and colorings have an impact on the hypothalamus gland and you become addicted. That's why a lot of people that have had eating disorders are obese; they cannot control themselves because that drive is just powerful. It's like the sex drive; it's the same thing.

The pharmaceutical companies have taken over, and the doctors are prescribing drugs or prescribing surgery, so they have a very unholy alliance here that's working out very well for them, but, as time goes on, it's not working out so well for the average person. With that said, I know many good doctors that are helping people. Diagnostics, emergency treatment and surgery are instances when a person would need a medical doctor.

I have come across people who don't want to know the truth; they're not interested in finding a way to become healthy by changing their diet or they don't have the understanding of what the impact could be. I've had people say some things to me that I believe are pretty ridiculous. I had one fellow say to me, "Well I'm not afraid to die," and, "I want to live my life, I want to do whatever I want, I want to do whatever I enjoy. I want to do some things that other people don't have the courage to do." I said, "Well, it's not that simple, my friend, because it's not like throwing a light switch where the lights in the room just go out; it might not be that way." Unfortunately, years later, I heard about him from a relative of his - that he got very sick, he actually got MS. It took him time to go into a wheelchair; he was in a wheelchair for a long time before he succumbed, so that's not really a good philosophy.

The food giants and the pharmaceutical companies have a tremendous effect on the lobbyists in Washington. They're actually subverting a lot of information that would be conducive to help the average person become healthy, aware and educated. Plus, the lobbyists have tremendous influence on laws that are being passed and the laws that should be passed, are not. We all should become aware that we are being taken advantage of and we have to educate ourselves.

Of course people are being fed statistics that say we're living longer and people are doing better and the quality of life is getting better. Well, that's not true either, because more and more people, though statistically they might be living longer, are spending a lot of time walking around with walkers, or they're sick, or they're on lots of drugs; their quality of life is very poor, they're depressed, they have anxiety, or they're spending the last years of their lives—5, 10 years or even longer—in nursing homes.

Now I've been through that experience; I had the misfortune to have somebody that I care about very dearly, it was my mother-in-law, spend time in a nursing home. Believe me, going to that nursing home was not a pleasant experience. I saw what was really going on there and it was just amazing. The disturbing thing about it is that there were people there for 10 or 15 years who were 90, 95 years old, and there were a few who were over 100. If you're using those statistics to say people are living longer—well I don't like those kinds of numbers.

It is unfortunate that many people think that organically grown foods don't make a difference. The truth of the matter is that they are tremendously important and they are a major factor in avoiding a huge number of different chemicals, hormones and other factors like GMOs.

To compound all of these issues, the confusion is getting deeper. I think a lot of that has to do with the Internet; everybody's got a website, everybody's trying to sell something—everybody's got some kind of a new diet. Everybody in the raw food community now is coming up with some new superfood that comes from the Amazon jungle or some new way where you could have the libido of a Mongolian warrior and look like Mr. America when you are eighty. There are people who buy into this information.

This has become a multi-million dollar business and a lot of it is just sheer nonsense. If you know the human body, in its highest biological form, when you provide all the nutrients that you need, connect all the dots, get enough calories, get enough sleep, drink enough clear water, think positively, live one day at a time, become spiritually grounded – then you're going to have a dynamic life. You're most likely going to live a long time and you're going to have a great experience.

Poverty is a big factor because so many people in the lower income group don't have the resources or the knowledge that they need, and they're buying the cheapest food that tastes the best. They're at a complete disadvantage. Of course, they don't really realize how bad it is for them. You can go into some of the playgrounds in New York City and see these fabulous looking athletes playing basketball, some young kid dunking a ball over the back of his head that has a fabulous physique and you see what he's eating is the best he can afford, which is mostly processed fast food. They have this fabulous natural ability and they're fueling themselves with processed food, which is a great source of fuel—before it kills you. They don't realize that when they get to be 55 or 60 they're going to be into chronic disease or something more severe. The poor are the victims; unless they become aware of their circumstances and make changes, they will be in deep trouble with their health.

It's really important that we get this message out and that we're not too dogmatic. In my opinion, we want everybody to be able to get something from this book. It's really not that complicated, the way I look at it. We really are our brother's keeper. We should be trying to reach everybody. If we could get people to leave out the processed food it would bring about unbelievable improvement in the health of this country. Raw food is the answer, but no processed food is more realistic to start with. There are many variables to being healthy. What you leave out is one of the biggest.

VIKTORAS KULVINSKAS

In childhood, mothers should be feeding children only breast milk. The proliferation of baby foods is troubling. There is no such thing as good baby food.

Vaccination programs, which require over 30 different vaccines by the time a child enters grade school, are having a negative impact on the state of children's health. Go to www.mercola.com to see how poisonous this infliction is and its connection to the development of degeneration.

The transhumanistic assimilation into EMF's, computer screens, cell phones and radioactive waves bombarding the senses have changed the way that people relate with one another. People don't connect and talk anymore, unless it's via some kind of technology.

Genetically Modified Foods are spreading like wildfire. The only sure way of having organic food is to know your farmers and know your resources. Get organic seeds and start growing your own food - fresh

"By becoming more alkalized on a raw food diet, you will have divine guidance." - Viktoras Kulvinskas

food. The GMOs will be eradicated, both by Mother Earth and the opposition at the marketplace through awareness of what we consume.

Over 60 different drugs have been identified in all city waters. These are medications that are spilled out by urine and defecation and are brought back into circulation after processing by water filtration. Unless you're using distilled water, there is not a single filter that will eliminate the drugs infiltrating our water supply. The only thing that will work is distilled water.

The first year that you live in a city, you can accumulate over a pound of inorganic matter in your lungs. You want to minimize that by getting yourself a quality air filter in your bedroom, as long as you continue to live within a city environment. Even the air in most people's homes is more polluted—up to five times more than it is outside, due to all the chemicals held onto within the home. Start using only natural and organic types of cleaners and solvents in your own home. Make your own.

But, going into the countryside doesn't mean you're going to be in a stress-free zone. We've got chemtrails and all the inorganic farmers that are spreading chemicals in the air. If you want safety, you'll have to move into higher and higher elevations. This is where the cleanest air is. This is also where you're going to be able to handle the difficult challenges that are coming up.

In our society, there is a deficiency of meditation. By becoming more alkalized on a raw food diet, you will have divine guidance. What to do, where to go and how to be happy, healthy and holy, no matter what is going on. That also includes the moment of leaving your physical body, which should be a very joyous experience, not a time for sadness and depression.

Start making your every action centered on this question: Is this a love act or is this something else? Start defining all your activities, both to yourself and to everyone else that you serve. Indeed love is the key driving force. Lack of love is the indicator of our addiction to prescription drugs, anti-depressants and levels of unhappiness.

9. WHAT IS A "LIFESTYLE" DISEASE AND HOW COMMON ARE THEY?

FRED BISCI

A lifestyle disease is an ailment that comes from living an improper lifestyle; smoking, drinking, not getting enough rest, recreational drugs, pharmaceutical drugs that are not necessary or over-prescribed and, of course, processed food—a bad diet.

There are a lot of people who are running tremendously long distances and the way they're fueling themselves might not be optimal but they'll be able to do it. That's not indicative that they're a healthy person. There are people who are into bodybuilding and weightlifting, and are able to put a tremendous amount of weight over their head and do heavy bench presses. They're huge and they're eating five or six meals a day with a lot of protein. They think they're on a perfect diet because the diet is producing what they're looking for; but is it going to produce long-term optimal disease-free health? No, I don't think so.

VIKTORAS KULVINSKAS

All diseases are lifestyle diseases. Not a single disease is due to any one singular contributing factor. Neglect of mental and emotional issues, which usually leads to behavioral alterations and comfort food addiction, as well as other addictive behaviors, eventually leads to the development of degeneration. So try in every possible way to be a happy camper, and that means becoming responsible for your life through loving actions toward yourself and others.

BRIAN CLEMENT

All major disorders are caused by a poor lifestyle—cancer, diabetes, heart disease, etc.

GABRIEL COUSENS

Lifestyle diseases are by far the most common ailments that I see. They are problems caused by our inflammatory lifestyles, which undermine all our regeneration and healing processes. Lifestyle diseases are extremely common. They are part of the emptiness which many people feel in their lives. In Ayurveda we call it *pratyprahara*—not following the natural laws of wisdom—or "crimes against wisdom."

10. DO THE YOUTH OF TODAY HAVE A BIGGER RISK OF DEVELOPING DISEASE THAN THEIR PARENTS?

BRIAN CLEMENT

The answer is, absolutely, yes. They eat more chemically riddled and addictive foods, breathe dirty air, drink dirty water, wear more manmade fibers, have greater stress, have less of the nuclear family in the sense of security—what you're going to see is more of what we are already seeing - the youth having a disease epidemic.

FRED BISCI

I say the answer to that question is, absolutely, yes. Everything is deteriorating. There is more stress and there are more and more people eating junk food. More and more people are not eating any fruits and vegetables. When somebody tells you that they don't know what a head of celery looks like—to me, that's pretty amazing. I had that happen to me. A young fellow told me he didn't know what celery looked like, he didn't know what brussel sprouts were, he didn't know what sprouts were. You ask some people if they eat any fruit.

They say, no, I have never eaten any fruit; they contain sugar. That's pretty amazing to me. Many people don't eat fruits and vegetables and don't have any idea what a plant-based diet really is.

VIKTORAS KULVINSKAS

The youth of today have a higher risk of developing a degenerative disease than their parents. We're living in a generation where the life expectancy of our children is shorter than those of our parents. This is a culture that has been immersed in ever escalating advertisements to addict children and adults alike to long shelf life, processed and comfort foods. It has made less than optimal choices sound normal and like a source of joy, vitality and happiness as well.

Our children, a generation later, are subject to more chemicals. The air and tap waters are more polluted than ever. The radiation levels have increased. The chemtrails within this generation have been phenomenal in terms of distribution of toxic products. All of these factors are affecting brain, as well as respiratory and immune function. We can all change the direction by upgrading our lifestyle habits. All of it is reversible. The genetic damage can be corrected in one generation.

GABRIEL COUSENS

Yes. The key to healthy living is to live with purpose, both with regard to one's individual sacred design and the greater purpose of life, which is to know God. Many youth have lost touch with these life purposes and have less motivation to eat and live in a way that maintains enough health to develop their life purpose.

HOW TO ACHIEVE OUTSTANDING HEALTH

"The answer is simple; understanding yourself, understanding how your biology, your body, your anatomy, and your mind work, and understanding history and true health." - Brian Clement

"All meals should include some form of green food, including supplements such as blue-green algae and spirulina."
- Viktoras Kulvinskas

"...how you achieve outstanding health is to leave out all the causes of disease and make changes, which include drinking clean water and getting plenty of exercise." - Fred Bisci

"The single most significant lifestyle change a person can make is to avoid or minimize sugar in all forms, including both glucose and fructose." - Gabriel Cousens

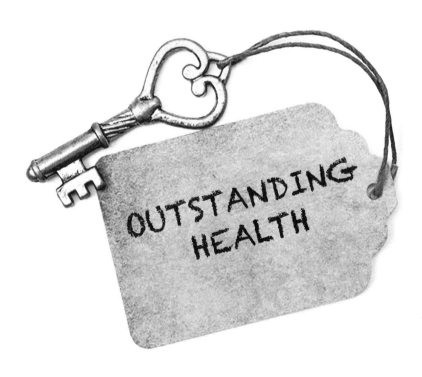

11. HOW DOES ONE ACHIEVE OUTSTANDING HEALTH?

GABRIEL COUSENS

What is the reason for achieving outstanding health?

The idea of health, for me, is to become functional on life's every level. This goes beyond how many push-ups we can do or how few hours of sleep we need. It is a total, integrated experience of health—physically, emotionally, mentally and spiritually - integrating and activating all of life's elements.

My view of health is a much more integrated, holistic view rather than simply a physical view. In this integrated approach, we're looking at becoming a super conductor of the Divine on every level. On a strictly physical level, an integrated approach of nature's seven healers is fundamental to the overall picture.

By the time people reach the age of 70, they usually have lost 50 percent of their lung capacity. It is good to have a PO2 of at least 97. Daily *Pranayama* exercises can help maintain lung capacity.

Also important is a proper amount of sun exposure. These days, I recommend 30 minutes of sunlight daily. Of course one can do the sun gazing and so forth; they are all added extras.

"It is a total, integrated experience of health—physically, emotionally, mentally and spiritually…"
– Gabriel Cousens

Proper sleep, between seven and eight hours a night on a consistent basis, is very important. Sleep is critical for general endocrine balance and resetting and rebuilding the serotonin levels, nervous system, and the immune system. People without adequate sleep have 40 times more depression and considerably more blood sugar disorders. Literally, a sleep-deprived person's fasting blood sugar may rise 10-15 points.

The optimal time to sleep is between 10 p.m. and 2 a.m., but I recommend at least seven hours of sleep each night. Unfortunately, some people in the Live Food Movement feel that they can ignore this rule. It is true that on live food, one does have more energy, and they can go longer on less sleep, but, in the long run, this is still skipping the regenerative times, and there will be a price to pay later. Many hours of meditation can substitute for some levels of sleep, but we still need to get adequate sleep.

Good water is fundamental to good health, and there's a great deal of research on the importance of hydration and being adequately hydrated. The easiest way to know that you are hydrated—depending on the different constitutions for adequate hydration—is to be urinating about every two hours.

Emotional health and spiritual health are part of the overall healers. There are a variety of people who have achieved some level of physical strength and vitality, but have not integrated the emotional. They have balance in the overall picture and so, operate with strong powers of *Qi*, but at the same time, they are not really emotionally integrated. To me, that's not a sign of health.

What I noted very early in the Live Food Movement is that people had certain levels of physical health, but they were often mentally imbalanced and very ungrounded in the overall picture. Integrated health suggests a person who lives in a way that they are constantly connecting the heavens and the earth. It is easy to maintain earthly strength with live food, and most of the Live Food Movement is focused on the earth plane. But the heavens, starting with the astral plane, which comprises the emotional, mental, and spiritual planes, tend to become imbalanced without a scientifically grounded live food cuisine. The shamanic walk is to walk in integration between the heavens and the earth. In Hebrew we call this "the walk between the B'limah and the Mah—between the Nothing and the Something."

Then, there's an issue of grace. Some people are simply blessed, genetically and chemically, with better health than others. We can just simply point ourselves in that right direction, and be happy with the results we have done all the right things – but it's important to be at your optimal no matter from where you start.

Another footnote is that people who focus their whole life on physical health often become obsessed with it. They're really missing the other higher planes, the heavenly part - the emotional, mental, and spiritual. This is, unfortunately, not an uncommon situation. For me, outstanding health is really an integrated picture of freedom and health on all levels.

BRIAN CLEMENT

The answer is simple—understanding yourself, understanding how your biology, your body, your anatomy, and your mind work, and understanding history and true health.

VIKTORAS KULVINSKAS

The most rudimentary step would be increased hydration. Most optimal is to consume at least one ounce of liquid for every two pounds of body weight. It should be distilled water, fresh vegetable juices and, occasionally, herbal teas. In addition, of utmost importance is daily exercise for a minimum of half an hour, combining cardiovascular, resistance training, and developing flexibility. Spend some time doing yoga or breathing exercises.

All meals should include some form of green food, including supplements such as blue-green algae and spirulina. I also recommend enzyme supplements and consumption of fermented foods and/or probiotics in the form of pills. Cut down on the size of meals, no more than two to three cups of food. Make a gradual emphasis on more and more segments of your nutritional program being made up of raw foods and fresh juices. Sprout wheatgrass, sunflower greens, buckwheat, and pea greens. Get some form of acupressure, reflexology and Chi and auric type of massage to keep yourself continuously at an optimum level of energy flow. Take a daily time out—either by doing a child pose three to five times a day, or a five to ten minute catnap a few times a day to decompress the spine. You may also want to take an herbal laxative at bedtime.

If you don't have any health challenges, mornings can be greens or fruit meals. If you work during the day, your noon meal should be nut or seed milks, as well as green juices. In the evening, have a more solid meal, which can be altered from day to day. One day emphasizing a protein meal, the next day soaked nuts and seeds, the next day emphasizing an avocado type of a meal. And, one day a week, fast on green juices, while also staying away from computers, refraining from a lot of talking, spending time reading sacred scriptures, and uplifting yourself through positive CDs and DVDs.

FRED BISCI

Well, as I touched on in all the previous questions and in my opening statements, how you achieve outstanding health is to leave out all the causes of disease and make changes, which include drinking clean water and getting plenty of exercise. You leave out all the processed food and gradually progress to a 100 percent raw living food diet. Even if you're just leaving out all the processed food, you're going to have a dramatic improvement in your health.

Of course, detoxify, get down near the ocean, run right near the ocean, get those negative ions and breathe the air that's been purified by the salt water. Get grounded with the earth. A lot of people don't realize that this actually helps people who have cancer.

Get out into the woods and near the ocean to exercise. Going to a gym is good, but it does not compare with exercising outdoors. Drink fruit and vegetable juices. Use your blender to make smoothies. You can be healthy without them, but they are a tremendous asset to help you. They are working for me. You will get more than enough fiber when you eat your fruits and vegetables. Exercise every day, if you can do it safely. Have true spiritual values. I believe in God. It works for me.

People have to educate themselves, and I hope that this book is going to be part of that. Expose yourself to information and then go on your own journey, and have your own experience, so that you actually become your own expert, rather than just going on the Internet and buying some product that someone is selling. You don't have to go to the Amazon jungle to get some exotic superfood to be healthy. Watch out for some of these superfoods, because they are going to wind your clock too tight; they're going to blow your adrenal glands and cause you to have some problems, so, be very, very careful. If you think you need stimulation, what you really need is rest.

12. WHAT IS THE SECRET TO HEALTH AND LONGEVITY?

GABRIEL COUSENS

There is more than one secret. Clearly, the research shows that on a vegan diet, men will live 7.2 years longer and women will live 3.4 years longer, as compared to meat eaters. There's a variety of research that points this out. The person who says, "Well, what if I ate the best food, the best organic meat?" is still going to live a shorter life and have more heart disease. Recent research published by the Harvard School of Public Health suggests that people who eat processed meat may lose 18-20 percent off their lifespan or have 10-16 percent more cancer. Even people who eat the highest quality of meat will have 32 percent more heart disease and 35-50% more diabetes than non meat eaters. According to a meta-analysis of 12 studies, meat eaters have 35 to 50 percent more diabetes. When we look at the world literature, it is incontestable that well-nourished vegans live longer and healthier lives.

"Healthy relationships are an important part of the longevity picture, and actually, in the weight of things, healthy relationships are perhaps more important than eating a perfect diet." – Gabriel Cousens

Now, one still needs to be a healthy vegan. In reviewing all the longevity factors, there are a few that stand out. One is low-fasting insulin, and another is low glycemic index intake of food. These seem to be the only significant lab measures for longevity. A live food cuisine of 1600 to 2000 calories per day seems to be associated with longevity. The average American has about 3800 calories in their daily diet.

Adequate clean water, as I've mentioned before, is very, very important for longevity. Another factor is adequate exercise. The Tierman Report, an 80-year study from 1910 to 1990, reflects a very broad understanding, addressing a number of contributors to longevity beyond the physical aspects. According to the Tierman Report, exercise is in the top 8. Other factors include connecting to one's life purpose, love, social connections, fastidiousness, spirituality, adaptability, and willpower.

What is very important is having meaning and value in one's life. In my terms, I put God at the center of my life and make God the context for my life. Being adaptable is extremely important. The ability to be free, to move in any direction, in a world with such chaos and confusion, establishes adaptability as a major longevity quality.

Willpower is very, very important. Again, these were rated in people from the age five until they left their body, and it turned out that willpower is connected with the energy and intent to live a healthy life. Being conscientious, surprisingly enough, was a major marker for longevity, as was prudence, persistence, and being well organized. These are associated with people who, in a sense, love themselves enough to care for themselves. People who are not as fastidious tend to have more accidents and do many things that compromise their health. Fastidiousness is actually pretty high up in the list of associations with longevity. Cleanliness is somewhat associated with the conscientious, with special attention to clean water, clean food, and good hygiene, which are all specifically associated with enhanced longevity in the study of over 900 people.

Knowing one's life purpose and working to be successful is associated with longevity. Also important is charity, receiving in order to share, and serving others. These have all been associated with longevity. Positive thinking—I would term it "thoughtfully optimistic"—is another factor that's associated with longevity. People who are thoughtfully optimistic live longer than people who are pessimistic.

It is good to aspire to the maximum of what we can achieve in our lives, but we must appreciate our limitations and not force ourselves beyond them. We're given certain gifts, and we need to operate at the optimum of those gifts. Avoid unnecessary risk and hurtful activities. People who are conscientious tend to do that. People who are a little bit wild in their life tend to create more damage and literally have shorter lives. Productive living is also important, and that means serving others, having a job, and doing work that's really benefiting the world.

The Tierman Report found that moderate exercise supported longevity. It didn't have the impact I expected, but moderate exercise was indeed an important longevity factor. From a Chinese perspective, maintaining our *Jing* (our primal essence) and not wasting it with excess sexuality and excess drug use, while maintaining a high life force on a daily basis by building *Qi*, are both important. Live food has the highest chi. Live food builds what we call postnatal *Jing* and *Shen*, maintaining a good spirit-heart connection with the world and balancing our emotions and spirit.

Using tonic herbs like gynostemma, reishi, goji berries, and ginseng on a regular basis is part of the Taoist system for promoting longevity. Some newer research suggests it may even build pre-natal chi by increasing telomere length up to 10%. Adequate sleep is extremely important for longevity because your body regenerates during sleep. According to the Teirman report, loving and respecting yourself was actually pretty important, as was not distorting your health with junk foods, cigarettes, alcohol, "recreational" drugs, and psychotropic drugs. These degenerative habits are all associated with decreased longevity.

Interestingly, the Teirman report suggests that, particularly for men, developing the feminine side, which is a more care-taking conscientious side, increases longevity. Being your life purpose is key. People who were being their life purpose tended to live longer than people who just took any sort of job, according to the Teirman study.

Maintaining a very healthy ecological environment supports longevity. Living in a natural dwelling with minimal noise and pollution, living in lower population densities, having low stress, minimizing TV (or not even having a TV), and maintaining access to a high *prana* ecology such as forests, rivers, and oceans are all important longevity contributors. Spending time in nature and seeking out community are vital. According to the Teirman report, social connections are important positive longevity factors. People who are involved in church activities and the like, actually tended to live longer. There's a variety of research that shows that when there's good family connections, people live longer.

Eating 100 percent organic, using natural cleaning products, avoiding all sorts of toxins, including chlorine and fluorine, minimizing radiation, and avoiding the use of drugs and excess alcohol all contribute to longevity.

There is research out there that shows that couples, whether or not they're happy, live longer. Happy couples live even longer than single people or divorced people, although that's a little less so for women than for men. Surround oneself with positive, loving influences is extremely important in the overall picture.

I want to emphasize the relationship aspect in terms of overall quality of life. People who are in relationships, who have healthy couple relationships, have less depression, and they tend to live longer. Healthy relationships are an important part of the longevity picture, and actually, in the weight of things, healthy relationships are perhaps more important than eating a perfect diet. The research on sexuality does show that, contrary to different Yoga and Taoism mythologies, men who have intercourse three times a week (not necessarily Taoist intercourse practices that preserve semen, but normal sexual intercourse) live longer. These men actually have significant less cardiac mortality - approximately 50 percent less cardiac mortality between the ages of 40 and 59. Three major studies in England and the United States have validated this point.

There are other factors to consider, including the quality of a relationship, and that includes vigorous sexual activity, as well as hormone regeneration. I don't think anybody has the exact scientific explanation for this, but the clinical observation is that people live several years longer with a balanced sex life. Men actually added two years to their lifespan and women added half a year with sexual activity. Even half a year is statistically very significant.

Surrounding oneself with a supportive community has been mentioned several times, but surrounding oneself with spiritually likeminded people is also very significant in the overall picture. I would say, live life in love, enjoy your world, and appreciate people. For women, the advice would be, "Don't worry, be happy." For men, "You've got to worry a little bit so you'll be more conscientious." That's what the research actually shows in the Teirman report. We clearly want to build the life-force or *prana*, which takes us back to the physical dimension with Yoga *Pranayama, Tai Chi*, ecstatic dance, and study to develop a quiet mind, with meditation and prayer, mantra repetition and chanting.

The research is fascinating in that actually, after the age of 45, there's a one percent decrease in brain size per year, that seems to be related to B12 deficiency and dehydration, and, fascinatingly enough, the research shows that prayer, meditation, and cardio-vascular exercise actually minimize and neutralize brain shrinkage.

The whole longevity question is a complex one and really the question, when we look at the whole picture is, "Longevity for what?" So longevity is also associated very much with life purpose and meaning. From my spiritual perspective, the life purpose is very clear—to know God and to live long enough to know God.

There are a few unique examples that are fun to consider. There was a famous yogi named Shriman Tapasviji Maharaj who did *Kaya Kalpa* until he became enlightened around the age of 180 or so. He lived to be 186, but once he attained enlightenment, then he stopped doing his practices because he had fulfilled the purpose of life. From a spiritual point of view, it is good to live long enough to become liberated. That doesn't mean that when you become liberated you stop functioning, but you also have a *dharma* and expression that has a time component to it as well.

People with a spiritual worldview will particularly want liberation and also will want to stay in their body until their *dharma* world service is completed, and they have that awareness. When these are completed, then they feel that they've completed their purpose on earth. The ideal is to be like Moshe, of whom it is said that at the age of 120, having finished his life purpose, his "eye had not dimmed, nor had his vitality abated." (Deuteronomy 34:7)

An additional longevity secret is not to view longevity as some kind of materialistic concept of "the number of years, the better you are, and the healthier you are." Life is more complex than that. There are many factors, such as destiny, that intervene in our life, and it would be rather naïve to simply think that you can eat and do all the proper things and everything is going to be just right.

Given that context, my position is to be totally viable—healthy in all aspects. Physically, this means no compromise in physicality and quickness, with healthy sexual function and mental clarity. The point is to be totally optimally functional at any age. That's a different view of longevity, but it's a not a new idea.

Whatever my age, my intention is that my eye be not dimmed and that my vitality be unabated. Rather than how many years I live, I am concerned with the intensity and quality of my life. Ideally one has energy all day long and with reserve, and one is able to do everything one needs to do. With age, there is more effort required to maintain optimal health and physical strength. They used to think that with age people got glycopenia, which is muscle wasting. This is not true, but if one doesn't exercise, one is more likely to have muscle wasting.

In my 69th year I decided to explore what would happen if I lifted weights. I put some energy into it, and I was able to gain six pounds of muscle within one month. I wasn't interested in doing that for a long period of time, because I was not interested in eating so much or the intense physical workout. However, the fact is that it can be done.

There are reasons to stay strong. In keeping one's core strength, one is less likely to fall down or lose balance. With age, people lose their core strength and are much more fragile in their physical beingness on the planet, and therefore much more likely to fall and hurt themselves. They basically aren't as grounded.

With age, people move more into the vata dosha (in the Ayurvedic system). So it's important that people, as they age, actually do more physical exercise to build their core strength, and to thereby maintain their core neurological and physical balance.

VIKTORAS KULVINSKAS

Happiness, being happy. To be happy means to be a self-realized being, which means knowing who you are and discovering through the help of numerology, astrology, and palmistry, as well as meditation. To identify who you are beyond the garbage that you have received from well-intended parents, society, and teachers. Be prepared to take risks and find out what you're like, what your passion is. What makes you feel alive? What makes you happy and be willing to change, because life is change.

We have very minimal nutritional needs once we get into light foods. We really are solar batteries. Like energy devices that handle solar, we're fed by our microbial cultures within the gastro-intestinal track. Engage in periodic fasting. Keep your body young and flexible through physical activity and spiritual practices like meditation. And, by meditation, I mean, still the mind, not the verbosity of guided meditations. It might mean initially you need to get your body into motion, get into the zone. It's a form of meditation whether it is dancing or being engaged in artistic expression. It might be a silent walk while being consciously aware of everything that is going on. Stillness is where your emphasis should be for longevity and health. Probiotics are essential, as are small meals and fasting.

Once you develop the practice of loving yourself, you will see that you will have tremendous amounts of surplus energy and you will be in a position to serve others. Do not get this in reverse. First, energize yourself, and then give surplus energy toward helping others who are seeking to be in the light as you are. Do not be sucked into the energy vampires who are prolifically present everywhere. You can only deal with such individuals when you have become strong enough so that they cannot touch you. Otherwise, they will taint you and can even destroy you. Avoid the negative people until you are strong enough to be a full light and a source of empowerment, but always go back to yourself, to your family, to your sanctity of positive individuals, and that includes nature.

BRIAN CLEMENT

Another very simple answer: finding your purpose and passion; fueling your body with raw, living organic plant-based foods; exercising on a consistent and regular basis; and falling in love with life.

FRED BISCI

It's lifestyle, all the things that I just mentioned—no processed food, raw or mostly raw vegan diet if you can. Remember, it's not all or nothing. Do the best you can, for everything you leave out, there is a reciprocal amount of improvement. Don't settle for mediocrity, and strive to be the most you can in all that you do. If you do this, you will do well and have a long and healthy life.

Clean water, proper rest, fresh air and a plant-based, whole food lifestyle. Try to eliminate as much of the stress in your life as you possibly can. Stress is a killer. It can damage brain cells and cause inflammation in the arterial walls, which can lead to clogged arteries. It can damage memory and lead to dementia. We have twenty-six chromosomes which are caped by telomeres which, when damaged, accelerate aging. Try to reduce and avoid as much stress as you can by slowing down and changing your lifestyle. Meditation and prayer both work very well. Leave out the processed food, and make sure you're connecting all the dots, getting all the nutrients that you need. Make sure you're getting enough calories to sustain your activity level. If you're a couch potato, you don't need a lot of calories. If you're running marathons, and you're training for the Iron Man triathlon, you're going to need more fuel. The calories for an athlete are like gasoline in the car. The further you're going, the more gas you're going to need. Do you have to keep filling up the gas tank if you're not moving anywhere? Of course not, it's just going to spill out into the street.

Most people are just trying to take too much of everything. It's kind of sad. People are taking all these protein drinks and all these super endurance drinks that are loaded with sugar, or are overeating on fruit and they're couch potatoes. That's not going to work. Get off the couch and start exercising. Fruit is a good source of fuel and calories. You don't have to go to excess—if you over do it, it won't work for you. Some people want you to leave out all the fruit. Other people want you to overeat fruit. There is another group that thinks everyone wants to exercise or train four or five hours a day. It is a shame that some people give advice that goes from one extreme to another.

13. WHAT ARE THE MOST SIGNIFICANT CHANGES I CAN MAKE TO PREVENT DISEASE AND MAINTAIN OUTSTANDING HEALTH?

VIKTORAS KULVINSKAS

If you make poor choices, the next day you'll do better. Don't worry about what has happened in the past. Einstein made many mistakes, so did Edison—over 5000 of them—before he found the way to make a light bulb. You are trying to light up your lifestyles so that you can be the light of the world, but first you have to be the light for yourself. If you're in darkness, you can't light up the world.

GABRIEL COUSENS

The single most significant lifestyle change a person can make is to avoid or minimize sugar in all forms, including both glucose and fructose.

In looking at the total picture, we have to consider the very negative effects of sugar. I want to talk about glucose first. I have defined the syndrome in my new book, "There Is a Cure for Diabetes" (Revised Edition), as chronic diabetes degenerative syndrome. This syndrome is not limited to diagnosed diabetes mellitus, but includes an increased fasting glucose followed by sugar spiking and pre-diabetes (which is defined as blood sugar more than 140, 60-90 minutes after a meal). Finally, full-blown diabetes is defined by a blood sugar of 180, one to two hours after a meal. There are enormous amounts of problems with a high-glycemic diet.

Unfortunately, at this point in history, we are seeing in people, particularly children, eating a high carbohydrate cuisine with such problems as chromium deficiencies, copper deficiencies, periodontal disease, and osteoporosis—because sugar pulls calcium, magnesium and other minerals out of the system. The high-glycemic cuisine is common in the live food movement, because there is a desire to compete taste-wise with the degenerative mainstream diet. At the Tree of Life Center US Café we have great, tasty, organic vegan entrees and freshly picked salads from our own gardens. With these quality ingredients, people are less likely to focus on high-glycemic live foods.

All these problems that I'm talking about really exist in the live food movement and amongst people eating a high-glycemic diet in general. I feel that my particular influence has made some degree of difference in shifting that, but it is a struggle, as people want to keep their "comfort zone" transition foods.

As we look at this whole issue of the high-glycemic diet, it is a problem. One of the biggest problems is the increase in advanced end products. This is the process where sugar binds the protein or fat molecules, which then creates an increased free radical problem and increased deactivation of our enzyme processes. Glycation, generally, without going into the biochemistry, accelerates aging, neurological problems, brain-degenerating senility, Alzheimer's, atherosclerosis, and kidney disease, and so forth.

A high sugar cuisine ages the skin by changing the structure of collagen, because sugar is also connected to the advanced glycation end products, known as AGEs. It also impairs the structure of the DNA. A high-glycemic diet, and I'm going to include fructose as well, is associated with cancer of breast, ovaries, intestines, prostate, and the rectum, as well as gout, high blood pressure, heart disease, obesity, and a variety of other chronic diseases. High fructose corn syrup is the biggest culprit, but excess fructose from any source can be a problem.

A high-glycemic cuisine stimulates insulin production. Insulin production may stimulate a hyperplasia that can get out of control and move to cancer. The organs particularly susceptible to this are the pancreas, breast, colon, and prostate. Sugar is carcinogenic. *The American Journal of Clinical Nutrition,* as of July 3rd, 2012, published a study wherein 11,576 women regularly consuming a high-glycemic load showed a 36 percent increased risk of estrogen receptive negative breast cancer.

The study concluded that carbohydrate intake was possibly associated with increased risk of developing estrogen receptive negative breast cancer, the most aggressive type of breast cancer. The sugar's quality is irrelevant. Sugar is not good for anyone. Sugar's suppression of the immune system is associated with multiple sclerosis, anxiety, and depression (the sugar blues). I find this very common in the people whom I see with a variety of mental difficulties, particularly depression, anxiety, and psychosis. The higher sugar diet is also associated with gastric and duodenal ulcers, Crohn's and ulcerative colitis, inflammatory prostate glands, kidney damage, arthritis, and alcoholism. Eighty-five percent of alcoholics have hypoglycemia.

There is a 275% increase in PMS, increased hemorrhoids, food allergies, saliva acidity, general acidity, weakened eyesight, and low enzyme function from the AGE effect. In children we see hyperactivity, anxiety, trouble concentrating, drowsiness, increased eczema, and lethargy. There is a competition between insulin and growth hormones. The more insulin that's being secreted, the lower the growth hormone secretion.

Sugar in any form is ultimately unhealthy, so it is generally good to avoid it and consume a moderately low-glycemic diet. Fructose is now considered to be a problem, particularly high fructose corn syrup. It is directly associated with causing diabetes. It isn't really safer than glucose. In fact, cancer cells need 10 to 50 times more glucose, and they need 10 to 50 times more fructose, than the glucose that they thrive on.

Problematically, fructose is primarily metabolized in the liver and has been associated with a very high level of non-alcoholic fatty liver degenerative disease. In fact, people with NAFLD (non-alcoholic fatty liver disease) usually eat two to three times more fructose than the average person. Fructose indeed, creates AGEs. In fact, it's 10 times more active in creating AGEs. Fructose has also been associated with 10 times more inflammation of the glia cells of the brain.

Fructose has also been associated with diabetes because it mixes up leptin and insulin signaling, resulting in increased food intake and weight gain. One of the problems is that fructose doesn't turn off ghrelin, (the hunger hormone), and therefore people keep eating. Glucose, on the other hand will suppress ghrelin. Additionally, fructose blocks leptin messages to stop eating and to decrease cravings for sweets. Instead, it signals, "keep eating and store fat," and this leads to obesity.

Part of the problem is that humans are designed to handle a normal amount of fructose, which is 15 to 25 grams daily. This amount is found, for example, in two bananas, two kiwis, or a few grapefruits. The average American takes in 81 grams of fructose daily. Fructose, whether from good fruit or junk food, is still fructose. There is a difference between these sources, but it is not a significant one in terms of metabolism.

When fructose intake is above 25 grams per day it is associated with a variety of problems: the chronic diabetes degenerative syndrome, insulin resistance, metabolic syndrome, diabetes, definitely increased heart disease, high blood pressure, obesity, gout, kidney stones, increased AGEs, non-alcoholic fatty liver disease, brain inflammation, increased cancer, and accelerated aging. These symptoms are particularly worse with high fructose corn syrup. Fructose is not a healthy sweetener.

Regarding glucose, again, people don't quite comprehend the seriousness of the glucose story. It is definitely associated with higher effects of a variety of problems. One study showed that people who had a fasting blood sugar of more than 86 had 40% more heart disease after 20 years. The study showed a 21% increase in fasting blood sugar; found 38% people were more likely to die from cancer of the digestive track; and showed a 58% increase in heart attacks, a 26% increase in cardiac failure, and a 27% increase in dying from stroke. This is blood sugar derived from consuming a moderately high-glycemic diet.

If your fasting blood sugar is above 88, which is the case in about 80% of the population, there is a 247% increase in incidents of heart attack, as compared to people with a blood sugar of 85 or less. People with a fasting blood sugar of 95 to 105, which is considered mildly pre-diabetic, have a 100% increase in developing stomach cancer. Remember, high glucose stimulates high insulin, which stimulates hyperplasia. People with a fasting blood sugar over 110 have significant increased rates of cancer. If one's fasting blood sugar is between

100 and 104, there is a 283% increase in developing Type 2 diabetes. It is a serious matter that the high sugar diet commonly found in the live food movement is a problem, regardless of whether it is natural sugar or refined sugar. In the end, the body still reads it as glucose or fructose. Sugar is detrimental to our health, wellbeing, and longevity.

Part of the longevity secret is being lived by the Six Foundations. The Six Foundations include spiritual nutrition and spiritual fasting. This includes an 80-100% live food plant-source-only organic cuisine. It is my experience that a seven-day fast twice yearly, with a series of enemas or colonics, provides very good maintenance. It clears the bowel, drawing toxins from the body in a consistent manner, and allows the body to rest from all supplements and food. Building chi/prana/nefesh, which includes moderate exercise, different varieties of yoga, pranayama, and some cardiovascular exercise, charges the body with oxygen.

"The single most significant lifestyle change a person can make is to avoid or minimize sugar in all forms, including both glucose and fructose. Sugar is detrimental to our health, wellbeing, and longevity." – Gabriel Cousens

This also includes not overeating. My teaching is that the less you eat, the longer you live. Here is the subtlety to that—when we eat live foods we literally can eat half as much because 50% of protein is lost in cooking. According to the Max Planck Institute, protein coagulates when cooked. We lose 60 - 70% of our vitamins and minerals and up to 95% of our phytonutrients when we cook food.

Service and charity compose the third foundation. Support from a spiritual teacher; seeing God in all things equally (equal vision); and perceiving the difference between the absolute reality and temporal reality, all make up the fourth foundation.

The fifth foundation is our focus on the Divine, which is activated by prayer, meditation, chanting, and repeating the name of God as a mantra.

The sixth foundation is to get as much shaktipat or s'micha m'shefa as possible for the awakening of the kundalini or ruach hakodesh.

These are the key elements. The overall result of the Six Foundations is a quiet mind, which helps us transcend the mind and experience the presence of God. They help us place the Divine at the center of our lives and lead lives of purpose. Purpose is valuable, beyond merely focusing on the materialistic view of how long one can live. The question of longevity is not at all my focus, but rather, "Longevity for what?"

Aside from the physical, emotional, mental, and spiritual benefits of the Six Foundations, the most significant dietary changes we can make in our life are to cut out all white flour, white sugar, and processed food, and to minimize our food intake.

BRIAN CLEMENT

Number one—begin, either slowly or abruptly, to remove all animal-based foods. Everything that comes from milk and the derivatives of milk, and everything that comes from the animal kingdom, from fish to poultry, through red meat, through pork.

Number two—hydrate yourself with the purer raw organic juices and pure drinking water.

Number three—exercise aerobically and stretch, as well as lift weights with your body weight or weightlifting mechanism. There's much more beyond that on the psychological realm, but I will leave it there.

FRED BISCI

Okay, I'll go over that again. Give up all the processed food and eat as much raw food as you can. Get plenty of exercise. You don't have to be an Olympic weight lifter or a marathon runner. I believe somebody can get enough exercise in just 20-30 minutes every day, just doing a mix of stretching and resistance exercises and aerobic exercise.

The body lives by natural law. In order to live a long and high quality life, you've got to use your body, and not abuse it. Eat clean food in its highest biological form, meditate, pray - whatever you have to do to maintain a tranquil state of mind. Don't be discouraged, don't pay attention to the news media with all their disasters, be selective about what you watch on television, because a lot of this stuff is so negative, it's depressing at times.

Challenge yourself. Don't settle for mediocrity; strive to be the most that you possibly can.

14. WHAT IS THE BEST WAY TO ACHIEVE HEALTHY BRAIN FUNCTION?

GABRIEL COUSENS

That's simultaneously a long and short discussion in the sense of the colloquialism, "Use it or lose it." The more we exercise our brain, stay creative, stay interested, stay vital, stay hydrated, and meditate and pray, the more we support our overall healthy brain function. There are brain exercises one can do, and there are whole brain gym programs people can utilize. Those are all good things, but in general, without going into detail, simply keeping an active, clear, healthy, meaningful, purposeful life is what we're talking about.

Often, people sustain brain injuries that they carry throughout their lives. I personally help people recover from brain injuries, and sometimes, there are specific homeopathics (beyond the scope of this book) that can help recover from long-term brain trauma. For example, I once helped a person who had been amnesic for seven years after a motorcycle accident, with brain trauma. After one dose of a particular homeopathic, his brain function returned to normal, and the amnesia disappeared. Generally, many of the people I see suffer from brain inflammation, and so I make an effort to test everyone for brain inflammation, which may be from severe toxic stress, radiation, or sustained brain trauma. All these need to be addressed to maintain active brain function.

Regular aerobic exercise is exceedingly important in enhancing brain growth and function. Diet is also important for maintaining ongoing brain function. I recommend a moderately low complex carbohydrate diet, avoiding all gluten and gliadin grains, and a low intake of even non-gluten grains. Grain induced brain degeneration is well documented, especially from gluten and gliadin induced brain inflammation, as is insulin resistance in the brain from all carbohydrates, including grains. Insulin resistance of the brain, as we may find in cases of diabetes, is part of a causal level of accelerated senility and doubles the rate of Alzheimer's. A slight ketogenic diet from a low carbohydrate intake can help to minimize this.

FRED BISCI

More people have dementia now than ever before. Alzheimer's disease is also more prevalent now. Stress is a killer. The latest studies show stress damages brain cells. Stress can affect our memory and is a factor heart in disease. We have twenty-six chromosomes, which are capped by telomeres. Stress can effect and shorten our telomeres, which can damage our chromosomes. This can possibly speed up our aging process. Of course, the best way to maintain healthy brain function is to follow a healthy lifestyle; live according to natural law, get enough rest, eliminate processed food and use better ways to deal with stress.

Your brain is like any other organ in you body. If you want to damage or kill it, follow the Standard American Diet. Eat a good diet, and don't overeat. With a raw living food diet you are on the right track.

BRIAN CLEMENT

I wrote a book years ago on longevity for a Swiss publisher, and I spent most of my time researching non-dietary factors. As time passes, nutritional science becomes a larger part of the medical world. We're finding certain nutrients effectively help brain neuron developments. In that book, what I pointed out was brain use—reading, crossword puzzles, participation with others; contribution was the one outstanding factor that permitted the human brain to constantly flourish, develop and grow, even well beyond 100 years old. When nourishing it with the essential fats - the bacterial forms of B12—this is an unbeatable combination.

As we move forward, we'll be able to validate further which nutrients are essential. As an example, a recent study out of Harvard University shows that elements in raw celery have the ability to maintain short-term memory. We couldn't have told you that 6 months ago. This is an ongoing development, and by constantly keeping up with the Elders on our web presence, much of this information can be poured in to you.

VIKTORAS KULVINSKAS

Fasting on liquid programs. Your brain requires alkalinity for optimization of its power electrical systems. Secondly, it needs oxygen. The best source of oxygenation is green foods, especially blue-green algae. The research has been done by a team of scientists in Nicaragua, who took over 2,000 children with the lowest academic performances and had them consume one quarter of a teaspoon of blue-green algae for one year. The children's academic performance went up by two and a half grades and they became the top school in the country. ADD, ADHD is overcome with the consumption of blue-green algae.

Meditation is the way to increase your mental power, as are small meals. There's an expression—full stomach, empty mind. When your energy is tied up in digestion, you can't have a clear mind. If you're going to be taking exams, or you're about to be involved in an important business decision, you want to stay on liquids like green juices, soaked seed and nut milks. The best thing is green juices and blue-green algae. Not spirulina, which is a big difference. Spirulina is good for bodybuilding and

"The best source of oxygenation is green foods, especially blue-green algae." – Viktoras Kulvinskas

many other things, as is chlorella, but they are not brain food. It is the blue-green algae (AFA) that is the only real brain food. If you want to see the radical impact of blue-green algae, just take about four capsules and chew them up. It will give you immediate delivery to the brain. This is called a sublingual nutritional feeding of the brain. Another thing that can help is gotu kola. Your brain's need for oxygen will also be helped by doing pranayama.

The high protein and fats in ones diet causes the red blood cells to clump together. As a result, the oxygen delivery just does not go adequately enough to the brain, and the volume amount of absorbed oxygen is diminished by 60%, according to science. With the combination of meditation and the practices I suggested, you can be functioning on 100% brain capacity where you have access to the total knowledge of everything that has happened in the past, present or future. That is the human potential. Under the practice of mindlessness and fasting for days, I was able to download all kinds of mathematical equations that no one else in the graduate school could solve. I just sat down and wrote out the perfect dissertations and all the answers without knowing the subject matter.

We have access in that fashion. Each one of us is a potential genius—so do not worry about your perceived limitations. As soon as you become a doubting Thomas about your potential, forget it. Keep realizing that you are a god/goddess with total unlimited mindfulness.

15. HOW CAN I ACHIEVE MORE ENERGY AND ENDURANCE, YOUTH AND VITALITY?

FRED BISCI

How you do that is to detoxify your body, especially your upper GI tract and your lymphatic system. That's what enables us to breathe on a cellular level. When you're breathing on a cellular level, you have a good oxygen uptake and you become more efficient. Everything's going to work better.

We are supposed to have between four and eight pounds of intestinal flora. If you don't have the intestinal flora, you're going to have gas, and your immune system will have a harder time protecting you against pathogens becoming activated and proliferating in your system. You can get the probiotics and the prebiotics from your diet. Inulins come from the fiber in your vegetables and glucosaccharides, which are critically important, as are the prebiotics that come in your fruit.

A lot of times, when a person first starts to eat well, they're not going to feel good, as we all know. They have bloat and gas, and that could be because the food that they're eating could be too efficient. It's releasing too much endogenous material and they don't have the intestinal flora and the system to deal with it. That's when they need colonics, and they need more rest. Rest is critically important.

"Detoxify your body, especially your upper GI tract and your lymphatic system." – Fred Bisci

If you don't know what to do, and you think your diet is okay, and you're not feeling good, go lay down and close your eyes. Remember simplicity. Don't drink a cup of coffee, or take some kind of stimulating herb, or some drink that's going to give you a lot of energy in 15 minutes, because all it's doing is pumping out adrenaline, working through your endocrine system and exhausting your adrenal glands. What you require is rest. If you're exhausted and you don't know why, and the doctor says everything looks good—just lie down, drink more water, and drink vegetable or wheatgrass juices, or E3Live. Clean your body up and follow a plant-based diet.

VIKTORAS KULVINSKAS

I'll give you an example. Dan O' Brien was just an above average athlete who competed in international sports. At best, he could work out an hour a day in terms of training, yet had aspirations to compete in the Olympic decathlon. Under the influence of Klamath Falls blue-green algae consumption, he was also given enzymes and probiotics and felt great. Within several months, he was able to exercise six to eight hours a day. He went to the 1996 Atlanta Olympics, competed with men ten years younger than himself, beat them all, and came home with gold.

Why did this work? It led to him re-alkalizing from the high alkalinity content of the blue-green algae. It helped overcome the limitations of digesting poor food choices by means of enzymes. It also empowered the immune system's high enzyme intake to recycle the tissue breakdown that is associated with extreme sports, and thus, have no downtime. Downtime is due to the lack of hydration and an acidic condition. It's diminished electro-voltage. There is also the fact that one's blood is flooded with incompletely metabolized proteins that are coming from the torn down tissues associated with sports activity. If you have a high enzymatic content, you recycle these tissues and they become amino acids, which means that they can be utilized by your body again. Thus, recovery time is reduced to minimal. Probiotics assure that you're going to have tons of enzymes manufacturing within your gastro-intestinal tract, as well as the production of very high resources of amino acids. If one wants to take it to another level, during the training phase, consume essential fatty acids, oily types of foods, green leaves, and seeds and nuts that have been soaked.

However, if one wants to be functioning optimally during the competitive phase, one should stay away from any kinds of fat for a few days prior to the event. Staying on primarily alkalizing green juices, taking enzymatic supplements, consuming blue-green algae, and adding a little bit of cayenne and/or gotu kola you will create the bloodstream of a winner during competition. Adequate hydration is key, preferably diluted alkaline juices from vegetables. Minimal amounts of fruit juices are fine to include, because you're going to benefit from the sugar, which you're going to burn off. The big emphasis should be on hydration in general. As part of the preparations for competition, one should practice meditation and see themselves as a winner. Practice auric massage, spinning the chakras and work with certain Kegel practices that will maximize your energy, remove blockages from the spine that will optimize the energy flow, and continuously keeping your mind still.

After the events, take more hydration and get back to your regular bodybuilding type of routine. You can consume during the bodybuilding, whatever level you need, a high volume of enzymes and green food smoothies, two to three cups in size every three hours. You could be consuming as much 3000 calories in a single day, as well as over 100 grams of protein. You can do all of those things yet do it on a raw vegan approach. This is in the preparation stage and the active stage. As I said, you want to have maximum oxygen, and that means no consumption of fatty foods, minimal consumption of sugary foods, because they interfere with oxygen delivery, and protein foods, which interfere with oxygen absorption.

BRIAN CLEMENT

I think this begins with attitude, considering yourself viable is the way we create vitality.

Number two is exercise and movement. Here at the Clement household, Dr. Anna Maria and I exercise six days a week. We lift weight three days a week, no matter where we are on the planet. We do aerobic exercise six days a week. We stretch every day and we also make sure that, beyond the gym, we are doing a variety of outdoor sports. This is one great way to keep yourself young.

GABRIEL COUSENS

In essence, it is the total lifestyle that I've been describing. It is a way of living in which you become a super conductor for the Divine.

16. WHAT REGIMEN DO YOU FOLLOW?

VIKTORAS KULVINSKAS

Come into functional foods. Whatever activity that I'm geared up for, I will eat and act appropriately in terms of nutritional and lifestyle habits. Whether I'm involved in bodybuilding, intellectual work, research, or spiritual exploration, I will be in a different kind of a nutritional program for each. In terms of a general nutritional approach, I'll usually drink four to six ounces of wheatgrass juice in the morning, but first I'll have some water or herbal tea, usually with cayenne and a little bit of sea salt. I would follow it up 30 minutes later with wheatgrass juice diluted with water and some cayenne added. It leads to quick absorption within a matter of 20-30 minutes, though I could just stay on wheatgrass energy for a long, long time. Then I follow it up with green juices, about two to three cups in size, made up of celery, cucumbers, kale, sunflower and other greens, herbs, spices and whatever else I might have on hand. Generally, I make enough juice to also use in the afternoon. Meals consist of greens, ferments and sprouts. I like 2 day sprouted grains. I would take a cup of sprouted wheat with half a cup of soaked sunflower seeds, blend them to a cream, add to it garlic or ginger, one chopped up small carrot, one cup of water, a pinch of sea salt to taste and I would eat it with some flax crackers on the side.

That could be my breakfast or I may have a fruit salad or a green smoothie. Generally my green smoothies are chopped up real fine in a Vitamix or food processor. I may take my green juice, mix it with the pulp and eat it as a meal as such. Usually during the day, I try to minimize my meals. Sometimes, I'll have another meal in late afternoon, which would be a wide variety of sprouts, baby greens and other greens. I always include sauerkraut or Kiamichi with some sea vegetables and avocado or, occasionally, some sort of a nut or grain pâté. During the day when my stomach is empty, I'll drink several glasses of water. I'll take blue-green algae and other supplements during the day, as well as enzymes with each of my meals. There are also times I may use ginseng, gotu kola and other herbals, depending on the kind of activity that I am setting myself up for.

BRIAN CLEMENT

Well, what I'm going to tell you is not something to mimic. Remember, this is decades later. When I began, I was an obese American who smoked three packs of cigarettes a day, and marijuana for 10 years, almost on a daily basis. I made a radical shift by giving up all animal-based flesh. Then, I struggled for two to three years to relinquish dairy foods, and, slowly, morphed into a raw, living food vegan. Slowly, but surely, I incorporated high-density nutrient foods such as sprouts and algae, and certain supplementation. In the early days, things like pollen would give me massive nutrients so that I was able to reduce the amount of food I was taking in.

In those early days, I didn't know that there were volumes of research to show that statistically, people live longer and have fewer diseases with lower caloric intake and high density nutrients. I eat very little and drink many raw juices—many are made of sprouts and organic green vegetables, lacking in high fructose. This is something one should aspire to slowly, but surely. One has to be doing this with a sound mind, and it must be tapered in such a way that it's not too rapid. Look at where you are emotionally, where you want to be, and if it takes you years to get there, that's fine. But, the person who is on a conquest of disease—that has to be done much more rapidly, in a clinical setting, at a place like Hippocrates Health Institute.

GABRIEL COUSENS

I have eaten a 99-100% live food cuisine for the last 30 years. My way of eating, organized according to my personal constitution, happens to be a lower protein intake (about 10% protein), 42% fat by calorie intake, and 48% greens, including leafy greens, sprouts and green vegetables, some colored vegetables, and also small amounts of berries and cherries. I have close to zero grains in my diet. I exercise and do yoga six to seven days a week. I do some degree of heavy muscle training one day weekly. I meditate several times a day totaling an hour to an hour and a half. I walk consistently for at least 40 minutes a day, uphill and down, 5-6 times weekly. I do regular breathing exercises (pranayama) every morning with my wife, Shanti. I do some work on the power plate as well. In total, I would say I'm meditating an hour to an hour and a half each day, I'm exercising by doing yoga and pranayama about an hour a day, and physically exercising (including walking) about an hour daily. I'm very active during the day and very creative, yet I still make an effort to get at least seven hours of sleep daily. I try to go to bed by 10:30 pm, at the very latest, and get up at 5:30 am regularly.

I create time for a relationship with my wonderful half side, Shanti, and we spend time together throughout the day. We have a date night at least once weekly and spend each Shabbat together. Shabbat is a complete break from all work, all phones, and all cell phones—for 24 hours. During this time, we don't use the car, choosing to walk instead. I try to be on foot most of the time anyway. My life is very active and creative, between teaching and being involved in the community, and traveling all over the world doing humanitarian work and spiritual teaching. It's a great mix. I also take a variety of supplements—mostly herbs—that support and balance the variety of environmental stresses I face in the world.

I do two seven-day fasts each year, with either colonics or enemas on a daily basis. I also have occasional cycles where I'll do a variety of colonics using super oxygen and iodine. It's very powerful and detoxifying.

I usually have two meals during the day and some sort of juice or soup in the evening. I usually have my relatively larger meal, a salad with nuts and seeds and maybe a half of an avocado, between 1 and 2 pm. I eat a small breakfast, with usually a little bit of chia seed porridge and some sauerkraut. Dinner is usually some sort of juice or in the colder weather, some sort of warm raw soup.

I make God the absolute center of my life and my life context, so I have no focus on longevity but focus all my energy on "seeing the name of God in front of me at all times and all ways," as it says in Proverbs 16:18. My life is involved with a regimen of love and great joy. The primary essence of my regime is the joy and love of God, and love in my life to all people, and most particularly, my wonderful partner Shanti.

FRED BISCI

I have followed a 100 percent raw living food diet for over 45 years. I don't have the desire to eat cooked food. It took me a number of years to get where I am now; it did not happen overnight. I felt good initially, but it took me quite a while to realize what was happening in my body and that I needed less food, not more. Every time I didn't feel good and thought I needed more food, it was actually just that I needed to rest more and do more detoxifying. I eat fruits, vegetables, sprouts, juices, blended green smoothies and a moderate amount of nuts and seeds, like chia, hemp and sesame. I use super green foods.

17. IN RECENT HISTORY, IS THE ALLOPATHIC COMMUNITY BECOMING MORE AWARE OF THE CONNECTION BETWEEN DIET, LIFESTYLE AND DISEASE?

BRIAN CLEMENT

That's a resounding yes. As I read medical journals, I'm seeing, slowly but surely, natural science research coming in and seeping into their literature. There's a long way to go, but I'm encouraged. Many doctors themselves come to Hippocrates to study with us, and this is a global trend.

GABRIEL COUSENS

My medical education at Colombia Medical School included only 1 hour of nutrition lecture. The allopathic community, over time, has become more aware of the connection between diet, lifestyle, and disease. It is a slow increase in awareness. I feel optimistic about this, in spite of the toxic influence from the pharmaceutical world.

FRED BISCI

I don't think so. I see a lot of doctors who are becoming holistic or integrative medical type of doctors, but they don't advocate what I think is a great diet. What they're really doing is substituting neutraceuticals for pharmaceuticals. People come in to see me taking 80, 90, 100 supplements.

A friend of mine told me that he saw a very well known person on television the other day who said he had the answer to living forever. He was taking 120 vitamin supplements. Well, I hope that he's right, for his sake, but that's not the way I look at it, to be perfectly honest with you.

I think that we've got to point science in the right direction, to support the body's function in a healthy way, rather than the way they're doing it now. I'm sure that everybody involved with this book wants to see new things happening; we want the research to support optimal health. When it is available and people become educated, they'll know what to do, and they won't need these neutraceutical substitutes. They'll be able to stay away from a lot of these pills and pharmaceuticals, and really enjoy their life in its highest form—simply.

VIKTORAS KULVINSKAS

Absolutely. In 1990, the *New England Journal of Surgery* published a study of the kind of choices that individuals made in addressing their healthcare needs. They found that over a 100 million more visits went to the alternative healthcare physicians than your typical allopathic. The Journal of American Medical Association did a study to look at the earning powers of the different healthcare management professions, and they found that the alternative healthcare practitioners were earning more on average than the allopathic personal family care physicians. They immediately made major changes in the medical schools, establishing alternative medicine departments where now hypnotism, herbology, acupuncture, reflexology, massage and many other modalities were included in the curricula of many medical schools. The group, PCRM.org - which consists of over 4,000 medical doctors - has taken the position that only a vegan diet is adequate and anything contrary to a vegan diet is contrary to good health. One of the most popular physicians on national television, Doctor Oz, advocates consuming raw green soups as a preventative to all forms of degenerative diseases.

The America Alternative Medical Association, The Integrative Medical Association and the Holistic Medical Association all place a great emphasis on the influence of nutrition. Their research is unquestionably showing the relationship between dietary choices and health. The greatest study was done by Harvard Medical School, which stated that 100% of the individuals on a Standard American Diet (S.A.D.) are saturated with incompletely metabolized proteins. This is creating an impact of inflammatory conditions leading to the immune system being continuously tied up in processing these viral-like structures called twisted proteins, all of which lead to degenerative diseases. The cause of this incompletely metabolized "twisted" protein is the cooking of food. Cancer, cardiovascular diseases, autism, Alzheimer's disease - every disease that you could list, is the result of this twisted protein. This was all confirmed via multiple studies and published on May 23, 2002 in The New York Times Science Section.

FOOD/DIET

"The preservation of our enzymes by eating live foods seems to play an important role in slowing the aging process"
- Gabriel Cousens

"Green juices allow you to rapidly increase your re-alkalizing without consuming a large volume of food." - Viktoras Kulvinskas

"Well, if you look at every single creature on earth that is not domesticated, they eat one food at a time. We're advocates of eating very simple and eating foods from the same family rather than mixing a variety of food." - Brian Clement

"I recommend that you design a diet that you can stay with for the rest of your life." - Fred Bisci

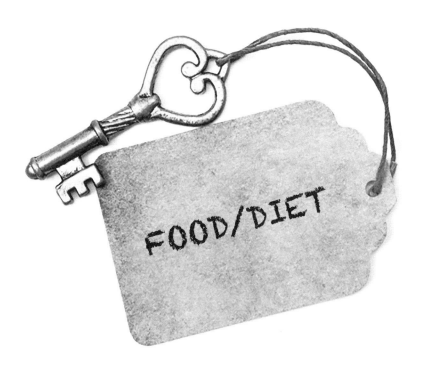

18. ARE THERE ANY DETRIMENTAL RESULTS FROM GOING BACK AND FORTH BETWEEN THE RAW LIVING FOOD AND COOKED FOOD DIETS?

FRED BISCI

Absolutely. I think that's a disaster. I've seen this happen over and over again. I have seen people that were on a raw living food diet for three years or more and, all of a sudden, somebody convinced them to eat raw meat or go back to animal protein, and then they develop a cancer. I'm absolutely positive that's where the cancer came from. I've seen other people get diabetes. Once you go on a raw living food diet or the vegan diet for any length of time, and you're doing it correctly, your body actually changes on the cellular level. It becomes less tolerant of processed food and especially, concentrated proteins.

I think the reason that I have done so well is that I never deviate. Keep it simple. Your body is a miraculous healer and it's the ultimate scientist. It is not a good idea to go back and forth from raw food diet to a diet with processed food. In the long run, it leads to failure. That's why I don't prescribe the optimal 100 percent raw living food diet for everybody that comes to see me, whether they could do it or not, because I know some people are not ready to do it, and I wouldn't want to see them do it for a year or two and go back, because it's not a good idea. A lot of people aren't aware of this because they haven't seen it. I've seen it in my practice because a lot of these people come to see me. I question people extensively and I can see why they got themselves into trouble. I don't like to see people going back and forth, especially from a 100% raw living food diet to eating cooked food. If you're going back to some vegan foods that are cooked, after you get through the initial adjustment, you're going to be okay, but I don't like the idea of going back and forth to animal protein from a 100% raw living food diet. Even if you weren't on a 100% raw diet, if it was 90% raw, I've still seen people get problems.

When people come to see me, I just tell them that if they want to be healthy, then they have to make sure to eat plenty of raw food, preferably 80/20. And if they can do a vegan diet, great. If they can't, then eat a moderate amount of animal protein that's clean, no hormones, no chemicals and no pesticides. If they're willing to go to a 100% raw food diet, great, I love that. A lot of people who come to see me are not willing to do that. I make sure people know that I'm against going back and forth.

BRIAN CLEMENT

I think it's best to slowly, but surely, maintain a raw diet, and if a person swings radically between a raw living organic diet and something as degrading as meat, it can be a big problem. I don't see a major problem if people stay mostly on raw food and then bring in some cooked food along the way.

The work that we did when we were still in Boston, about 30 years ago, when we had colleagues from the university there and the capacity to use their laboratories, showed that people—once they had developed good health and conquered a disease such as cancer, diabetes, or heart problems, among others—could literally eat up to 20% of their diet as organic cooked food without it having a negative effect on the immune system. We're not people who believe in a zealot fashion that one must maintain a 100% raw food diet. But, I think our aspiration in most cases, should be to embrace the 100% raw diet.

I know that in the early days, emotionally and psychologically, that's what I needed, because I have had in the past an all-or-nothing attitude. I'll never forget, when I would open up a cookie bag, I would eat the entire bag. That is maybe what happens to a lot of us, emotionally and psychologically, so it's probably best to maintain a raw diet. Then as you become confident in yourself, your diet becomes a part of your health, not the central part of your life.

It's your life that we're really trying to get together and to get you to look at food as energy to fuel a happy and healthy existence. Once you're at that place, eating a little bit of cooked vegan food is not problematic and not detrimental. Again, swinging radically from one place to another back and forth is not such a great idea. But I don't think it's that harmful compared to going back and eating a horribly bad western diet.

GABRIEL COUSENS

The body likes consistency and the more consistent we are in our cuisine, the more it can stabilize and organize. People who try to go back and forth between these cuisine approaches do not do as well as people who fully assess where they are in terms of percentage of live food and cooked food and slowly move to 80% raw, with clear honesty about what they can really do at a given point in time. I strongly recommend people transition slowly in their dietary approaches, which helps moderate the amount of physical and emotional detoxification that occurs. This also helps to maintain gradual balance and, therefore, will improve their ability to succeed. I strongly recommend one small step at a time, unless one has a particular health emergency, such as diabetes or cancer.

"I strongly recommend people transition slowly in their dietary approaches, which helps moderate the amount of physical and emotional detoxification that occurs."
– Gabriel Cousens

VIKTORAS KULVINSKAS

No, it's all a matter of what kind of cooked food. If you're going to go in and out of doing raw food by consuming processed food or animal proteins, then yes, you're going to run into some serious problems. Your body has the job of adapting itself to every kind of dietary habit. However, if you're going to be consuming probiotics and enzymes with your meals, you're going to find that there's a great deal of tolerance and most often, no difficulty whatsoever.

Processed types of food can cause respiratory problems, so even when you're taking enzymes, they can create complications. If you're going to consume processed foods, just make sure you take an adequate amount of quality enzymes. Also optimal is to always bless your food, whether you're eating raw or cooked. Your attitude and vibration means a lot. Are you saying, "This food is killing me. This food will make me unhealthy?" Forget it and enjoy your cooked food meal and take the enzymes. If you feel like you're heavy and dragging, take a mild herbal laxative at bedtime. Just see what motivated you. Why are you doing this? What's causing you to be driven into this kind of lifestyle behavior? What motivated you? Is it some kind of emotional storm that you're not addressing? If you're looking for comfort, that's what cooked foods are all about.

So, just keep doing the best that you can and gradually, you'll find that you feel totally comfortable on a 100% raw food diet.

In our experience at Hippocrates, you can maintain a very healthy condition if you're taking enzymes with all your cooked food and you make your diet about 70-80% raw. At the same time, be sure to eat organic and make simple cooked meals not elaborate dishes with all kinds of bad food combining, because then of course, you'll be running into problems. And it's not even an issue of raw food versus cooked. If you go out to a restaurant, even a raw food restaurant, and you pile up big huge meals of all kinds of raw foods, and then you add dessert and everything else—well if you take enough enzymes you might be able to get away with it, but it will cause tremendous stress. Small meals well chewed and well combined, this is really the best direction there is. Don't be so hard on yourself, enjoy your life, enjoy the process and you will find that less and less you're being driven into the cooked foods syndrome.

Before you eat a cooked meal, it's good to just imagine what will be happening in terms of your own self. In terms of the biochemistry, the digestion, the reduced energy, vitality and clarity—you're just not going to be fully yourself. You're a happy camper who's high all the time and, all of a sudden, you consume cooked food and you're on a downer trip. So what do you need a downer for? Just get some rest, communicate, write a diary, process thoughts and emotions, call a friend, a raw foodist friend and just talk things through.

19. CAN I EAT FRUIT IF I HAVE CANCER?

BRIAN CLEMENT

More than 3 decades ago, by sheer mistake, we discovered that fructose feed cancer. This happened in an interesting way. In 1980, I was asked to become director of Hippocrates after coming back from several years in Europe, where I was developing the raw food knowledge in countries there, although in modern times, the raw food movement began in Denmark with Dr. Kristine Nolfi. She had the very first living raw food clinic there about a century ago. I had the great distinction of directing that center for a year and also lived in Switzerland, helping to develop centers. I went from Israel to India, all over, and I came back in 1980, and was asked to become the director.

I studied why people came to Hippocrates then. I found that it was through one person, in a book called, *How I Conquered Cancer Naturally*, by Eydie Mae Hunsberger. Eydie and I became friends and colleagues. Eydie was assisted by a fellow who was helping run and develop the Linus Pauling Foundation back in those days. He followed and monitored her with great interest, to learn how she had reversed, on a raw food diet, stage 4 breast cancer. She called me and said her tumors were coming back, but not her cancer. This went on for several years, until she finally concluded that it happened when she was eating large amounts of dried fruit. When the dried fruit was not available, because the season was over in Southern California where she resided, the tumors would go away. This put a big red flag up and an alarm on, and we then did an in-house study in Boston in which we divided the small group in two, half off all fruits—carrot juice, beet juice, any fructose—and half on. About three decades ago we removed fruits from the diets of those with cancer and, in short order, we discovered the same was applicable to viruses, molds, yeasts, fungus, bacteria, and later, Lyme's Disease.

We clinically showed in humans that fructose contributed to all forms of disease, and removed it. As time passed, even mainstream medicine started to recognize all forms of sugar-fed diseases such as cancer. This is a common voice of wisdom and science validation that you hear often today.

Now, do we think fruit is problematic for all people? We discovered there is a level of fruit that one can take organically and ripe, but the preface here is that all fruit, including organic fruit, is picked unripe. Unless you go to an all-you-pick place and it's on the ground or you shake the tree and it falls easily, all fruits are picked unripe. That, in and of itself, manifests acidity because all fruit is acidic when unripe. Your body now becomes an incubator, whereas, nutrients are taken from the bones and the cells etc., by the fruit that is searching for the nutrients that were gained from being on the mother tree, plant, bush, shrub, etc. We don't want that to happen. One can eat, once they're healthy, up to 15% by weight of your diet in fruits and fruit juice. But, only organic ripe fruit and fruit juice.

One of the things that we suggest when drinking fruit juice, is to put 5% to 10% organic fruit juice in the bottom of the cup and then add water. In very short order you're going to prefer that over 100% juice, which is a little overwhelming once you get away from the sugar.

VIKTORAS KULVINSKAS

It's not advisable. The sugars do interfere with the healing process, the oxygen delivery. However, we need to look at everything in perspective. There is such a thing as an optimal nutritional program for someone who is in a recovery associated with cancer. Doctor Max Gerson's program included carrot juice, which is no different than fruit, and they were drinking like six glasses a day of carrot juice. Mind you, the program actually led to healing many individuals who had cancer. However, in reality, one needs to take a look at the whole program, and the overall observation is that on such a program it takes a long time—forever, in terms of recovery. That's number one. Secondly, the individuals are re-enzymized, which is a key driving force in the relationship to cancer that leads to recovery. Doctor Chin Po Kim, without any dietary alteration and with a five year follow up, published results which showed that with enzyme saturation, he had 79% recovery in all forms of cancer. The Gerson program is comprised of just vegetables, which are low in enzymes in comparison to sprouts and wheatgrass or fermented foods. This is the key emphasis at Hippocrates Health Institute Holistic Program and in conjunction with enzyme supplementation, they get total recovery in the shortest amount of time. The Gerson program not a very effective approach. I haven't really seen too many individuals who are regenerated on the level they would have had they followed the Hippocrates program.

The Hippocrates program is basically oriented predominantly on greens, which leads to hyper oxygenation. Dr. Otto Walburger showed that if you reduce the oxygen level in the vicinity of normal reproductive cells by as low as 30%, the cells will mutate into cancer cells within a matter of 48 hours and what they do is have an absorbed capacity for circulatory protein. That is not amino acids, but circulatory and completely metabolized protein, which should not be there in your blood stream. And I show from research and science news that the circulatory protein causes a reduction of oxygen absorption and circulation by as much as 60%. That is critical in terms of triggering the mutation of normal cells into cancer cells.

Other risk factors have been referred to as nitrogen traps or protein dumps. They basically are capable of absorbing circulatory protein to up to 20 times faster than normal cells, thus enabling the transport of normal oxygen and every chemical reaction. As I said, you have 10 followed by 27 zeroes number of chemical reactions occurring within your body every second and this oxygen dependency is very key. You'd die of asphyxiation if it weren't for cancer cells. They help to clean up your environment, and if you stop abusing yourself by eating raw predigested and digestible protein resources, not cooked animal protein, you will not have circulatory proteins. At Hippocrates, we address all the causes of cancer, namely re-alkalizing—which if the body is acidic, it causes normal cells to breakdown rapidly, and at a rate much faster than the body can absorb these broken down cells.

FRED BISCI

Fruit is not really the problem. It's the processed food, especially the processed carbohydrates and animal protein. In the years of my youth when I was a competitive weight lifter, I never saw anyone build muscle to the degree that it is happening today, without excessive protein. Elevated blood sugar stimulates the production of insulin-like growth hormones. Without the protein, cancer cells or tumor cells will not grow as well—they'll just grow like normal cells. The purpose of a cancer cell is just to replicate itself. It doesn't do that well on a diet of low, but adequate protein. Even with animals such as dogs, I have seen tumors shrink with a reduction of animal protein. With that being said, glucose in plants requires insulin. Fructose in non-starchy fruit does not require insulin. The sugar is actually diffused into the cell. I have seen many diabetics that are told not to eat fruit and when they do eat fruit such as cherries, berries and such, their blood sugar goes down. There are some sugars in vegetables, because they contain fructose, and they could actually raise your blood sugar. But, on a raw vegan diet, it is very easy to control your caloric intake by including exercise.

"Cancer is a lifestyle disease. It's not caused by one thing or one food."– Fred Bisci

Most people think that when you're eating fruit, the sugar is going to make you more vulnerable by feeding the cancer. That's not really true, unless you're a diabetic. If your blood sugar is between 70 and 80, and it's under 140 two hours after you eat, it's not really going to have an effect on your cancer.

The reason why people are thinking this is because they're looking at what Otto Warburg said when he won a Nobel Peace Prize. And of course, what Otto Warburg said is basically true, that a cancer cell is an anaerobic cell and it doesn't utilize oxygen. That's why doctors think you have to kill a cancer cell. Because of what Otto Walberg said, a book was written that recommends a diet with no fruits and vegetables, and high in animal protein. There is no sugar in animal protein, but your blood sugar is still going to end up between seventy and one hundred. I would not want to try that. There are a lot of people out there in the nutritional field that I think really don't understand the nature of cancer. I don't want to sound arrogant in any way, but they really don't understand it.

My personal belief is that all disease, including cancer, really begins in the GI tract and the lymphatic system, and most people are focused on the lower GI tract, which is very important. But they need to focus on the upper GI tract, where there are 16 to 20 feet of intestines with all kinds of folds. Your upper GI tract is like a second brain. It has tremendous effect on your whole chemistry.

A lot of people, even if they're moving their bowels three times a day, are really suffering from constipation of the upper GI tract, because what you ate four or five days ago is just finally coming out today. It's passing through the upper GI tract very slowly, especially if you're eating meat, and especially if you're eating meat that has hormones, added chemicals and pesticides from whatever's in the animal feed. Even methane gas is transferred from the upper GI tract into your blood through the villi. A lot of people have this indigestion, which is really a rotting fermentation process, taking place in the upper GI tract, for years.

Everything that is going through your mouth is absorbed through the villi and the upper GI tract, or is eliminated as waste. We have to remember that what happens when people who have cancer eat fruit, and they don't have a clean GI tract, is that the sugars actually stir up more of a discomfort in there, because they cause more fermentation. Every case is different and should be treated as such. Fruit is a healthy food that is loaded with vitamins, minerals and antioxidants. The latest research is showing that, actually, the most powerful antioxidants are in fruits.

As far as the sugar is concerned, there is more sugar in some vegetables than in some fruits. IGF-1 and 2 are insulin-like growth factors, which enable a cell to divide and multiply, and that includes the cancer cell. Surges in your blood sugar cause them to promote growth. It's the protein that is the problem. Processed food and animal protein are the problems, not fruit. A diet that is high in calories, high in processed carbs, and processed food in general, along with animal protein, is the main problem.

Of course, there are other issues. Cancer is a lifestyle disease. It's not caused by one thing or one food. I believe that people should know the whole story and then make their own choices. Some of the best results I saw with cancer patients were people that were actually including some fruit in their diet, but they were doing lots of colonics and lots of cleanses and taking lots of enemas and probiotics.

GABRIEL COUSENS

As I pointed out earlier, all cancers love glucose and fructose, and so this is the prime food of cancer cells. Therefore, in cases of cancer, I strongly do not recommend having any fruit or, for that matter, any high-glycemic vegetables. Cancer cells use about 10-50 times more fructose than glucose for their metabolism.

20. IS IT EVER TOO LATE TO INCORPORATE THIS DIET/LIFESTYLE?

FRED BISCI

No, it's never too late. But, older people who change to an all-raw diet definitely should have professional guidance. You just can't go by the philosophical explanations you're hearing out there on the Internet, because you could put a person into a radical remedial detox, and that could be damaging.

GABRIEL COUSENS

It is never too late. The research, such as Dr. Kallath's from Sweden, as well as my own clinical experience, show that, at whatever age one starts, one is able to reap life-sustaining benefits in just 1-2 years.

VIKTORAS KULVINSKAS

It is never too late. We have many young men and women in their 70s, 80s, 90s and later who have either health challenges or actually want to improve their lifestyle habits in order to have more mileage and start reaching for the Methuselah potential. These individuals not only overcome what are considered by the medical profession to be incurable diseases, but at the same time, take on a much more youthful predisposition. A good example is Noella Johnson, who was an old man of the '50s who began gradually pursuing a holistic lifestyle, eventually getting into grazing live food, then ended up writing a book called "Dead at 70...Stud at 80."

As we grow older, it becomes easier, because we have much more free time and make a full-time job commitment to the idea of rejuvenation and youthing. Start taking baby steps, a daily commitment to a ten minute walk, drinking more water, using tapping or some other technique to get rid of the negative emotions, or, whenever you are negative, get your body in motion and the negativity will disappear.

"Love yourself unconditionally. Forget the past. The future is yours. Be daring. Be young. Be healthy. Be happy and holy." – Viktoras Kulvinskas

Start eating at least one meal a day of live food. Chew your foods well. Eat smaller portions. Organic, organic, orgasmic. Whole food based. Stop eating breads and pasta and all that starchy spaghetti. They are processed foods. Reach for whole grain, cooked and sprouted legumes, sprouted grains.

Visit speakers who are discussing positive lifestyles. Go to potlucks, raw food potlucks, and get rid of that pot. Keep a daily log of your future, both commitment and progress. Don't judge yourself. Just keep on making an effort. "Every day, in every way, I am getting better." Keep saying that to yourself. Love you. Love yourself unconditionally. Forget the past. The future is yours. Be daring. Be young. Be healthy. Be happy and holy.

BRIAN CLEMENT

We don't have "too late" in our vocabulary. Hippocrates is noted for people coming to us at the gate as you say, and we have seen many of these people render up enough self-respect, love, and responsibility to reverse their own diseases. Of course, here in the United States, in Florida, there are certain kinds of people we cannot work with since they need hospitalization. There are clinics worldwide that have hospital facilities and do a far more natural protocol and approach than do mainstream allopathic hospitals. I would search them out for bedridden hospital patients. People who are viable and can walk, talk, think, know that here they can be educated and supported—centers like Hippocrates are the places you should come.

"We don't have "too late" in our vocabulary." – Brian Clement

21. EATING FERMENTED FOODS—ARE THEY HELPFUL AND NECESSARY? WHAT IS THE BEST KIND?

BRIAN CLEMENT

Well, about 30 years ago, we did some research with a colleague who was at the University of Massachusetts, and found that many of the fermented foods had unhealthy bacteria in them. We used to have something called Rejuvelac, which was fermented grain in water with our belief being that it had healthy probiotics in it. Because it wasn't under controlled conditions, it also had unhealthy bacteria in most batches. So, we relinquished that from the Hippocrates diet.

We found food like sauerkraut with its high sulfur content was able to rid the body of the unwanted bacteria. For half of the population, things like sauerkraut, eaten alone as a small meal or in between meals, is appropriate. The other half can choose for it to be eaten along with their food, without it being potent in creating further gas.

Consuming the right fermented food under the right conditions is fine. There's lots of history to show populations that consume this predigested food with high enzymatic quality live a little bit longer too.

VIKTORAS KULVINSKAS

The cultural studies that have been done on the nutritional impact of longevity found that countries that had the lowest incidence of infant mortality, premature deaths, and degenerative diseases, as well as high longevity, all, as a general pattern, consume some form of fermented foods on a daily basis. Fermented foods are the major source of enzymes within your gastrointestinal tract, B-complex, B12, as well as being a very tasty food that adds a great deal of gusto to the meal itself. The best choice is the one that you like the most.

Our friendly bacteria are extremely important. Not only do they create a hostile environment to the pathogenic microbes within which you are immersed, but they can be the resources for 30 grams of protein by fixating nitrogen from the air and making it available to you on a daily basis. In a healthy individual, over 60% of the fecal matter is made up of friendly bacteria. So if you have difficulty in expelling your waste, it's a good indication that you are not only acidic so that your peristaltic action is weak, but also you have very low number of friendly bacteria creating the bulk and fiber component. The documentation and a reasoning is found in my book *Survival*.

On my YouTube channel, Viktoras Kulvinskas, you'll find how to make almost instant sauerkraut with kimchi and other beverages in twelve hours, more or less, through techniques that I have innovated by conversing with the microbes. They directed me during the last 35 years on how to get it right. Also through my fermentation process, you maximize the enzymatic content. You'll not only have an extremely high source of probiotics, the friendly bacteria, and also you'll have extremely high resources of enzymes.

When should you eat it? Definitely never with starchy meals, because it interferes with the metabolism of starch. Starch digests well in an alkaline environment, not in an acidic environment. If you have a history of migraines or severe aches and pains, chronic fatigue and chronic pain, you definitely would be better off just consuming probiotics in moderation. Test it or introduce it gradually, in very small amounts, because they do increase the acidity; however, an individual can handle more when they are healthy, when they have alkalized their body through fresh green vegetable juices and green salads, sprouts, etc. You can have a diet that is made up of 20% from the acid category, such as fermented food.

The least of all recommended, though if you have a high tolerance, go for it, but in moderation, is Kombucha tea. That is made by utilizing a mushroom. It's a beautiful beverage, but it is made, as a rule, with some form of sugar and also with caffeinated teas. You can make it yourself. Get the mushroom on the Internet and you can avoid these particular components, or minimize their presence. In the fermentation, alcohol is also produced. Continue to explore, experiment, including developing cheeses of all sorts, from every seed and nut, even from some of the legumes that are going to be adding the life of source of protein, predigested amino acids, and enzymes.

GABRIEL COUSENS

There is some research that suggests that sauerkraut and kimchi are the best way to supply the body with healthy probiotics, and the body definitely needs a regular input of probiotics. Personally, I use primarily kimchi—being a kapha constitution physically. I tend toward spicy foods and do better with them, and so I like kimchi or spicy sauerkraut. This, of course, should be raw and eaten daily. The fermented foods have advantages. Some people say they give you as much

"...sauerkraut and kimchi are the best way to supply the body with healthy probiotics." – Gabriel Cousens

as ten times more the amount of probiotics that you can get or sustain with supplements, and they are able to sustain themselves in a more healthful and stable way in the body. Keeping a good probiotic base is very important for many levels of health.

FRED BISCI

Fermented foods are helpful, but I don't believe they're necessary. I do eat some fermented foods and they are a good form of probiotics. I would say a good kimchi and raw sauerkraut are the most useful for everyone.

22. WOULD YOU ADVOCATE A 100% RAW LIVING FOOD DIET, AND, IF SO, FOR HOW MANY YEARS? IS IT NECESSARY FOR OPTIMUM HEALTH?

BRIAN CLEMENT

Well, we certainly advocate a 100% raw living organic diet for everyone who's in the conquest of disease, or who wants to radically turn around the free radical damage and the degradation of their own health that's not going to sustain a long life. For the early stages of even "non-diagnosed" healthy people, yes 100% raw. Again, to repeat—for those people who are as I was for most of my life, that is all or nothing, you're probably best eating a 100% raw diet. To repeat again, up to 20%, even 25% of your diet by weight as cooked vegan organic food would not really impact your health in one way or another and, in my observation has been very, very good psychologically and socially for people because it allows them to be with their families or friends without anyone feeling awkward.

VIKTORAS KULVINSKAS

In the wild animal kingdom, from which we all evolved, nobody questions what percentage of the diet should be composed of living foods, raw foods and cooked foods. Neither should it be an issue for people. However, considering the practical issue—that you are an addicted individual who is trying to return to a natural state of consciousness, lifestyle and resources of energy and nutrition—what percentage of your dietary habit would be desirable to be composed of raw and living foods?

If you are an individual who is suffering from some form of what is medically stated as chronically incurable disease, or medically treatable disease, which it really isn't, then all they are doing is turning you into a drug addict and continuing to siphon off finances out of your pocketbook until they have you at the mortician. However, if you want to take control of your life and be your own doctor, then, our favorite thing by our Reverend Ann Wigmore, would be to go on an all raw food diet that would be about 85%-90% of your diet made up of baby greens, wheatgrass, sunflower greens, buckwheat, all forms of sprouts, some fermented foods, a little bit of seed cheeses, and also baby vegetables. You would emphasize immature vegetables, especially the spring greens and emphasize overall greens, which are mature plants with much less enzymatic composition, as well as pursue all the other modalities of a therapeutic lifestyle - enemas, days of fasting, as well as intervention through noninvasive forms of therapies that accelerate the process of rejuvenation. If you have already moved into a healthy condition, and if you so wish to continue to indulge in some form of cooked food, go for it.

The resurge of Pottenger has very significant indications with animal experiments. By having a diet made up of 80% enzymatic nutrition, you find that they had healthy reproduction, no changes in genetic makeup, and of course, longevity was not compromised, fertility was not compromised, and no degenerative diseases appeared.

"….using it as comfort food, which shows that you have some old emotional stuff coming that you are not processing." - Viktoras Kulvinskas

They appeared to have a normal pattern of aging. On the cooked food diet of 80%, they found degeneration such that the first reproduction led to individuals living now with anticipated reduced longevity, and already exhibiting old-age diseases at middle age. Those who were able to still be of reproductive quality on this 80% cooked food diet were followed by the next generation in which the degenerative conditions appeared in the teenage years, and most of them had lost their reproductive capacity. With a raw food approach, they were able, within a period of several generations, to return their pattern again to normalcy. Remember, they were working with raw foods—not high enzymatic activity of the germinated, fermented and soaked seeds, and nuts—the kind of foods that are extremely high in enzymatic activity and in a predigested plan base.

If you want to maximize your quality of life and increase your longevity, then in the words of Dr. Gabriel

Cousens, in his book *Spiritual Nutrition*, you'll find that raw food is a prerequisite for the soul journey traveler who wishes to align himself in a most rapid and deep way to the cosmic creation process and has overcome all addictions, including the addiction to cook food. I wrote the introduction to the book and I highly recommend it.

Certainly as you can see, eating enzymatically active foods is going to be part of the solution to whatever question you ask, as long as you wish to continue to live in this sacred temple and, as has been expressed, cleanliness is next to godliness. Cooked foods will leave many more track marks, much more residual waste products, and that starts piling up the patterns of aging, showing up on your facial features. What you don't digest, that is enzyme-less type of food, you wear it on your face, you wear it on your skin. It ends up plugging up your capillaries, your arteries, your brain. Fasting and cleansing will help, but it's much better to minimize the waste products and to go more and more towards the 100% raw food dietary orientation.

At the same time, don't get into orthorexia, where you become addicted to doing everything right. Be very forgiving if you slip back and end up having something marginal that is cooked food. Take plenty of enzymes and your body will hold no record of this transgression. However, if it becomes habitual, then you are using it as comfort food, which shows that you have some old emotional stuff coming that you are not processing. You need to address and get rid of it, erase it out of your blood pattern, so that you are continuing to stay as a happy camper who is handling all the stresses that come as part of living in a civilization, without any reliance, escape or suppressive mechanism. Escape can be in the form of a Tombstone pizza and tranquilizing yourself into oblivion, or you might take the next gaff, which would be caffeine, drugs, cocaine, marijuana—all the kind of stuff that, again, is part of the escape because you're so acidic and you need to temporarily reduce the acidity and make yourself feel a little bit happy or a little bit more active. But, it's an indication that you need some radical changes. Don't judge. Love yourself unconditionally and move on by improving your lifestyle habits. Goal setting, focus, creating a timeframe schedule, and anticipate results. Keep a log, a diary, hang out with raw foodists for support and go out as a missionary among the cooked food tribes that badly need your advice.

FRED BISCI

I don't advocate one specific dietary philosophy for everybody. I advocate a diet that's the best for each individual's optimal health. The only thing that I'm very specific about, that everybody that comes to me should really try to achieve first, is to give up all the processed food. As far as the length of time it takes to achieve optimal health, I can't give a time on that because everybody's a biochemical individual. For some people, it happens very quickly. For others, it takes years before they really feel super—the way people are capable of feeling on this type of a diet.

A 100% raw diet is the way to go, if it can be done. It certainly seems that many can't do it. Sometimes people on a 100% raw food diet might have to use some kind of supplement, like Super Green Food or blue-green algae. Wheatgrass also works very well. I'm not very fond of wheatgrass personally, though I do use it sometimes. I use blue-green algae; the E3Live BrainON is very good.

GABRIEL COUSENS

I advocate a minimum of 80% organic live food cuisine as a cutoff point. I find that people who are able to sustain an 80% live food cuisine, after a few years reap the same health benefits as people who go on a 100% raw food diet, although those on a 100% raw food cuisine attain these benefits more quickly. They also take a risk of more intense detox, both physically and emotionally. However the difference between 80% and 100% live cuisine is significant in terms of its spiritual impact. A 95-100% live food cuisine helps one become a more consistent and more powerful super conductor for the Divine in a shorter time. However, I want to point out that on a live food cuisine we can eat half as much and get twice as much nutrition, so generally, just eating less will also support spiritual life. Remember, from a spiritual perspective, one cannot eat their way to God, but an 80-100% live food cuisine supports one's ability to become a super conductor of the Divine.

I have been eating a 99%-100% live food cuisine since 1983. This is over 30 years. I have no intention of changing that, as it seems to be a successful cuisine for all aspects of my life, physically, emotionally, mentally, and spiritually. Is it really necessary for optimal health? I think that an 80% live food cuisine, properly balanced, works well for most people.

23. GREEN SMOOTHIES VS. GREEN JUICE—WHICH IS BETTER AND WHY?

FRED BISCI

I believe they both serve two completely different purposes. The green juice is a very powerful alkali and it gets into your system very quickly. It helps reduce inflammation and provide additional nutrients, and it's useful in situations where people can't masticate well. I also encourage people to use smoothies made in a blender where they can control the RPMs so they keep the oxidation to a minimum

GABRIEL COUSENS

I recommend green juice, because it is a much more powerful food concentrate. It is more cleansing and more alkalizing than green smoothies. Green smoothies, on the other hand, can undermine the overall eating process. When we blend food, there is some question about them being oxidized, as their cellular structure is broken up and disrupted electromagnetically in different ways, with all blending machines. Green smoothies change our eating patterns. Many years ago, I read a report out of England where they gave mentally disadvantaged kids all their food via smoothie. After two years, they saw that there was degeneration in their digestive tract.

Chewing food well is very important. Although people will certainly iterate that, even with smoothies, one can chew their food. However, it is less likely, because the body senses that it has already masticated, so trying to chew a smoothie takes a lot of discipline. Why is it important to chew our food?

1. Chewing stimulates a five-fold increase in serotonin production.
2. Chewing stimulates all the meridians in the teeth.
3. Chewing prepares the body and acclimates the body for digestion.
4. Chewing activates a great deal of saliva, and there's a tremendous amount of energy in the saliva itself.

There are whole disciplines where people just practice chewing and generating saliva. Chewing is an essential macrobiotic practice. The more we chew, the more we activate our whole digestive system. The more we build saliva, the more we activate our teeth and our jaw muscles. These send off all kinds of healing signals to the body. I recommend chewing each bite at least 50 times. When one drinks smoothies, it is far less likely that they will do that, and I think it sets up a slow and subtle degeneration process. People haven't been doing smoothies long enough to really see the results over the decades, except the research with the developmentally disabled children, which only suggests that there could be a problem, because the context is different.

Green juice is directly absorbed. It is clean, clear, and it really comes into the body as distilled water and supports our overall intake of particular minerals and nutrients. For this reason, I feel that green juice, at least once daily, is a very good thing, and I strongly support green juice fasts.

Those are the main differences between juice and smoothies. It is vital to create balance in our manner of eating by establishing a stable pattern. When we move to prolonged blended foods, and then go back to eating just raw food, I think it's a little more confusing for the body. I recommend chewing food well, having two meals a day according to one's constitution, and adding juices, which yields an increased concentration of nutrients and supports detoxification. Juicing, because it is concentrated, helps minimize nutritional deficiencies. Raw juices help us to quickly assimilate nutrients. They are powerful for nourishing and regenerating cell tissues and organs.

It need not be an "either/or" for blending verses juicing. Simply understand that blending is not a substitute for juicing. Juiced foods are easier to assimilate. Juice is a fully cleaned liquid, whereas blended food is essentially a more broken up food and is an advancement on the digestion process. My long term observation at the Tree of Life Center US, in people trying a 2-3 month blended diet, is that they don't lose any more weight than those on a 2-3 week juice fast on which I have seen people lose up to 46 lbs. My theory, based on some research, suggests that on juicing the body stays in fasting mode, and on blended food it goes into more of a food deprivation mode and holds onto the weight.

VIKTORAS KULVINSKAS

Most people come into the raw food lifestyle enzyme-less, severely depleted enzymatically, extremely acidic, and with digestive and allergic conditions. As you very well know, the only foods that are alkalizing are the raw foods and the raw juices.

You need the alkaline juices to accelerate the whole process of re-alkalizing. That will help prevent rocklike crystals from building up that can be marginal to the point where they're already causing pain, or pain under active pressure, or pain on walking. You can get rid of these crystals with salt baths as I have described in other places. Also, I recommend consuming at least a pint twice a day of green juice. Use celery, cucumber, kale, baby greens, possibly some sunflower greens and other green herbs and spices. If you find this initially highly unpalatable, add a carrot or two, or one small apple, for a different flavor. Experiment, and you'll find very desirable overall results.

Green juices allow you to rapidly increase your re-alkalizing without consuming a large volume of food. It takes approximately one pound of greens, carrots or apples to produce ten ounces of juice. If you eat one pound of vegetable in the form of greens or fruit, it will take a long time to digest, process, and pass through your system. In the form of juice, it would be assimilated within thirty to sixty minutes, so you would able to consume a much larger volume of alkaline components into your system.

The green smoothies can be an excellent source of protein. You can choose from spirulina, a mixture of greens that include blue-green algae, chlorella, as well as all forms of grasses in a dried form, which are 40% protein, and algae are about 65% protein. It's a much better choice than all the protein powders in the world. You can have your protein powder resourced from soaked seeds and nuts, which, once they've gone through soaking, become predigested, low in fat and also very high in enzymes and amino acids. They are better alternatives to any of the soy, whey, or rice proteins.

Protein smoothies are good for those with hypoglycemia, or those on a body rebuilding mode trying to add extra lean muscle mass, as well as for individuals who, due to compromised dental situations, aren't able to chew their foods too well which places stress on the digestive process. A smoothie meal, if you're consuming about two cups, is usually digested in a short period of two to three hours, so you could have many frequent meals of that sort. The more you consume at a single sitting, the longer it's going to take to digest. It is not good to take anything beyond three cups. Two cups is going to keep your mind clear and your energy high, without tying up a lot of your energy into the digestive process.

When you're creating a blended preparation, start off by blending the soaked nuts and seeds and concentrated greens with your liquid medium, preferably water. If you can add a little bit of fruit, add some berries, or an apple, or some papaya. Finally, just add in as the last measure, some of the greens—fresh raw greens like kale, spinach, sunflower—and just marginally, for a few seconds, chop it up, but don't run it any duration of time. It diminishes their nutritional value by a very significant amount the longer you blend them.

Such nutrition is great for office workers, athletes, as well as philosophical thinkers. They're having the most efficient and productive day, by having liquid forms of meals, whether they're in juice or smoothie forms. Using them throughout the day and then having more complicated, chewy meals in the evening within a family setting or a business meeting works well.

BRIAN CLEMENT

Well, a smoothie is not a juice and a green juice is not a smoothie. In recent years, smoothies have become prominent, and I'll give you the history of the "green smoothie," which is interesting. Back in the very early 1980s our founder, Ann Wigmore was never much interested in the economics of the operation of Hippocrates. She covered the bills for what it was costing us to buy green vegetables with which to make green juice, and, at the time, it was thousands of dollars. Now, we spend multiples of thousands of dollars a month buying these organic vegetables to make green juice. She then personally came up with an idea that she could instead, blend up the vegetables, thinking it would be less expensive. Later, other people decided to also blend in fruit.

So, it was all really initiated by a concern over economics, and God bless Ann, she was an Eastern European and went through very, very hard times herself, and I understood. It was never really out of the sense of health or digestibility.

Now, one area of health that does enter into this is, at times, we have people with Irritable Bowel Syndrome, Colitis, all of these terms. In such cases, we use these green smoothies, as they're called today. Certainly with food combining, not with fruits and vegetables and nuts and seeds and avocados and coconuts and all the things people put in—including the agave syrup—but just blended up green sprouts and veggies. So, it would be easier without the roughage concern for these gastrointestinal problems.

We also had a colleague of mine, who as a favor, ran a little subtest at a university here in Florida, where we went in with the highest speed blender and found out that, in 90 seconds of blending, you're losing about 90% of the nutrients, for obvious reasons. The blending process oxidizes the cells and opens the cell walls, while blowing air through it, and in that manner, it breaks down the nutrient factors. That was a pretty easy test. So, a green smoothie is not nutritionally at the same level as a fresh, immediately consumed green juice.

The blender manufacturers try to tell you that you need the roughage in the juice, or you need it in the liquefied food. But, roughage requires chewing. Why? It's nature, the evolutionary, process that requires it. Chewing activates enzymes that break down the fiber of that food and brings the nutrients out. Can you imagine what happens when you liquefy food and drink it, and then it completely bypasses the enzymatic activity? 90% of the nutrients are gone. It seemingly ferments in people's bodies at that point and, I find the true advocates of blended food to be either emaciated, very thin people, or obese people. It's what's happening. The food doesn't interact with metabolism, enzymatic processing and channels of the system, and ferments while creating a really slow metabolic, obesity or overweight issues, and with fast metabolism, a thin body.

Juices have a problem too, if you use a proper augured based juicer and drink the juice immediately, you're getting most of the nutrients, but we found out a long time ago that if you let that juice sit for 15 minutes, it's more than 90% dead. We always joke and say get two people: one juicing and one drinking under the juicer and then switch back and forth.

We're big believers in juices, we've been using them successfully for almost 60 years. We've watched the results on a clinical level. We can take pounds of highly dense nutritious foods and get you to drink it, where nobody would be expected to, nor should they be, consuming pounds of food to get nutrients. Drink it fresh.

Is there anything wrong with taking blended food, providing that all of the things blended are appropriate together? Absolutely not. We use blended food as a bridge, as a recreational food, but not as nutritious food. Again, as food must be employed in many cases for people with really bad intestinal problems, and as slowly as those problems get better and resolve themselves, then they can go to more roughage.

24. WHY DO YOU RECOMMEND A RAW LIVING VEGAN DIET?

FRED BISCI

I've been doing it myself for 45 years, so I know how miraculous it can be, and what it can do to alleviate the aging process and keep you healthy to a very advanced age. I believe it to be the best diet for a person who understands it and is willing to commit to it for the remainder of their life. The commitment is key, because I have seen too many people follow a 100% raw living food vegan diet for years and then go back, and a lot of them had a disastrous experience. I encourage people to make the transition gradually and then to stay with it. To go back to eating animal protein is not a wise thing to do; it can cause disease and failure.

> *"...to alleviate the aging process and keep you healthy to a very advanced age." – Fred Bisci*

BRIAN CLEMENT

Well quite simply, it's because we've seen, with hundreds of thousands of people, the resulting effect of eating the raw diet on a biological, physical basis, and we are morally committed to the idea that this is the diet humans should be eating, since it protects fellow creatures and protects the very planet we live on.

All serious environmental scientists that look at the area of diet show us that, minimally, 40% of the problems we have with greenhouse gases and the breakdown of the environmental ecosystem on planet earth, have to do with meat and dairy consumption.

VIKTORAS KULVINSKAS

Because it's the most compassionate way to eat for humans and all other life forms. You submit to your quantum electromagnetic body fuel that creates the highest energy and highest corrective, rejuvenating, regenerating effect on the human organism. It is the way of creating a sustainable planet, whereby we can easily feed and nurture a much larger biomass than even the seven and a half billion people on planet earth, without any kind of ailments, existing in a happy, harmonious, healthy, and holy way. With disorganized foods, we create disorganized physiology by the use of fire, by the use of radiation, by the use of frying—we create something that is going to place high stress on the organism which accumulate with incompletely metabolized products being retained within your system and creating the aging process.

Even within the wild animal kingdoms, dietary choices that are appropriate to a particular species and structural orientations, such as the anthropoid apes, certainly fit into the category of a human similarity. They are the strongest animals in the world and live exclusively on greens, just like other mammals live on greens, and they present strength, wisdom and a peaceful predisposition. By consuming heat-treated animal protein, you are looking at ingesting the pain and suffering of tortured animals that have gone through the slaughterhouse, and you take on the vibration of fear by way of their pituitary excretions and their adrenalin excretions, and in this manner, there can never be a planet of peace. War is very disorganizing and, interestingly enough, the opposite of the word war is R-A-W, which is right.

Basically, we have a solution that will give us not only freedom from disease, freedom from war, and much better usage of resources, but a peaceful planet as well. Vegan as a starter, and eventually raw food, as we progress in consciousness and awareness—you'll finally come to the idea of cooking vulgar like smoking.

GABRIEL COUSENS

Let's begin with the philosophical aspects of the vegan cuisine before we discuss the living raw aspects. Eating a raw living vegan cuisine goes back to the time of Genesis (6000 years ago), where it was the primary cuisine given to humans. There is a historical component to live food veganism. This is not a New Age fad diet.

According to Herodotus, the Pelasgians ate 100% live food, and their average age was 200 years. They lived 3000 years B.C. in southern Greece. Then we have the evidence of Akhenaten and Nefertiti (the pharaoh and queen of Egypt) about 1351-1334 B.C., advocating a live food diet for all of Egypt, and particularly for the priest class. In at least the inner circle of the Essenes, who emerged 600-500 B.C. and existed in community until 70 A.D. until they were dispersed by the Romans, they were said to eat

"A live food vegan cuisine brings peace with the body, peace with the mind, peace with the family, peace with the community, peace with the culture, peace with the ecology, and peace with the Divine." – Gabriel Cousens

vegan live food. Pythagoras, who lived 570-495 B.C., was said to have been taught by the Essenes, and became enlightened on Mt. Carmel, where he trained with them. Until the time of Donald Watson in the 1940s, a person eating a plant-based diet was called a Pythagorean.

The live food diet was lost over time and re-emerged in 1890s with Dr. Bircher-Brenner, who used it for healing, and read much of Pythagoras' work about it. In the 1920s Dr. Max Gerson initiated the healing of type 2 diabetes with live food by curing Dr. Albert Schweitzer, and wrote the famous book, *50 Cured Cases of Cancer with Live Foods*, in 1937. It was published in English in 1957. Between 1940 and 1970, Dr. Edmund Bordeaux Szekely, who reignited the Essene movement in 1929, was said to have treated 133,000 people in Mexico. Ann Wigmore did remarkable work in the '60s, followed by the current Live Food Elders today; namely myself, Brian Clement, Viktoras Kulvinskas and Fred Bisci—who have been working with this clinically for 40 years plus. The whole history of live food literally goes back 6000 years.

Today, feeding lower on the food chain with only plant source cuisine is important for the survival of the human species. As Dr. Abraham Hoffer, Ph.D. wrote, "Recent intergender durational research in animals and people have shown that on an uniformly poor diet, the offspring of each generation deteriorates more and more. This continues up to eight generations. We do not know what the final stage will be in the human deterioration. I shudder to think of the final outcome."

Today, we are overwhelmed by environmental toxicity. There is increased radiation exposure coming from Fukushima, and there are many pesticides. We know that animals have 15-30 times more radiation in their tissues than vegetation, and not only radiation, but also 15-30 times more pesticides and herbicides. This is not just I-131 and depleted uranium, but over one hundred radio-nucleotides released from Fukushima, in addition to the radiation released 25 years earlier from Chernobyl. These are very significant exposures.

Preserving the germ cell for viable reproduction is vital. Both Pottinger's cat research and Weston Price's research (which was not about ingesting meat, but rather about the bad effects of a diet high in white flour, white sugar and processed and cooked food) showed a degeneration of germ cells and a decrease in viability. Holistic veganism and live food is best suited for the protection of the germ cell and survival of the species.

That's one major reason why I am in favor of live food veganism. We know that live food veganism preserves and protects personal health, vitality, and energy. The meat-centered cuisine hoards resources. The food that feeds 100 cows could feed 2,000 people. If all the people in the world ate plant-source only, we would have enough to feed the entire human population 7 times over. If everybody ate live food, plant-source only, there would be enough food to feed the world at least 10-12 times over. The only thing that stops that flow is human greed.

It is important to eat low on the food chain. This means plant-source only nutrition. It prevents cruelty to animals. It also preserves the ecology and the global community. It preserves the topsoil, and it preserves the water. Animal agriculture uses 50-75% of the water and 85% of the land, and requires 10 to possibly 29 times more energy to bring the food to your table. A vegan diet minimizes the pollution of the environment. This includes carbon dioxide, which now has gone from 280 parts per million to 382 parts per million, making it harder and harder for us to get adequate oxygen. An animal-based diet produces methane, which contributes up to 30 times more global warming, and ammonia, which creates up to 300 times more global warming.

A vegan live food diet maintains and protects the human bio-computer mind, so that one may go beyond the five-sense bio-computer mind to know God as the purpose of life. By this, the mind is able to move out of the matrix. It is able to experience the consciousness of sovereignty.

The Ten Speakings, known as the Ten Commandments and the Yama and Niyama in the Yogic system, are fulfilled and protected by living a lifestyle that includes live food vegan cuisine. The result is a calm mind and inner peace. A plant-based diet clears the nadis, which are the body's subtle energetic channels, and the koshas, which are the layers of the mind through which spiritual energy moves. Thus, by eating a live food vegan cuisine, we become superconductors of the Divine. It is no accident that the vegan live food cuisine is the cuisine most associated with spirituality and enlightenment in almost all traditions. We know that the ancient Taoist masters and the ancient Rishis several thousand years ago ate a live food cuisine. The Torah teachings of Genesis 1:29, recommend a live food cuisine for spirituality.

As we look at these aspects, it is important not to take a righteous, moral viewpoint, or a superior viewpoint, but instead, to understand that we are responsible for the total impact of our actions. A live food vegan cuisine brings peace with the body, peace with the mind, peace with the family, peace with the community, peace with the culture, peace with the ecology and peace with the Divine. A live food, vegan cuisine brings seven levels of peace. In Genesis 1:29, God said, "Behold, I have given you every herb yielding seed, which is upon the face of the earth, and every tree, in which is the fruit of a tree yielding seed; to you it shall be for food." That is a very clear statement of a live food vegan cuisine. Then, it is interesting to note that Genesis 1:30 recommends "for every beast in the earth and to every bird in the heavens, and everything that creepeth upon the earth, wherein there is life, I have given every green herb for food: and it was so." Even the animal kingdom, in time, will no longer be carnivorous.

In the Yamas and Niyamas and the Ten Speakings (Ten Commandments), we have ahimsa, which is nonviolence or at least minimized violence, or "Thou shall not murder," which is the 6th Speaking, and this of course, applies to killing animals. Then we have satya, truth; and "Thou shall not bear false witness." The flesh-eating world creates a myth that the animals are just happily giving their lives so we can eat them. For example, Elsie the Cow is so happily giving milk, that she doesn't mind being milked to death. Dairy cows used to live 30 years and produce about 2,000 gallons of milk a year. Now, with all the hormones and other ways of extracting milk, they're giving about 50,000 gallons a year and dying in three to five years. This is the kind of lying that goes on. The meat just appears in the store. The third is asteya, non-stealing and "Thou shall not steal." When one is killing the animals, they are stealing their life; they are stealing the fur; they are stealing the flesh; they are stealing the milk; they are stealing their eggs; and they are stealing the animals' soul function.

Now, the 9th Speaking is, "Thou shall not commit adultery," which in the Yamas, is brahmacharya (control of sexual energy). "Adultery" in the Torah means sexual perversion. The artificial insemination of the cows and chickens is a cross-species sexual perversion. The bulls' semen is collected by humans who stimulate the bulls. This is another cross-species perversion. All those who eat meat are participating directly or indirectly in this sexual perversion. Finally, "Thou shall not covet," the 10th Speaking, which in the Yamas is aparigraha, non-greediness, is violated in animal agriculture. The people who are driven, trying to extract as much out of the Earth as possible, create ecological pollution because they don't see their connection to the whole. In Deuteronomy 23:10-15, it says, "Thou shall not pollute the public commons." We understand that meat eaters use 5-10 times more water than vegetarians. One vegan saves 1.5 million gallons of water a year, as compared to a meat eater. Eating a vegan live food cuisine will decrease animal farming and decrease destructive practices and reduce deforestation. We lose about 50 million acres of trees each year, and about 20 million acres each year are turning into desert. Animal agriculture consumes 50-70% of the grain and petroleum. We are literally skinning the Earth alive through topsoil depletion.

From a spiritual perspective, yoga is "chitta vritti narodaha" meaning "quieting the mind." This is often translated as, "Yoga is the quieting of the mental activities of the mind." When one eats meat, they're taking in the pain, cruelty, misery and fear of that animal, and that agitates the mind. That pain affects your consciousness, affects your mind, affects your thoughts, and affects your actions. Food is a love note from God. When we're eating death, it's hardly a love note. Some people say, "Well, the ancient yogis had milk," I would quote Srila Prabhupada, founder of the International Society of Krishna Consciousness, who said, "If you can maintain it, raw food and vegetables are the best cuisine for a human being." Even the founder of the Krishna Consciousness Movement has said, "We don't need dairy."

One of my spiritual teachers, Swami Prakashananda, an enlightened being, said, "When we kill animals, we create pain, misery and fear. When we eat the flesh of these animals, that pain, misery and fear enters us and creates illness and disease."

Diabetes is an area of particular interest to me. A vegan diet, according to Neil Barnard's research, gives people a 46% reduction in diabetes medication in 12 weeks. In my 3-week program, 97% of type 2 diabetics came off all medications; 61% of the non-insulin dependent diabetics were healed; and 86% were off oral medications among the insulin dependent type 2. That's a 24% cure rate. For type 1 diabetics, we had a 21% cure rate in 3 weeks. That means off all insulin, and their fasting blood sugar was less than a hundred. There was an average insulin drop of over 67.5% in those who weren't cured. Thirty-one percent were off insulin, but not less than a fasting blood sugar of one hundred.

These are factors in understanding the importance of veganism. The survival of this planet depends on the consciousness of holistic live food veganism, because it supports every level of our evolution. In each generation, we are given the medicine to repair the world. Holistic, organic, live food veganism is the medicine for healing today's world. Holistic, organic, live food veganism is the way for the present and the future on every level. Those are the philosophical overviews for understanding live foods. Now, I'm going to focus more specifically on the aspects of live food veganism, as opposed to cooked food veganism.

The essence of understanding living food is, "If it's not broken, don't fix it." In this context, I define living foods or raw foods as, those that have not been cooked, processed, pesticided, herbicided, microwaved, irradiated, or genetically engineered. In that context, live foods represent an unbroken wholeness that is the original creation and nutritional gift of the Divine. Live food is an energetic whole, greater than some of its parts.

Research done by Dr. Brekhman of the Soviet Union found that animals fed whole live foods increased in endurance by 2-3 times than when given the same food cooked. From a nutritional perspective, theoretically, there shouldn't be any difference between cooked and raw foods, as they contain the same amount of calories and, therefore, the same amount of energy. Dr. Brekhman's research gives us a way to understand the negative effect of cooking the whole food. Cooking destroys the ecological balance of the food. If it's not broken, don't fix it. Cooking destroys 50% of the protein by coagulating, according to the Max Planck Institute in Germany. Cooking destroys 60-70% of vitamins, up to 96% of B12, and up to 100% of phytonutrients, which are needed to bring superior health to the body and boost the immune system. Cooking the food also disrupts its bioelectrical structure, the bioelectrical transfer power, and the bioluminescence. All these factors are important for building and maintaining lifeforce and health in general.

Now, there are many ways to understand cooked food. Cooking is commonly believed to destroy the enzymes in a food, and this of course, is true. Our enzyme reserves seem to be connected to life force, health, and longevity. In this way, enzymes are living biochemical factors that activate and carry out all the biological processes, including digestion, nerve impulses, detoxification processes, DNA/RNA functions, bodily repair and healing, and even the mental function of building neurotransmitters. There are natural enzymes in live foods that maximize the enzyme pool for digestion because they self-digest, allowing the body's enzymes to be converted and used for such processes as detoxification, repair, and overall healing.

The preservation of our enzymes by eating live foods seems to play an important role in slowing the aging process. With age, if we are protecting our enzymes, we minimize the drop in the enzyme reserve. There's also a drop in the enzyme reserve with all chronic diseases, which is ameliorated to a certain extent with live foods.

The word cooking is a little unclear, and there's often a lot of confusion. Some people say anything above 105 (F) degrees; some people say 110 degrees; and some people say 118 degrees Fahrenheit. It appears to vary on enzyme systems. My general impression is that if you go for a minute or two or even three at 118 degrees, you probably will have insignificant enzyme loss. Some of this research was done long ago and has not been repeated. The research was done with certain sets of enzymes that have certain sensitivities. Other research has shown that other enzymes even endure up to 157 degrees for short periods of time without destroying them. In humans, it is my observation that when people overheat their personal enzymes, by fever, their systems begin to break down. (In India, I saw people with temperatures of 106 degrees.)

My feeling is that cooking and heating food above 118 degrees for a few minutes is as high as I would recommend going, as it probably causes very little enzyme destruction and nutrient destruction. Dr. Paul Kouchakoff in the '30s had research that suggested that cooked food causes leukocytosis because the food begins to look like a foreign body, and this is worsened with cooked junk food. One of my Spiritual Nutrition Masters students actually did research to validate this, and she didn't exactly find this to be the case. Her research showed that, except for packaged meats, hotdogs, and that kind of meat—where indeed there was leukocytosis—in most cooked food there was not a significant amount of leukocytosis.

Another aspect of the importance of live food is the work by Dr. Hans Eppinger of the first medical clinic at the University of Vienna. He found that with chronic disease, the micro-electrical potential of the cell would decrease, and so in a sense, the cell would become a less effective battery. This compromised the ability of chronically diseased people to absorb nutrients into the cell and impaired the elimination of toxins. Interestingly, he found that live food was the only type of food that could restore a healthy micro-electrical potential to the cell. The electrical potential of our tissues and cells, in other words, the battery potential, is a direct result of the aliveness of the cells. Live foods enhance the electrical potential in our cells because they are great active electron donors. When the cells have the proper micro-electrical potential, they have increased power to rid themselves of toxins, and they maintain that battery charge across the membrane. This gives them a selective capacity to absorb healthy nutrients and proper oxygen.

Dr. Eppinger's work correlates with the work of Dr. Kollath of Sweden. Dr. Kollath found that when given typical cooked food cuisine, to simulate an affluent Western lifestyle, animals would go into what they called "mesa-health." This was a condition in which the animals looked healthy, but died sooner than the animals living on the live food diet. These animals had less resistance, and developed chronic degenerative diseases at an earlier age, than those animals on a live food diet.

Dr. Kollath found that the ingestion of raw food was able to restore health and slow the rapid aging process. We find this to be true today. It's very clear to me that the live food cuisine, for a variety of reasons, is regenerative because it increases the vital life force. It actually turns on the positive healing genes, because what we eat or don't eat communicates to our genes, for better or for worse. Foods don't change our genotype, the structure of our genes. Instead, the food we eat changes the way the messages in the genes are expressed in the phenotype. Raw foods upgrade the epigenetic expression.

The food we eat turns our genetic epigenetic program either off or on. We can turn off negative messages, or messages that result in disease, and turn on messages that result in health and wellbeing. How we live directly affects our optimal epigenetic expression. A corollary to this is that genes do not give rise to disease, but disease rises when lifestyle and cuisine alter the gene expression to create disease.

One of the best researchers in this field is Dr. Spindler. In 2001, Dr. Spindler found that when he fed a mouse a 40% calorie-reduced diet, there was a 400% increase in the expression of the anti-aging genes, anti-cancer genes, the oxidant genes, and anti-inflammatory genes. What he also found was that 60% of the age-related changes in gene expression from calorie restriction occurred within a few weeks after the start of the calorie-restricted diet. He found that this calorie-restricted diet specifically produced a genetic anti-aging profile and was actually able to reverse the majority of age-related degenerative diseases. He found a four-fold increase with short-term caloric restriction and a 2.5 fold increase with long-term caloric restriction, and this was 95%

reproducible. This is very, very important research. He noted that the caloric restriction did not only prevent deterioration or genetic change, but actually reversed some of the aging process.

I consider Dr. Spindler's research as perhaps the first to show that caloric restriction could actually turn on the youthing genes and reverse the aging process. He found that weight loss from calorie restriction decreases insulin resistance, decreases blood glucose levels, decreases blood insulin levels, decreases heart rate, and improves blood pressure. He also saw a potential anti-cancer effect. There was a significant decrease, again, in the inflammatory gene expression. To summarize his finding, relevant to understanding live food, no matter what one's biological age, one can create an anti-aging effect through calorie restriction. Anti-aging effects can happen quickly with a low calorie diet. Calorie restriction of only four weeks in mice seemed to partially restore the liver's ability to metabolize drugs for detoxification, and, finally, calorie restriction seemed to quickly decrease inflammation and stress, even with older animals.

On a live food diet, calorie restriction happens naturally and safely. As I stated earlier, when we cook food, we lose 50% of the proteins, 70-80% of the vitamins and minerals, and 95-100% of the phytonutrients. Simple math shows us that when we eat live food temperately (not overeating), we require 50% of the calories required with cooked cuisine.

By this measure, we do better than Dr. Spindler's research, which was a 40% decrease, so we have at least a 50% decrease, if we're able to eat appropriately. A live food cuisine is a pleasant and fun filled natural way of calorie restriction, which turns on the anti-aging, anti-cancer, anti-inflammation, and in my opinion, anti-diabetic genes. For me, this is the first real scientific explanation of the youthing and health effects of properly eating a live food cuisine, which I've observed in thousands of patients since 1983. Clearly the only proven fact we know is that live food has an anti-aging effect due to caloric restriction, naturally achieved with live foods.

Another way of understanding live foods is the idea of subtle organizing energy fields, which I first read about in 1986. These are the energetic matrices supporting the physical materialization of the body. Rupert Sheldrake's history of the morphogenic field, in essence, states that we're in a field we share with our species. The subtle organizing energy theory adds one more piece to that. It says that that field becomes more or less coherent depending upon the coherence of the subtle organizing energy fields. If they're subtle, they're organizing the morphogenic field.

When we eat live foods, the life force energetic power of the food comes in and organizes and structures our subtle organizing energy fields. When we eat junk food, and we live an imbalanced lifestyle, we disorganize our subtle organizing energy field. By this, we may define aging as increasing chaos in the field, and youthing as increasing order in the field. By like manner, we have a definition of disease as increased chaos in the field, and a definition of health as increased order in the field. Live foods bring order to the field and therefore health, viability, and anti-aging effects.

Clearly, from a dietary perspective, as I mentioned earlier, there are many aspects that create longevity effects beyond diet. From a dietary point of view, the longest-lived people—such as the Tahera Humera and the Pelasgians—all had a lower calorie diet. This was approximately 1600-1800 daily calories. The research of mice, rats, and earthworms all show that when you decrease the amount of intake in the diet, the animals live longer.

Wild live food increases vitality and health, by ordering the subtle organizing energy field. Biophoton energy, which is, in essence, the living field, was studied by Dr. Popp from Germany. He found, with his devices for measuring biophoton emissions, that junk food eaters put out about 1,000 units of the biophoton energy. People eating organic cooked food put out 20,000 - 23,000 units of biophoton energy. A newborn baby puts out 43,000 units. People eating organic live foods put out 83,000 units of biophoton energy. That's 83 times more biophoton energy than a person eating junk food. A person fasting and consuming different herbs, in addition to live foods, could be putting out up to as much as 116,000 units of biophoton energy. Biophotons are part of the larger cosmic field and, by increasing biophoton energy, as live food does, we move into resonance with the larger biophoton field. Therefore, we are tuned in spiritually and psychically.

Finally, we must also consider the increased alkalinity that comes from a live food cuisine. To review, history goes back at least 5,700 years to the Garden of Eden; the Pelasgians in 3000 B.C.; and then the Essenes, the Pythagoreans, Bircher-Benner, Dr. Gerson, Dr. Szekely, and Ann Wigmore. Additionally, we see that Dr. Brekhman's work supported the idea that live food increases our total life force energy by 2-3 times. Dr. Eppinger's work shows that it increases the electron flow and the membrane potential. Dr. Popp's work supports live food in the context of biophotons and the idea of increasing general vital life force and bioluminescence. The enzyme work by Dr. Howell supports the importance of protecting against enzyme loss. The calorie restriction work by Dr. Spindler's demonstrates the anti-aging effect and anti-inflammatory effect. Alkalization and mineralization generally improve all biological functions.

We know that inflammation is the driving force for most chronic degenerative diseases including heart disease, Type 2 diabetes, and cancer. We also see that the vegan live food organic cuisine is best for optimizing spiritual life and the life of all humanity on all levels on the planet

Having now discussed the advantages of the raw living vegan cuisine philosophically, emotionally, mentally, and spiritually, I want to address some possible places where people can get discouraged.

Firstly, in my experience, if people are properly focused, I have seen 99.99% success with live food cuisine. I have actually had one person in 40 years who sincerely wanted to do it, but was from the Arctic Circle and really had to have fish once a week. In 40 years, there has been only one person I've seen who wasn't fully successful on at least an 80% live-food cuisine. The key to success is eating according to one's constitution. There are some people who need a higher protein diet, and others who need a higher complex carbohydrate diet. My clinical estimation is about 70% of people need a higher protein, slightly higher fat diet, lower complex carbohydrate, and about 30% need a higher complex green carbohydrate, lower protein and fat macronutrient ratio.

Recent research at Stanford University actually found the genes that literally determine constitutional types. They found that 75% of people need a higher protein diet and 25% need a higher complex carbohydrate diet. The key, however, is determining what that is and paying attention to it. There would be no dramatic failures in people who try to be fruitarian, which is obviously a higher complex carbohydrate cuisine. These people don't thrive, and then they have a steak or something and think they've found heaven, when really, all they've discovered is that they're a fast oxidizer (parasympathetic). They really haven't discovered anything objective, but they get very enthusiastic about meat and attempt to deter people away from vegan live food cuisine. There's no morality connected to these things; it's just whatever makes people feel good. Certainly that speaks to a whole lot of people, but in terms of intelligence, in terms of wisdom, finding one's constitution is absolutely important. No matter the cuisine, one achieves an optimal macronutrient balance.

Additionally, there is a certain amount of detox that may occur when one transitions to a live food diet. That phase can last from a few months to a few years. Then, increased sensitivity begins to diminish and people become very stable, strong and able to tolerate toxins in the environment. There is a belief that once one is on live food, one is more sensitive. From my perspective and experience, once one has gone through the detoxification phase and one's body is functioning at a high level, in a toxic environment (which is really the whole world at this point) this doesn't impact as much. Individuals still thrive because all their detoxification systems function unimpaired. The ability to handle levels of toxicity from air and food grows strong. But even perfect organic food still contains a certain amount of toxicity from global pollution, as long as the food is grown outside.

At the Tree of Life Center US, we grow much of our organic, veganic food in greenhouse settings, as this cuts down on the amount of radiation exposure and external pollution by about 500% and completely eliminates GMO exposure. Even organically grown food does not offer adequate degrees of protection. As a world traveler, I find that my body and its detoxification systems are so toned that they can throw off many of the toxins, and I am relatively unaffected by them. However, in the beginning stages, or if one has not properly detoxified so one's system becomes clear, one may feel more sensitive to environmental stresses.

To properly detoxify my own system, and I don't necessarily recommend this for everyone, I did a variety of weeklong fasts six times yearly for a few consecutive years. I used colema boards, enemas and colonics, which certainly helped the detoxification process. These are things we can do to speed up detoxification and move into stability.

Certain supplements are necessary. Largely, after 6 years, 80% of vegans or live food vegans develop a B12 deficiency. I strongly recommend using a B12 supplement. Carnosine is also very important and will be discussed in detail when we get to the nutrients. Basically, carnosine only comes in meat, and carnosine is connected with longevity and anti-inflammation of the brain and the body and protection of the heart function as well. It also is associated with glycosylation reversal. Glycosylation is the inappropriate combination of glucose with protein enzymes, and also fats and lipids. Carnosine also slows telomere shortening, as well as providing general antioxidant effects. Both B12 and carnosine are longevity protective but also generally protective.

People do not get, even with the highest quality live food, optimal amounts of minerals. The food at Tree of Life Center US is highly mineralized. We use ocean water solution for all our veganic farming. I also recommend a minute dose (1/8 teaspoon total per day; depending on one's constitution) of scalar salts to increase natural mineralization. I encourage the consumption of as many sea vegetables as possible. Iodine is another common nutrient deficiency, with 97% of all Americans deficient in iodine. Live fooders are no exception. I have yet to meet a live fooder, or anyone for that matter, whatever their diet, who is not iodine deficient. I use a particular iodine called Illumodine, which is scalar activated. I'll discuss this more in the nutrient section.

Those are some fundamentals for being 99.99% successful with live food. One should progress at a pace that doesn't require sacrificing physical, mental, emotional, or spiritual stability. One may slowly transition into a moderately low-glycemic, 100% live food cuisine as a healing phase, 1.0. The next step, phase 1.5 of my system, includes low-glycemic fruits and the option of adding some cooked beans or some non-gluten, non-gliadin grains. Again, I'm not an advocate of these, and I personally really enjoy the 99% live food cuisine, which is phase 1.0 with the occasional addition of berries and cherries. You want to enjoy whatever you're doing. My own diet, as it has evolved, because I am metabolically a slow oxidizer, is really only 10% of my calories from protein, 48% from carbohydrate, and 42% from omega three fatty acids. Everybody needs the right macronutrient mix that works for him or her. That's key in the big picture, finding your optimum macronutrient ratio.

When I first began to work with live fooders in the early '80s, several problems were obvious. Many of them were omega-3 deficient and had a variety of mental and emotional imbalances. This was because of the then pervasive myth that a 10% low fat diet was healthy for everyone. The current extensive scientific literature, in addition to my research over the last 30 years, overwhelmingly states that this premise is completely false. Women actually live longer with higher cholesterol. The research suggests that cholesterol between of 160 to 260 produces no increased incidence of heart disease. There was a Norwegian study done with approximately 52,000 people that showed women with a cholesterol of 273 lived 28% longer than women with a cholesterol of 193. Like most of the medical and vegan world, people bought the popular propaganda and didn't study the science. I am committed to the science, whether it is popular or not.

Low cholesterol, that is, below 159, is associated with increased suicide, increased accidents, increased mental imbalances, and increased depression. At the lowest levels of cholesterol, there are six times more depression, suicide, and reduced mental function and wellbeing. This negative mental and physical effect has also been found with low long-chain omega-3s. Not only are these needed for building ojas in the Ayurvedic system, but also, adequate omega-3s are important for mental functioning. Recent research from Iraq showed that the people who had the highest rates of suicide had the lowest omega-3s. While low omega 3s are indeed associated with increased suicide, deficiency is also associated with decreased cognition, poor memory, inability to handle stress, increased accidents, increased emotional liability, depression, decreased neurotransmitter function of serotonin, GABA, dopamine, and acetylcholine, and decreased ability to manage cortisol, the death hormone.

Low omega-3s are also associated with increased cancer, and adequate omega-3s literally cut your breast cancer risk by 50%, as well as helping to prevent skin cancer. My research with diabetics is showing that 25-45% of calories can come from fat. The premier study, from the Archives of Internal Medicine in 2009, using both randomized and controlled studies, found that there was no evidence to support the widespread mythical belief that limiting saturated fat intake is beneficial or protective for heart health or for longevity. As I mentioned, low cholesterol is also associated with not only increased suicide, depression, violent behavior, stroke, accidents, hormonal imbalances, but also with memory loss, Parkinson's disease, increased neurodegenerative disease, and decreased brain repair and growth.

Adequate omega-3s provide significantly improved brain, emotional, and mental health, including less bipolar disease and depression, and increased serotonin production as well. Adequate omega-3s help minimize impulsivity, hostility, aggression, and they also help balance and moderate cortisol, epinephrine, and norepinephrine elevations, while reducing the risk of Parkinson's disease. People with atrial fibrillation, on adequate omega-3s, have an 85% lower risk of dying

"The less one eats, the longer one lives." – Gabriel Cousens

from all causes. Clearly, we need adequate fat intake, and we need to focus on omega-3s, because we get plenty of omega-6s. Again, at least 25-45% of calories should come from fat. The people that I observe in my diabetes program who really do well follow this percentile.

A low fat cuisine can definitely undermine success with a vegan live food diet. As for protein, the optimal range for consumption is somewhere between 10-25% of calories; the average being about 15% of calories from protein. Considering these factors, plus eating according to your genetic and Ayurvedic constitution, yields my 99.99% success rate among people thriving on a live food cuisine.

Once you understand how easy it is to be successful on a 100% live food cuisine, it is easy to dissect the rather intellectually and scientifically weak discussion of ex-live fooders who maintain that a live food cuisine did not work for them. One basic defect in their discussion is the lack of distinction between the terms "cuisine" and "diet". "Cuisine" refers to culinary style, i.e. French, Italian, Cooked Vegan, and Live Food. "Diet" refers to macronutrient ratio. One's particular cuisine has little to do with their success or failure. Any failure to thrive on a diet is determined by macronutrient ratio imbalance—protein: fat: carbohydrate. This ratio is determined by individual constitution and basic science. For example, because of lack of soil strength and vitality today, supplementation, beyond B12, is a contributor to success. While some grains may be balancing for vatas, they create a much higher glycemic intake, and the correlative inflammation has been associated with gluten and gliadin found in many grains besides wheat.

"What's the secret to health and longevity?" Summarily, what one eats is just a part of it. Keeping God at the center of one's life and love in relationships are both very important. I cherish my relationship with my wife, Shanti. We're still, after many years of marriage, writing love notes to each other. Love has been shown to enhance longevity, and part of that is appropriate sexual activity. Our research with 525 people shows that, with live food cuisine, sexual activity became normal. If it was low, it became normal. If it was high, it became normal. Over the years, on a live food cuisine, there is no compromise in sexual function, even at the age of 70. This is one of the benefits of live food cuisine—it supports full functional ability in every aspect of one's life.

The less one eats, the longer one lives. On live food cuisine, the calorie intake is at least less than 2,000 calories per day. Mine is somewhere between 1,600 and 1,800 hundred per day, and again, as I pointed out, on live food cuisine we can eat half as much. Many call this calorie restriction, but for me it's not a restriction. On live foods, one finds that they eat less and less, while still maintaining optimal weight and health. One moves to the optimal set point in their life for that.

For longevity, it is necessary to have meaning and purpose. When I ask the question, "Longevity for what?" I don't just mean to know God. While knowing God is our primary purpose, living life with a specific personal purpose is crucial. This may mean humanitarian work, teaching, or any number of creative contributions to the world. Purpose adds meaning and value to life and is clearly emphasized in the Tierman study of longevity. They found the hard-working people who have purpose and meaning in their lives live longer because they're working with meaning.

Proper hydration is essential for longevity. As we age, we tend to shrink in size. By the time they are age 60, most people have lost as much as two inches off their height, on average. Now, at age 70, with proper spinal hygiene, which we've worked out at the Tree of Life, this shrinkage does not need to happen. I'm at least as tall as I was when I was twenty, possibly a quarter of an inch taller. Instead of shrinking with age, with proper spinal hygiene and with proper hydration of my discs, I'm actually at least as tall as I was in my youth. Proper spinal hygiene and lengthening the spine are very important for nerve health, lymphatic health, and circulatory health.

Another important longevity factor is a particular quality that the Tierman report talks about - fastidiousness. One loves themselves enough to want to heal themselves, and one loves themselves enough to want to pay attention to their wellbeing.

Good social connectivity is something that specifically supports the longevity. This happens through service, through charity and through being part of different spiritual groups.

Another supportive longevity factor appears to be not living in the city. People living outside the city, in the country, live longer. These are the kind of key factors in the overall longevity process - in essence, a summary of the total secrets to longevity.

I want to make a point about protecting the brain. What is the best way to achieve a healthy brain function? The simplest thing, from a nutritional perspective, is actually to minimize sugar, including a variety of grains, which are both a carbohydrate stress, as well as a potential inflammatory stress. A number of recent studies have shown that sugar in the diet does affect cognition. Researchers from the Mayo Clinic just published a study in

"Limiting sugar is the single most important approach to protecting the brain." – Gabriel Cousens

the Journal of Alzheimer's Disease showing that people 70 years and older who eat a diet high in carbohydrates have nearly four times the risk of developing mild cognitive impairment. Also, any diet that's low in sugar - those with a diet high in fat and protein with lower carbohydrate - are less likely to become cognitively impaired.

Researchers observed 940 people, aged 70 to 89 years, and four years later, they looked at the people who had begun to show mild cognitive impairment, about 200 of the 940. They found that people who had the highest intake of carbohydrates were 1.9 times more likely to develop cognitive impairment, as compared to those with the lowest consumption. Individuals with the highest sugar intake were 1.5 times more likely to have cognitive decline, compared to those with the lowest consumption. Those with the highest fat intake were 42% less likely to face cognitive impairment. That's important because one of the "group think," "conventional wisdom" mistakes made in the vegan and/or live food cuisine is based on the myth that low fat is healthy. Adequate omega 3s and cholesterol are needed to support optimum brain function. As I said before, those with the highest fat intake were 42% less likely to face cognitive impairment. The highest intake of protein reduced the risk by 21% for cognitive impairment.

The increasingly high carbohydrate diet that is euphemistically called "transition food" amongst live fooders is a problem. The "transition food" term would be more properly termed "early transition" diet. My emphasis on a low grain (I have essentially no grain in my own diet), moderately low carbohydrate, higher fat intake, and moderate protein emphasis—depending on one's constitution—does not get me invited to many vegan or macrobiotic workshops.

This confirms what I've also seen in studies: Type 2 diabetes (chronic diabetes degenerative syndrome) can be reversed by eliminating or drastically limiting refined carbohydrates and sugars. This significantly lowers the risk of cognitive decline and dementia. Limiting sugar is the single most important approach to protecting the brain.

25. WHAT IS THE BEST SUGAR ALTERNATIVE? WHY IS SUGAR BAD FOR YOU?

BRIAN CLEMENT

Here's where I switch the channel and tell you that I'd rather have you eat processed Stevia, where they take away the green leafy bad tasting part and pull out the sugar-tasting complex carbohydrate that's literally, gram for gram, is three hundred times sweeter than white sugar. Because it really tastes the most like sugar, doesn't interact at all with the pancreas and there are lots of studies that show it actually helps to regulate pancreatic functions. So, Stevia helps control blood sugar rather than create it, unlike agave syrup, maple syrup, xylitol and all of the other fancy exotic forms of sugar. Sadly, most people are not really serious about getting off sugar, they just want to change the name of the sugar they eat, so that they get their fix without being guilty.

GABRIEL COUSENS

My clinical experience with diabetics and non-diabetics shows that Xylitol and Stevia are the best sugar alternatives. Stevia doesn't affect blood sugar at all.

There are many reasons why sugar is bad. Sugar accelerates cognitive decline, and aging in general. Alzheimer's disease is associated with insulin resistance in the brain. To defend against cognitive decline and Alzheimer's disease, increase dietary fat intake, particularly of coconut oil, which converts to ketones that are able to give your brain up to 90% of the necessary energy. Many of the people with Alzheimer's have significant improvement because they are getting ketone energy to the brain via coconut oil. When the brain is insulin resistant and glucose can't get in, the result is deficient energy in most of the brain centers.

FRED BISCI

Sugar is the ultimate junk food. It's very acid forming. It's just empty calories. It's addictive. It just does not contribute anything that's beneficial to the human body. If you're eating a raw living food diet, you really don't need a sugar substitute. I use them very, very rarely. My diet is simple; it basically revolves around fruit and vegetable juices, raw salad, nuts, seeds, avocados and sprouts. I eat sprouts just about every day and I include seaweeds in my diet. I believe in eating a variety of different raw foods.

We've got to realize that sugars and fats don't work well in the same meal. About 20 years ago, when I was distance training for marathons, I ate plenty of fruit to give me energy and drank juices to increase my caloric intake. I knew not to eat fat and sugar in the same meal, so for about a three-month period, I didn't eat any fat, and I experimented to see how much sugar from fruit I could include in my diet. I was so energized, because I was exercising so much; I probably had a lot of insulin in my blood and probably had a lot of sugar as well. My energy levels were absolutely unbelievable. In fact, my wife thought something was wrong with me when, one day, I actually tried to see how long I could run up and down stairs. I ran up and down the 22 steps running off our deck down to ground level for almost six hours and all I did was sip on a little bit of fruit juice with a little bit of celery in it. I finally stopped, not because I got tired, but because it got dark out. I did not want to fall down the stairs.

Then, I completely stopped eating fruit and switched to eating fat. I started by eating half of an avocado, because after all that fruit, if I ate more than half an avocado, I wouldn't have felt good. I would have felt a little lightheaded, a little nauseous. I'd had cramps in my fingertips. Over a period of about three or four months, I gradually increased the fat, to the point where I was eating six avocados a day. It takes approximately two weeks for your body to start to switch from burning sugar for fuel to burning fat to convert to glucose as fuel, and I was able to do that.

The amount of fruit that you're eating should be based on the amount of exercise that you're doing. If you're not exercising, then you certainly don't need a lot of fruit. If you're a sedentary person, you can have more than enough walking around energy not eating any fruit and you won't be bone-thin either. The main thing, if you're eating a plant-based, diet is to get plenty of leafy green vegetables, and you've got to make sure that you're doing that.

VIKTORAS KULVINSKAS

All forms of concentrated sweets should be avoided with everybody who is on any kind of therapeutic nutritional lifestyle. If you are a healthy individual, marginal usage of sweet concentrated food can be part of your recreational indulgence and part of a healthy lifestyle habit. The best way to eat sugars is through consuming whole foods—ripe fruit, and, to a lesser extent, dried fruit. This is especially true for individuals who are on a weight gain program, of course, to gain lean muscle mass, not fat.

"When you are enzymatically deprived, you'll have great cravings for sugars and frequent meals." - Viktoras Kulvinskas

For smoothies, stick to the food that comes from the grass family, and add the sugar cane juice powders that are available to minimize the desire for desserts. A good suggestion is to always add shredded beets, carrots, squashes or non-GMO corn to your salad type of meals. All of them provide a slow acting boost in sugar and reduce the likelihood of cravings for desserts, which is due to the drop in sugar that usually takes place during the early portions of a meal. If you include these wonderful root vegetables, as well as the squash family, you'll find that there will be none of that kind of desire.

For those who want something that is clean and natural to create a sweeter taste, Stevia, which does not affect your blood sugar level, would be an excellent choice.

Why should persons avoid concentrated sweets, especially during the early stages of this lifestyle change? It's because the sugars increase the likelihood of the proliferation and growth of yeast within your gastrointestinal tract, which will then produce alcohol and overall toxemia. Your body thrives best on low glycemic foods. On the other hand, processed food and concentrates of sugar end up putting a major stress on converting and processing sugars. They end up becoming triglycerides, which reduce your oxygen absorption, because they cause red blood cells to clump together and they do not travel well into the extremities, such as muscles and the brain.

When you are enzymatically deprived, you'll have great cravings for sugars and frequent meals. Hypoglycemics are a good example of this. Get yourself on a high enzyme saturation and you'll see the conditions clearing up in a matter of a month or two, and cravings will disappear. Also, when the cravings come, go for greens, whether it's chlorella, blue-green algae, Spirulina, or grass powder.

Again, it comes down to how often and how addicted are you to this pattern. An occasional birthday cake made out of raw chocolate, xylitol, agave, coconut sugar, a succinate from sugar cane, juice powder or dried fruit, in a small serving—if it doesn't create an addictive pattern—is something that you are not to be judgmental about. Indulge in it, if you so wish. Definitely, it's not a requirement for healthy living.

As a matter of fact, our celebrations of the future, you can be assured, will include none of this junk. Instead, we will be drinking elixirs of wheatgrass, green juices, and Spirulina, Aphanizomenon flos-aquae, often referred to as E3Live or AFA, sometimes adding to it a little bit of fruit juice. Beyond that, we will have no need of any other way of socializing and will be having the best time ever.

The future is very bright and sugar-free. You will be getting it in your whole food, and your body will be converting more than an adequate amount when you are enzymatically inactive from your bad starches, which you will eventually not be consuming either. They are not required. Instead, you'll be consuming predigested sugars as found in sprouted grains and root vegetables.

26. WHAT IS PROPER FOOD COMBINING AND DO YOU RECOMMEND IT?

GABRIEL COUSENS

I've seen people get obsessive compulsive about proper food combining. Firstly, don't combine lots of fruits and vegetables together. Since we aren't overeating, we won't overwhelm our digestive systems, and we needn't be so concerned with proper food combining. Secondarily, there are a few who have weak digestion and need to follow all the food combining rules until they strengthen their digestion.

VIKTORAS KULVINSKAS

Yes, there is certainly a need for it in individuals going through therapeutic healing programs. I will give you the highlights, which are extremely simple and to the point. Namely, if you are consuming any form of starches, you had better be taking some enzymes, because most people just don't have the enzymatic reserves to digest starches effectively. But, if you're consuming some form of starch, you will do well to avoid combining it with any form of protein, because starches need an alkaline environment for digestion and proteins need an overall slightly acidic environment for digestion. Protein foods, such as nuts don't do well, even when they're soaked, with fruit or dried fruit. Likewise, a lot of people believe that nuts and sprouted grains should not be included together, and I am of the same mindset. These combinations will create a gassy situation.

Of course, starches should never be combined with anything acidic. So, if you eat a sprouted grain in a meal, or the somewhat starchy foods like lentils, mung bean sprouts, adzuki sprouts, or chick pea sprouts, you definitely should not have lemon, tomato or vinegar in that same meal, and definitely no fruit. Otherwise, you're going to be gassy and feeling uncomfortable for a few hours, if not a few days.

Seeds such as quinoa, chia, flax, buckwheat, wild rice, amaranth, and others, are great cooking sources, as well as having no starch component. They combine very well with dried fruit, proteins, and starches.

FRED BISCI

I do recommend proper food combining because it certainly can't hurt you and it can help you. If you have poor digestion, or you're just getting into a raw food diet, or if you're elderly, proper food combining will definitely help you. Years ago, when I started to get into endurance training, I always had pretty good digestion and I could mix my food up—it didn't bother me. But then I realized what was happening when I started doing long training runs and had to train consistently. What I found out was that when I combined my food correctly, even though I was getting

"Proper food combining is very simple...Take a good look at a food combining chart..." – Fred Bisci

fewer calories overall, I was able to go farther in my long runs. That made an impression upon me.

Proper food combining is very simple. You can mix the protein vegetables and the starchy vegetables with the leafy green vegetables and light starch vegetables. Acid fruit and sub-acid fruit can be combined, and sub-acid fruit with the sweet fruits are okay. Melons do not combine well with any other fruit. Take a good look at a food combining chart and you'll see how it works.

There are people who say it's totally unnecessary to follow food combining rules. If you're not into endurance sports, you may not notice as much of a difference, but it is still beneficial.

BRIAN CLEMENT

Well, if you look at every single creature on earth that is not domesticated, they eat one food at a time. I personally began to see this years ago, how my health flourished, how my digestion improved, how my elimination improved when I ate simple foods, and simple foods from the same family. I also, as a nutritionist, understood that when you mix certain nutritional compounds together it was counterproductive for the digestibility of the food.

We're advocates of eating very simple and eating foods from the same family rather than mixing a variety of food.

27. DO YOU RECOMMEND A NATURAL HYGENIST DIET?

VIKTORAS KULVINSKAS
No.

BRIAN CLEMENT
Well, one of the great contributors since the mid-19 century to the raw living movement was a natural hygienist named Herbert Shelton. Certainly, I think that any of us who look back through history would say resoundingly that we've all been influenced in some way, small or great, by natural hygiene. So, congratulations to the original hygienists.

I think that what we knew 150 years ago or more doesn't always apply today. The organic plant-based foods then were radically different and more nutritious than in the present day, with only a few varieties, none being hybrid. Today, with the multitude of hybrid varieties and lack of good soil, we have to look at superior nutritious foods, like sprouts, to make up what we would have gotten a century and a half ago. So, congratulations to the hygienists, but, as we move on, develop, morph and change, and disprove as well as improve, we have to alter some of these ideologies.

GABRIEL COUSENS
This is an issue of individual constitution. A certain percentage of people who go on a fruitarian diet are successful. I personally do better with a higher complex carbohydrate percentage (approximately 48% of my diet). I tried fruitarianism for 2 years. I couldn't eat more than 4 bananas daily, but I basically ate only fruit, and I did okay. However, as I approached my 60th birthday, I was intuitively aware that I was not as strong as I could be, and so I switched to a relatively low fruit, high vegetable diet, and was able to do 601 consecutive push-ups on my 60th birthday. That feat was not accomplished on a fruitarian diet. On my 70th birthday, I did 29 consecutive chin-ups, as compared to 10 consecutive chin-ups at age 20. This is on a primarily phase 1.0 cuisine for 30 years.

There are a few people who can do fruitarianism successfully, and I honor them, so I wouldn't say that natural hygiene cuisine is off. I have seen many people who get more focused on a theory of what is "ideal," than on practical and scientific reality, and have failed to reach robust health as a result of that. Individualizing one's macronutrient ratios by constitution is important, as is mineral and vitamin supplementation. Everyone I have seen over the past 40 years of my clinical experience (live food, vegan, or meat eater) has had some level of mineral and vitamin deficiency beyond B12 deficiency.

FRED BISCI
Not really. Natural hygiene brought a lot of attention to the raw food movement, but the only thing is, the natural hygiene movement was never open to change. There were people who did very well in the beginning, but I don't know any natural hygienist on a 100% raw food diet who did well over a long period of time. Some of the leaders didn't do well at all. Many years ago, Dr. Christopher Gancaursio supervised a large group of people in upstate New York. I believe there were more than three hundred people involved. They were very dedicated natural hygienists.

In the beginning, they did wonderfully. The children were very bright, very sharp, and they looked very good. They were very energetic. They behaved like mature adults. But as time went on, they started to run into problems. By the third generation, birth defects started to pop up. There was a girl by the name of Dee Robins who was 28 years old, a very beautiful girl, and she was Miss Natural Hygiene. She died when she was 28. I was told that her cause of death was fractures due to osteoporosis.

I think the basic premise behind it, that fruits, vegetables, nuts, seeds, and avocados are the basis of a raw food diet, is valid—but there are people who need other things. They might need Vitamin B12. Natural hygienists are totally against colonics and enemas. In the past they didn't believe in drinking juices or blending. They thought that you needed the fiber and they didn't think anyone should eat more than 4 ounces of nuts a day. They did not believe in sprouts or super greens. Everybody is notthe same. You can't clone people. After Dr. Gancaursio added blended salads and protein to the diet, people did well.

28. WHAT ARE THE 10 MOST IMPORTANT FOODS TO EAT?

BRIAN CLEMENT

Well, the top three I'll start with are the very first foods that were on this planet. The very first life form on this planet was blue-green and then green algae. Blue-green algae is 54% predigested protein, green algae is 52%, and both have a spectacularly high amount of essential fatty acids, the same type that the brain is made of. Also recognized—these foods literally have every element in them that came after them. Since they were the very first life form, they're foundational foods, or essential foods and we have massive research to show that they correct chromosome damage, fix DNA, which relates to longevity.

Number 2—sea vegetables. A wide variety of sea vegetables from dulse to kelp. This is a second primitive life form, and we recommend using these sea vegetables for the mineralization and elements you get in their structure.

Number 3—grasses and their related sprouts. So, at the core of the Hippocrates Program are the first, second, and third life forms on this planet - fresh water algae, sea algae, land based superior foods, sprouts, grasses and their juices. With that said, then it would be organic green leafy vegetables, the fresh ones, and equally important, if not more important, would be edible weeds. Edible weeds are quite primitive and highly nutritious foods. No cost worldwide, when it's warm enough for them to grow. I know people who sustain pretty much their entire diet on edible weeds during the times of the year that they're available.

I would also include nuts and then, next in line would be seeds, always germinated. Nuts and seeds are powerhouses, condensed nutrients that sustain energetic outreach over a long period of time, hours, and provide a lot of these basic nutrients that a body maintains on.

Next, I would say ripe organic fruits, starting with, if we were in the tropics, tropical fruits. If you're in the very far north, whatever fruits are available—apples, pears, in their ripe organic form. To sustain a little bit of fruit in the diet, is it essential and necessary? You can live without fruit, but it's a great thing to include in the diet when you are not ill.

I would probably say after that, other forms of plant-based foods are good for you, but the ones that were just mentioned are the most important foods.

FRED BISCI

I encourage people to eat a large variety of different foods. From a raw food perspective, I recommend a diet that includes fruit (if you don't have a problem that would preclude it), vegetables, nuts, seeds, sprouts and avocados. Use your juicer. Make green smoothies. Get your fatty acids.

GABRIEL COUSENS

These are my personal preferences. I like the Klamath Lake E3Live powder as my favorite all-around protein and for enhanced brain function. I have personally found it very good for mental clarity and creativity. I eat the full range of vegetables and the full color spectrum of vegetables. I eat all varieties of sprouts. Low glycemic berries, particularly blueberries, are good. I eat plenty of nuts and seeds, particularly the omega-3 focused nuts and seeds. These are walnuts, hemp seed, chia seed, and flax seed. I also consume oils, such as coconut oil, to improve conversion of short chain omega-3s to long chain omega-3s. Coconut oil, particularly, yields a higher conversion rate of 1:3 up to 6-10% and, thus, greatly increases DHA/EPA in the body. Coconut oil also converts to ketones that give your brain energy.

I would also include a variety of Chinese and Ayurvedic herbs that build the Three Treasures, which are the deep *jing, qi*, and *shen* energies. Finally, I would also recommend all sea vegetables and avocados, which are actually a great food for bringing a variety of fats into the body and improving protection against heart disease. Those would be my key foods.

VIKTORAS KULVINSKAS

Fresh, organic, preferably locally-grown, non-GMO, and relying a lot on your own greenhouse apartment or home gardens, potted plants as well as hydroponic systems. With the changes and uncertainty of our times, I recommend strongly that all of you should have at least 100 pounds of seeds stored for each member of the family for long-term survival. My book *Survival in the 21st Century* gives recommendations on ways to go about doing this.

Number one: Wheat. Most of you think in terms of wheatgrass, which is great, when grown at home. However, you should give consideration also to growing sprouted wheat. Brother Benet Luchion, who is now in his 80s, has, for over 50 years, lived exclusively on sprouted wheat and wheatgrass. No other food. He's a tantric priest, has a Ph.D. in Biochemistry and Comparative Religion. He has several dozens of followers who have lived on such a dietary regime for 10 years and more. He says it makes him blissful, happy, full of joy. I think the foods contribute. However, his tantric practice has a lot to do with it also.

A perfect meal for breakfast would be a cereal of sprouted wheat, soaked sunflower, a cup of one, half a cup of the other. Blend it with one carrot, some garlic, one cup of water, and sea salt to taste, eating it with flax crackers and some bells.

Number two: Sunflower. Sunflower greens, sunflower seeds, and growing to maturity your sunflower. Thus, you would be able to harvest from one seed, 100 to 500 seeds at the end of the season. In 1969, I discovered sunflower growing in my compost heap. I saw a wonderful idea and it became the foundation for the sunflower greens that are ever so popular, not only at Hippocrates Health Institute, but also worldwide.

Accidents are gifts of God. Do you notice the gift or do you just walk by? Share it. Gifts are meant to be shared, and that's what I did, instead of withholding. The sunflower seed itself, shelled, can be soaked and eaten, added to solids or made into milks. It can also be blended into milk, unsoaked, thus maximizing the fat content and then predigested by the probiotics that are in the air. Or you can use sauerkraut for its probiotic properties, a couple of tablespoons in the milk as a starter, blending it together. This makes an excellent foundation for veggie burgers, nut milks, and crackers.

Number three: Buckwheat. It's another seed I discovered as a cover crop and domesticated it, and it became part of the Hippocrates program, though it's not as popular as the sunflower. It is part of the rhubarb family and it should be eaten in moderation, so a quarter a pound to a half a pound per day. It's something that will cause no difficulty. In larger volumes, it could end up diminishing your red blood cell count. It is a great source of lecithin and a blood thinner. It can be also grown to full maturity, harvesting the seeds at the end of the season. Many others also grow pea greens, which was a contribution from the Hippocrates Health Institute.

Number four: Sprouts in general. From all kinds of seeds, from vegetables to grains or legumes, they are the most powerful alive fresh food. The Bible talks about Daniel and his brothers being given pulses to eat, as an alternative to king's meat. Within 10 days, by eating the pulses, which were either lentil or mung bean in a soaked form and sprouted for a day, they proved to be wiser than the astrologers and the magicians of the king's court, as well as bulked up as warriors and showed no nutritional imbalance. Because of the ritual practices at a certain time, they were forced to do fire-dancing within the pits that the king created for them, as well as to be fed to the lions. However, the lions became their brothers and sisters instead of devouring them. It has to do with the Essene way.

The lentils can be grown for two days. Mung beans can be soaked in very warm water, up to 160 degrees for four hours and then soaked in much warmer water for another 24 hours and then just germinated for 12 hours and eaten, in the tradition that you find normally in the oriental restaurants. The quick approach will give you maximum calories and also a high bioavailable-concentrated form of protein.

Five: Fermented vegetables, sauerkraut and kimchi. I strongly recommend that you add to your ferment batch at least a half a cup, if not more, of sunflower seeds that have been soaked for a few hours and drained. The reason for this is that now, all of a sudden, your probiotics, your airborne bacteria, will have for food something that has a high amount of fat and protein and as a result, they will produce a high volume of protease and amyl and lipase, supporting the regeneration of your body.

When you have only cabbage and other vegetables, which are low in fat and protein, and high in carbs, you will have a product that will be rich in amylase. Thus with the system, you will be growing your own digestive enzymes. Considering its sour nature, it should never be used to support the digestion of starchy foods, because starchy foods such as sprouted grains don't digest well in the presence of acid. Otherwise, all the other foods will be supported, as will the regeneration of your enzyme reserves. A time will come when you will not be in a position to purchase enzymes in a capsule. In this way, you can grow enzymes in your own home, empowering not only your digestion, but also your immune function and metabolism.

Number six: Sea vegetables. Dulse is one of my favorites. However, kelp will give you the full spectrum of minerals. I also suggest Himalayan salt. Many will say that this is an inorganic food and I will not argue that issue. However, the bioavailability of the minerals is perfect for the microbial cultures, which are extensive within your GI tract. They will consume the inorganic minerals and release them in the form of organic minerals, so there is a wonderful tradeoff with the flora and fauna within our gastrointestinal tract.

By using the full mineral spectrum in your diet, you will be creating a new cellular environment, the genetic code will be moving into higher and higher octave of manifestation of the source, DNA, which exists as a hologramatic electromagnetic imprint in the cosmos that your DNA downloads, depending on the nutritional and the toxic environment of the cellular environment. So, consume the full spectrum of minerals on a daily basis.

Seven: Grow your own weeds, as well as harvest weeds from forests and fields, and learn how to identify them and use them depending on their potency and the time of the year that they are harvested. For example, dandelion could be used abundantly during the early spring, when it has a succulent taste. Just like lettuce, it does get old and has a very bitter trace when it reaches post-maturity. It can be added in small portions in your juice regime.

My favorite is purple lambsquarter, in memory of Reverend Ann Wigmore. I have purchased the seeds on the Internet and I will plant them wherever I see empty land. You can plant it yourself, using the hydroponic www.gardens.com system, and be harvesting it all season. Lambsquarter is very unique among plants in that it does not turn bitter as it grows into maturity. You can use it in blended soups, salads, and even drink it as a juice. At the end of the season, you can harvest the seeds as a source of high protein and use them as such, and at the same time, save them for replanting.

Eight: Moringa You can purchase the seeds on the Internet. It is often referred to as the salad tree. In the tropics, it will grow to 16 feet in height within one year. It can be a good border plant. It can be harvested and cut back as a hedge for easy access. Each one of the branches can be replanted, thus starting a whole colony. You don't need many seeds in order to get your own edible hedge. Plant these seeds everywhere. There are many websites showing the many ways of preparing it, but as a raw foodist, you would do the same thing as described for the other greens.

Number nine: All kinds of green smoothies, green vegetable soups, and green juices. These are a less-than-optimum type of food because they are old. However, they will create alkalinity within your system. Drink organic juice made out of celery, cucumber, and all the other greens you have access to, and during your transition, if you need to, add some carrot or apple in order to sweeten it up.

I also like adding many of the herbs, so I add to my green juices and smoothies, herbs such as parsley, cilantro, basil, mint, ginger, garlic, hot pepper, as well as a little dab of sea salt. If you don't like the taste, add a few drops of stevia to sweeten it further, as an alternative to apple and carrot.

Ten: Sweet foods. That is, shredded carrots, beets, and squashes, added to salad to satisfy your desire for desserts. This desire for sweets stems from the fact that most people have a lowered blood sugar in their system during and after a meal, due to inadequate enzyme levels. Eventually, the blood sugar level rises, and this uneasy feeling goes away.

The other sweets that you should be giving consideration to, if you don't have degenerative diseases or a yeast problem, is fruit. You should consider growing berries and fruit trees on every public piece of land, or on your own property, and that also includes growing nuts, sunflowers, and buckwheat. You have to become your own resource. Soon, you will have to be relying on what is available locally.

A very delightful food is the artichoke. It produces beautiful sunflower-like flowers. Very tall, very small, with bulk roots like the potato, except that it's non-starchy. You should also consider growing other vegetables—carrots, beets as a winter crop—then cover it in autumn. Then, as soon as you see that sign of first frost, cover it with hay and a tarp and you will be growing not only greens and tops, but also, at the same time, be able to harvest these sweet vegetables from the soil. Fresh white potato can be quite tasty. I've eaten it many a times. Remember, during World War I, many nations lived exclusively on potatoes. It's a very powerful food.

29. IF I START INCORPORATING JUICING, RAW LIVING VEGAN MEALS AND SUPPLEMENTS INTO MY DIET, HOW LONG UNTIL I SEE CHANGES?

FRED BISCI

Everybody is a biochemical individual. I can't tell you how long it's going to take. It might take some people days, and others might take months. Another person might see changes much more quickly, especially if they're doing a lot of cleanses, going for colonics, doing enemas, going on a supervised fast, doing juice cleanses and taking enzymes and probiotics.

GABRIEL COUSENS

This, of course, depends on the individual. The more chronic disease one has developed, the less healthy one is. While, one may see changes early on, full radiant health may take up to 2 years to cultivate, depending on age and starting point. At any age, one will see changes with positive shifts in diet and lifestyle. I had a woman come to one of my Diabetes Recovery Programs at the age 92. She had diabetes, high blood pressure, wheelchair-confining crippling arthritis, and she was on 11 different medications. After three weeks on our Diabetes Recovery Program of 100% live food cuisine, she was out of her wheelchair, her diabetes was gone, and her blood pressure was normal. She has remained so in the year since she finished the program.

"At any age one will see changes with positive changes in diet and lifestyle."
- Gabriel Cousens

VIKTORAS KULVINSKAS

First of all, we'll talk about supplements and juices. The juices should be green, as described earlier, and taken on an empty stomach. Add a little cayenne for increased circulation. The supplements we're going to be talking about are very few, but they will create dramatic effects, and I will share a story or two.

Take digestive enzymes of plant origin, with each one of your meals. In the first week also take enzymes, one or more capsules between meals, thus allowing them to clean out your bloodstream, acting as a detoxifying agent. Also, most people, unless you're having three or more bowel movements per day, you are somewhat constipated from the primitive high-fiber diet point of view. Initially, you might take a cascara sagrada-based herbal tonic, whether it is Internal Cleanse from Hippocrates, or some of the others found at health food stores. Take one at bedtime and increase the dosage until you start having increased bowel evacuations or loose bowel. If you have loose bowel, cut back. That will fix your gastrointestinal tract.

Then, the other one for superior nutritional impact is E3Live blue-green algae. I suggest taking capsules or adding it to your green drinks. I personally like to consume it sublingually, where it immediately feeds the brain and you see an increased mental acuity and increased energy.

Then, the last item would be probiotics. If you consume these four, you'll see miracles occurring in your physiology. Also, add cayenne for increased circulation and to accelerate the cleaning out of your blood vessels.

Under such a regime of supplementation that I've just mentioned, my grandmother, who I was asked to be the caregiver for, who was bedridden, could not walk and also had Alzheimer's disease. Within a period of five weeks, she was out of bed at normal brain functioning. For another three years, she refused to make lifestyle changes and died of toxemia.

If the only changes you make are consuming enzymes and a mild herbal laxative, you will see radical changes within a matter of one to two days, not only clearing up digestive problems, but also increasing energy, vitality, and brain function. Within a matter of a month, your skin conditions may start clearing up. You will start looking younger.

Of course, the most important supplement that I neglected to mention is water; distilled water taken during the day, at least one ounce for every two pounds of body weight, initially. Eventually, you will cut back and balance the amount of fluid intake with the intake of green juices and herbal teas.

There was a study in which I was a participant within the medical community, submitted to the University of Illinois' Medical School. 200 cases of incurables were treated successfully with three superfoods. Within a matter of four months, subjects with many of the degenerative conditions, ranging from asthma to bronchial emphysema, as well as some forms of cancer and diabetes, were found to be free of those diseases.

As we observed the individuals for many years, I found that, eventually, the supplements were inadequate and the people returned to their early symptomatology, due to the fact that you can take all the supplements you want, but unless you make lifestyle changes, toxemia will eventually get you.

On a short-term basis, supplements can have a radical impact, allowing you to continue to enjoy your addictive relationships to the foods that you have chosen, whether it is cooked vegan, involving animal protein, or even processed foods—but eventually toxemia will destroy you.

In the studies of longevity, the key driving force is a balance between optimized nutrition and removal of toxins, not only metabolic waste, but toxins associated with the foods. You will not in the long run, be able to eliminate the toxins. It's better to work with supplements initially to overcome whatever is going on, that is, deficiencies in your system, and at the same time, work toward dietary and lifestyle changes, exercise, attitude modification, meditation and spiritual practices.

BRIAN CLEMENT

Well, this is frightening news. Now, if you come off the western diet and start this, you're going to feel sick, weak, nauseous, and it's hard, unless you're supervised or around very supportive knowledgeable people, to think that it's a healthy thing.

I'll never forget my own experience; I felt I was going through an exorcism. If it weren't for the support of one very strong, committed vegan, I would have turned around and gone back to hamburgers, as sure as I'm sitting here. The people around me kept saying, "This is part of the elimination process." The exorcism, as I called it—where you have to be forgiven for your sins before you raise your health—is difficult without community. When this is conducted at the Institute, with professionals around to guide you, you're going to see a difference within a matter of a week or two.

Again, at the Hippocrates Institute, we generally have a 21-day program. When people commence, 100% of the cases, out of the thousands of people every year, have radical improvements and change within this short period of time. The vast, vast majority, 95% of them, recognizes the physical and psychological improvements, and report it to us. You may want to get on the Hippocrates website to see some of the on-the-spot interviews.

30. HOW CAN I TELL WHAT NUTRIENTS I'M MISSING?

GABRIEL COUSENS

There's a variety of testing techniques to determine deficiencies. There is no "average you". Each person is unique, so what may be adequate B12 for one person's body may be inadequate for someone else's body. We have to be very careful about the standard laboratory values approaches in analyzing deficiencies, and one may need to do more subtle electro-diagnostic or O-ring testing to determine specific, individualized needs.

BRIAN CLEMENT

We use a sophisticated method called Cyberscan and SpectraCell testing that is slowly becoming more available worldwide. Most nutritional testing, even as a nutritional scientist, I don't submit to. I don't think it's good. The SpectraCell, for instance, takes your white blood cell, leukocyte, and opens it up to see what nutrients have been absorbed by the body. What matters to me is not what you're eating, but what's absorbed, and in that way, we can determine what you really have and what you don't have. We then fulfill your deficits with whole food nutrition, either the nutrition itself or whole food nutritional supplementation.

VIKTORAS KULVINSKAS

Get a book, David Hawkins' *Power Versus Force*, and look up kinesiology or muscle-testing on the Internet. This will enable you to ask questions, such as, for optimal wellness and long-term health, should you be adding more Vitamin A? You do muscle-testing and you will be able to determine that.

Now, as a general rule, 99% of people are deficient in enzymes and water, or hydration, so you better start increasing hydration and enzymatic reserves. Until you have your enzyme levels as those of a teenager, or preferably an adolescent, or preferably an infant, you are enzymatically depleted. Once you move into high enzymatic reserves, you have optimization of the functioning of digestion, immune function, and metabolism.

The nutrient that is most pronouncedly deficient in everybody is oxygen. Remember, if we go back a few hundred years or more, the planet was more or less covered with greens, and the oceans were not depleted of phytoplankton, which produce practically 80% of the oxygen. The air oxygen level was closer to 40%. Right now, in cities like New York and L.A., the oxygen levels are closer to around 10%, 11%. In the countryside, it might be as high as 15% in some areas.

Most people are anemic by the standards of regulations of 100 years ago, in terms of red blood cell count and hemoglobin. You want to increase your oxygen level by doing pranayama, or having an oxygen unit for yourself, and by also consuming green foods. My book *Survival* shows how, over a period of 10 years, all forms of anemia, including pernicious anemia, anemia of unidentified origin, Vitamin B12-induced anemia, were all treated successfully with chlorophyll-rich greens. This study was done by medical doctors. Now you'll maximize your oxygen level.

Furthermore, you want to clean out your lungs through detoxification. The worst culprits are dairy products and white flour products, as well as unsoaked seeds, nuts and grains. They will congest your lungs. Even consuming such products as cooked beans, cooked starches, organic whole food-based pasta spaghetti will congest your lungs. Minimize the usage of these foods.

Everyone is enzyme-deficient, so take enzymes with meals, as well as between meals. I have been consuming enzymes for over 35 years. I have stopped taking enzymes for as much as a couple of months and consumed cooked foods, and I had no difficulty in digesting anything, because I'd built up my enzyme levels to those of a teenager.

The fermented foods will supply the complete B complex nutrient profile. Many people feel concern about Vitamin B12, and with good reason, especially if you don't do any detoxification, which means that you will continue to have sludge and blockages and phlegm saturation of your stomach and intestinal tract. As a result, you will have poor absorption of the Vitamin B complex. That's why sublingual Vitamin B12 is desirable for most individuals, at least until they have gone through detoxification.

Why you need to consume enzymes, even if you're on a raw food diet, is that it's protection. None of you are consuming organic, raw air. All of you are consuming cooked air, cooked by automobiles, cooked by stoves, microwave ovens and all kinds of electromagnetic machines. Air contains proteins in the form of pollens, as well as of fragrances and fatty substances, all of it having gone through some level of heat-treating. And you are absorbing these. As a matter of fact, there are studies that were done which showed that individuals who were living within 500 feet of greasy restaurants that had exhaust fans shooting out into the air, had something like 500% higher incidence of cardiovascular diseases. Airborne stuff is pretty nasty. Try to grow a lot of greens within your own home.

Other more specific vitamin and mineral deficiencies are not an issue. Primarily, get your meals from the consumption of sea vegetables, whole sprouted seeds and Himalayan sea salt, and you will get all the needed type of foods. Don't become obsessive-compulsive with trying to identify some missing nutrient.

Don't be sold by all these vitamin companies, mineral companies. That's a lot of BS. More often, what you have is a deficiency of joy, happiness and self-love. Start meditating. Start moving your butt. That's some of the kind of deficiencies most of you have. It's called procrastination. You have a lot of it. Don't put it off. Get on and move on into the divine Garden of Eden nutrition that is taught by the way of the Hippocrates Health Institute.

Before you start running around and getting into this nutritional program and start reading all these prevention and supplement-preaching magazines, read *Supplements Exposed* by Dr. Brian Clement, because only whole food-based nutrient supplementation is essential.

Many of you are probably indoor-living. Go out and get a tan; it's free. But most of you live indoors and develop cancer of the skin. What a joke. Then they blame it on the sun. Then of course, the Omega-3 and all the other oil supplements, what nonsense. Get them from whole foods and you'll get much more than enough. One of the highest sources of Omega-3 is blue-green algae. The others are chia seeds or flax seeds. Don't worry. Don't start buying fish oil. Read the book *Killer Fish* by Dr. Brian Clement.

FRED BISCI

The best way to do that is go for a blood test. I don't guess about anything, and I don't base anything on philosophy or hearsay. I'm not a medical doctor, so I don't diagnose or prescribe anything for people. I want to see their blood tests.

31. IT CANNOT BE DENIED THAT A HIGH CALORIE, HIGH SUGARY FRUIT DIET IS BECOMING VERY POPULAR WORLDWIDE, AND THERE ARE MANY CASES OF HIGH FRUIT EATERS EXCELLING IN MARATHONS, BIKE RACES AND OTHER ELITE COMPETITIONS. IS THIS FOOL'S GOLD? LONG TERM, DOES THIS TYPE OF DIET CORRELATE WITH A LONGER LIFE THAN THE STANDARD AMERICAN DIET?

GABRIEL COUSENS

It is a mix. Athletic competitive ability is not demonstrative of true health, as many athletes often die at earlier ages. Carbohydrate loading is very important for athletic events, but life is not an athletic event. We don't need carbohydrate loading unless we're competing athletically, so we have these bursts and an ability to sustain energy. Any more than 25 grams of fructose a day is unhealthy in the long run, creating a variety of chronic disease processes. Fructose is obviously associated with fruit as well as high fructose corn syrup. With a high fructose setting, there comes a variety of problems. Chronic diabetes degenerative symptoms, insulin resistance, metabolic syndrome, and full-blown diabetes are all directly associated with high fructose. Heart disease, high blood pressure, obesity, gout, kidney stones, AGEs (glycosylation process), non-alcoholic fatty liver disease, brain inflammation, and cancer are all associated with excess fructose. A high fructose diet does not correlate with longevity. Correlative with longevity is a low-calorie cuisine, and the only two things we know, in all that research, are that the less one eats the longer one lives, and that there is some correlation with a normal or low fasting insulin and longevity. Neither of these scientifically established points are supported with a high fruit cuisine in most of the population.

VIKTORAS KULVINSKAS

The high fruit- and sweet-oriented diet is leading to quite a bit of new successes in the Olympics and other competitive sports. Is this going to have a long-term impact on this generation? Well as a starter, unless they're having it in the form of apple pies and frozen peach smoothies, I don't think so. If they're consuming it in light food form and are into athletic performance, I think they're going to do extremely well as far as overall longevity, but the aging process is definitely going to be accelerated.

Now, what are the benefits, first of all, and then what are the alternatives? The benefits are that yes, you can have heightened sugar access, which is very quickly bioavailable and will be burned very fast. However, this leads to a kind of fatty cellular makeup, as seen by the natural hygienist templates, which is the triglyceride formation out of the sugars that are stored up all over your body and can be readily utilized. It certainly is not a problem. It does diminish your red blood cell oxygen transport capacity because it is quite mucousy and causes stickiness of red blood cells. You can see this impact. Eat a whole meal of fruit and then observe the red blood cell count on a live cell analysis, a dark field microscopy.

On that level, it's not really desirable. You're getting a sugar rush. You can get an alkaloid rush, for instance, if you go to cola and consume caffeine. Many athletes have performed outrageously. You can increase your performance by 10-20%, and as long as your system is intact, you can keep going.

The strongest animals in the world are the green eaters, not the fruitarian animals. If you want Olympic performance, go green. You can also write to me for personal guidance towards Olympic championship. Most of the fruits that people consume are acidic and unripe, so it has a burnout impact on your system. You want alkalinity. You want to maximize your power.

Go for the green juice, blue-green algae, superfoods from the green category, grasses, as well as spirulina and chlorella. Take enzymes with meals and in between meals for a quick recovery, a regeneration of your torn-down muscle tissue.

The champions of the future will be all green. We have the decathlon winner in the Atlanta Olympics, Dan O'Brien, sponsored by Cell Tech, consuming eight grams and more of blue-green algae as well as enzymes and probiotics. We have Venus Williams, who was down for the count and regenerated herself on Hippocrates' green food-oriented diet and went on to win the women's category at Wimbledon in 2012.

FRED BISCI

I ran 18 marathons and two 50-mile races. I also pushed a person in a wheelchair through the New York City marathon from the 4th mile until the end, and in order to do that, I had to eat more fruit. You need extra calories to sustain daily training.

If you're training 60-70 miles a week and you're doing cross training with your bike and you're doing some resistance exercise, you need more food and fruit is certainly not contraindicated if you're doing this correctly. If you're a sedentary person, then you don't need the fruit.

As I said previously, a lot of fruit can be really toxic. It is going to have a negative effect on your upper GI tract; the results will be bloat, gas, and discomfort. After you're clean and exercising a lot, you can eat more fruit and not have any of those symptoms, because your GI tract most likely is clean. I have never seen any body that was on a vegan diet, and training hard every day, who did not make up the calories with fruit or cooked starches.

BRIAN CLEMENT

Well, quite simply, when you pose the question about athletes eating a high fruit diet, it's probably not the worst thing in the world. If the athlete is seemingly healthy and without any disorder, viral microbial disease or mutagenic cancer disease and they're athletic, they can burn up this enormous amount of calories in fruit without a whole lot of breakdown of their body. One wants to do this without mitochondria being affected, without the chromosomes being damaged, etc. Whereas the other portion of the population, the vast majority who are not elite athletes, when they take that high amount of sugar into the body, it actually bonds with protein and starts to break down the chromosomes in the body, so, it shortens life span.

"...take that high amount of sugar into the body...it shortens life span." - Brian Clement

In a new series of books that I published for the academic community, Food is Medicine, we addressed how sugar, including fructose, shortens lifespan. This is based on real science, good science—experiments that have been conducted a couple of thousand times since 1930. People on low caloric, high-density nutrient diets live longer and have less disease, and this I echo with scientific data out of major universities in my series of books *Food is Medicine*.

A little bit of fruit is not a problem. Today, unfortunately, all the fruit has been hybrid. So, the average increase in sugar, in the average fruit is 30 times more—not 30% more—but 30 times more than the original fruit would've had in it at one point.

32. MANY OF MY FRIENDS SUBSCRIBE TO THE BLOOD TYPE DIET, BUT IT DOESN'T MAKE SENSE TO ME. WHAT IS YOUR OPINION OF THIS DIET?

FRED BISCI

It's not something I would recommend. I believe that what you leave out is the key; that's the common denominator amongst every diet that works. Of course, there are some biochemical individualities with people, but I know plenty of people who are type O and are vegans and are doing very well. I know some other people who said that they couldn't go vegan. They tried for a couple of years and they said they couldn't do it. They wanted to eat some animal protein, but remember, if you come from an area of the world where people have been eating a heavy animal protein diet for 1,000 years, getting into a vegan diet takes more time, and possibly more work. With that said, I know plenty of people who want to eat a small amount of animal protein within a primarily plant-based diet, and they are doing well. Omitting all processed food is were I begin, and then try to go to a vegan plant-based live food diet, if the person is willing

I don't want to consume anything that comes from an animal for my own reasons, but I don't subscribe to or recommend only one dietary philosophy. It all depends upon what the person wants to accomplish and what they're able to do; what medical condition they have and how active their lifestyle is. If somebody's a competitive weightlifter, and they want to eat animal protein, I could show them how to do that. You can get more than enough protein for anybody from a vegan diet, if they are willing to try it.

BRIAN CLEMENT

Well, number one, we have to give a lot of respect to Dr. D'Adamo, the father, who was persecuted decades ago for practicing naturopathic medicine in the State of Connecticut. He had to flee his homeland, and for at least a period, resided in Canada so that he could practice good medicine. His son, thank goodness, brought his father's theories forth, wrote a very successful book and it became a worldwide bestseller, *The Blood Type Diet*. These are good men who believe in what they're doing, but they have no biochemical basis or scientific validity to support their theory.

The Hippocrates Health Institute, 60 years later, can tell you that we've put every kind of person, hundreds of thousands of people, under clinical settings, in clinical research on a very similar diet. We varied the diet, depending upon each individual's particular circumstances— nutritional deficiencies, state of mind, blood test analysis, bio-frequency testing, etc. At its core, though, we offer a raw plant-based vegan diet and we have never found blood type to be of any significance. I congratulate the D'Adamos, because they're advising people to get into a better lifestyle, a better diet, than we have here in the West, and they have helped millions of people do that.

But, as far as the blood type diet being valid, it's not valid in any significant way and the debate is over for anyone who really wants to listen to the truth, since we debunked it by the mere fact that we have this illustrious long history, with data and research to show that blood type has nothing at all to do with what you should be eating, but has to do with your biochemistry.

GABRIEL COUSENS

The blood type approach really has some major difficulties. It's based on a series of mythological beliefs that are not scientifically accurate. First is the belief that type O people need to have a high protein diet. I, myself, am a type O, and I certainly don't need to eat meat, and I certainly don't have a high protein diet. Many people in the live food movement who are type O are very healthy without a high protein or a meat diet.

"...bogus science on every level." - Gabriel Cousens

Not only am I a type O, but so is Brian Clement. Recent research has debunked the claim that type O people produce more stomach acid. All blood types produce the same amount of stomach acid.

The problem with the general hypothesis is that the blood types existed before humans and animals, and there's no anthropological evidence, according to Dr. Steven Bailey, a nutritional anthropologist at Tufts University, that all the prehistoric people were type O. Contrary to the theory that Type O was the original blood type, the Japanese have definitively shown Type B to be the original blood type. A vegetarian program has definitely been shown to reverse heart disease in all blood types. These facts make a strong statement against the idea of *Eat Right for Your Blood Type*, and the idea that blood types O and B require animal protein to be healthy. The other faulty theoretical foundation is that the Cro-Magnons living 40,000 to 20,000 years ago were all type O and ate meat. The paleontologist, Robert Leaky, who is acknowledged worldwide as an authority on evolution, states that the Cro-Magnons did not have canine teeth, and therefore, would not have been able to use food sources that required canine teeth, such as large amounts of wild game. He thinks that the Cro-Magnon cuisine was probably similar to that of the chimpanzee, our closest genetic relative. But even the chimpanzees have canine teeth and eat primarily plant-source diets.

To sum up my opinion, John Robins, in *The Food Revolution*, quotes Frederick Stare, M.D., founder and former chairman of the Nutrition Department of Harvard School of Public Health. Dr. Frederick Stare said, *"Eat Right For Your Type"* is not only one of the most preposterous books on the market, but one of the most frightening." Early humans did not have Type O blood. Early humans were perhaps eating a 97% plant-source diet. The sliver of truth in the blood type diet theory can be found in another book, *The Answer Is In Your Blood Type*, written by medical doctor Steven Weissberg and physical therapist Joseph Christiano, a fitness trainer. These two showed that it is recommended for people with blood type A to be vegan, as type As who are on a meat eating diet, tend to die around age 61 of cancer or heart disease, and it appears that they can add an extra 15 years to their life if they go vegan. This is what I do recommend to people.

There is an additional piece regarding lectins. Lectins are part of the antigens that are in food, and when we take those foods with the wrong lectins for us, they act like we're eating for the wrong blood type if we have more than 5% of these particular foods in our diet. However, D'Adamo, et al's recommendations of lectins did not correlate with the world scientific literature on lectins. Currently, in our live food masters program, we are doing a study, spanning the last few years, in which we are determining which organic foods have known lectin potential and which have lectins. I hope, in the next few years, to be able to determine, out of about 100 different foods, which foods have a negative impact due to lectins and which have a negative impact because of herbicide and pesticide residue. *Eat Right For Your Type* is bogus science on every level.

VIKTORAS KULVINSKAS

There is no scientific foundation for any of the relationship between blood type and dietary recommendations. I know many individuals who are of exceptional health who are blood type O and who have lived for over 30 years on an exclusive vegan and/or raw food diet. The seeming benefits of the blood type diet come from predominately from the lifestyle change recommendations and not from the prescribed dietary choices for a specific blood type.

33. ARE COOKED GRAINS HAZARDOUS TO YOUR HEALTH? WHAT ABOUT SPROUTED GRAINS?

FRED BISCI

If you've been eating an all raw diet for a while, and you decide to go back to eating cooked grains, I think you're going to have some problems—but there are people who do it. As far as labeling them a hazard to your health, no, I'm not going to go that far, because I know plenty of people who eat some cooked grains and are very, very healthy in the context of a plant-based, mostly raw diet. If they're having a juice or salad, some steamed vegetables and then, for example, a small bowl of rice and peas—that's doable. I have seen numerous Mediterranean people eat some grains and live beyond 100. Some were members of my own family.

You can eat sprouted grains. I don't; I never cared for them. I tell people to try it. If it works well for you, and you want to eat a moderate amount, go ahead and do it. I know sprouted wheat is very good for people for endurance, but it was never my food. I never enjoyed it and I usually don't bring it up to people unless they bring it up. I'm not dogmatic. Look at other cultures. Look at other people in the world that are healthy. It is not the same. Do the best you can.

BRIAN CLEMENT

There are radical differences between a sprouted grain and a cooked grain, one being that a sprouted grain becomes a plant again. A cooked grain, as we all love it of course, is made into a powder, yeast is almost always added to it, as well as some form of sugar, and it becomes a bread, a cake, a cupcake. All the things we grew up loving, and why we love them, is they all breakdown within minutes to sugar. That's another way to get our sugar fix. It's not a very healthy food for you. If you sprout the grains and then cook them, they are much, much healthier. The less sugar you have in it, or no sugar at all, the healthier.

When you're fighting a disease, we don't want to create something called the "leukocytosis" that we reconfirmed again, not too many years ago, by doing some work up in Boston in a laboratory setting. The original work, done at the beginning of the 20th century, showed that when you eat even a plant-based cooked food, the immune system attacks it and it weakens the immune function, allowing diseases to flourish and to grow and to be attracted to you. So, we don't want that to happen. Sprouted grains in their raw form become things like wheatgrass, barley grass, spelt grass and kamut grass, etc. This makes the grain

"There are radical differences between a sprouted grain and a cooked grain..." - Brian Clement

far more digestible, plant-based, enzymatically rich, having a massive amount of phytochemicals. If you look at the research that's been done on phytochemicals, it's just outstanding and astounding that in plants, inherently from the beginning of the life itself, millions, hundreds of millions of years ago—encoded into these plants were phytonutrients or phytochemicals that were there to protect humans, to give us longer lives, and to protect us from diseases that didn't even exist. We didn't show up until 7-8 thousand years ago. Phytochemicals fight cancers, diabetes, cardiovascular disease.

So yes, sprouted grains are very good. No, we're not in support of cooked grains and we don't think cooked grains in any case can be healthy for you. If you are going to cook the grain, just use the sprout that's been germinated. But, if you're fighting a disease, please avoid cooked grains completely.

GABRIEL COUSENS

Generally, I don't recommend cooked grains for a variety of reasons because, again, they really drive up your carbohydrate intake, and the gluten and gliadin in many of them are inflammatory for the body and brain. I personally eat almost no grains at all. However, I will have some sprouted buckwheat in salads. I think some sprouted grains, such as buckwheat, quinoa, and millet seem to be safe, but they're very different than cooked grains, which are higher in sugar than are vegetables.

VIKTORAS KULVINSKAS

All cooked foods are detrimental to your health and exhaust your enzymatic reserves. Considering that they're so high in starch, and so prevalent in our culture because they're the cheapest food available, cooked grains predominate in processed foods. What it leads to is the exhaustion of your amylase starch digesting enzyme, leading to sourness in your stomach and a burning sensation eventually requiring antacids. This is a poor choice. It leads to bone degeneration. It is acidic on your system.

Sprouted grains are a different food all together. There's no comparison between consuming sprouted grains and consuming cooked grains. When you sprout, you increase the nutritional value, especially in the B complex, with some individual B vitamins increasing by as much as 1500%. The vitamin E increase is 300%. It is one of the strongest, most powerful libido regenerators. There's a good reason why they call wheat the "staff of life" and why they say, "sowing your wild oats." These are all very powerful foods in terms of generating the reproductive system, and I have all this documented in my book *Survival in the 21st Century*. Sprouted grains are excellent and should be consumed by everybody who wants to have a wonderful time in the evening with their favorite mate.

Many individuals, when they get into this raw food oriented program, are severely deficient in enzymes, especially amylase. For these individuals, I do not suggest, under any situation, consuming sprouted grains except with enzymes. The other thing is, grains are made up of lots of starch. They should never be consumed with anything from the fruit or acid category. That's also true when you're eating a salad that includes tomato, lemons or some form of vinegar—if you consume, for instance, sprouted grain cereal or sprouted grain crackers with this kind of salad, you'll find that it will cause digestive problems because acidic foods interfere with the digestion of starches. Those are important considerations, but otherwise it is one of the most powerful foods.

Grain that was grown in the Nile by Cleopatra created one of the strongest militaries, because they had full spectrum minerals in the flood plains soil where the grains were growing. They created one of the strongest armies as well as also some of the most brilliant citizens in the world. They constructed the pyramids. They also created some of the great mystical schools.

34. IS THE RAW LIVING FOOD DIET APPROPRIATE FOR ALL PEOPLE? ARE THERE CERTAIN HEALTH REASONS WHY A PERSON WOULD NEED TO INCLUDE COOKED FOOD IN THEIR DIET?

GABRIEL COUSENS

During the last 40 years, I have encountered only one person, someone who grew up in the Arctic Circle, who was not able to successfully do a 100% live food cuisine, and that person had to have fish once a week. All people can be successful on a live food cuisine, if one includes eating to balance one's constitution and the macronutrient elements, which are oxidizer,

"...some people are very, very toxic and need to move to a live food cuisine carefully over a period of a year or two so that too many toxins don't come out all at once and create a healing crisis." - Gabriel Cousens

parasympathetic/sympathetic, and also kapha, pitta, and vata doshas. All of those have to be balanced in the big picture. The other consideration is that some people are very, very toxic and need to move to a live food cuisine carefully, over a period of a year or two, so that too many toxins don't come out all at once and create a healing crisis.

FRED BISCI

This might upset certain people, but my answer to the first part of that question is no, it's not. People bring up names of some of the old timers, like Norman Walker, Paul Bragg, Bernarr Macfadden—but they were not on a 100% raw living food diet. There are some people who can't or do not want to do it. A raw vegan lifestyle helps in all health conditions. With that said, it's not a panacea. I would not give a blanket answer to a question like that. Every person is a different case.

VIKTORAS KULVINSKAS

Individuals with gastro-intestinal ulcerations can have some difficulty with roughage, and it can make them feel very uncomfortable. The direction to take in such individuals is to eat blended soups and some cooked foods initially, because eating only raw foods could trigger cleansing reactions and excretion of a lot of internal acids by way of the gastro-intestinal tract. Such individuals might feel discomfort—so blended soups containing some sweet potato or squashes will basically slow down the overall cleansing reactions.

Cooking food is associated with nutritional destruction and loss of roughage and fiber, which feeds the friendly bacteria. As a result, we need to consume much more food and you'll never get a Kirlian auric feeling—

the vibration of therapeutic value—from the cooked food as you would from raw food. You eat vibrations, that's it. You eat vibrations. Once you apply heat, you have destroyed the vibrations structurally. The only reason that cooked food eaters are alive is because of the friendly bacteria along the gastro-intestinal tract that keep them alive by providing live enzymes, live protein. The friendly bacteria provide live protection against pathogenic microbes. They provide live vitamin B complex and many other vibrational components.

The raw diet is the cheapest diet. It's the one you can do all organic by just buying your own seeds and growing them at home, by making some fermented foods and utilizing sea salt and sea vegetables and all of a sudden, you've got complete nutrition in a most cost effective way. Anything else just does not do it.

BRIAN CLEMENT

I don't know why anyone would be silly enough to consider that cooking food would make your better. I mean, it doesn't make any sense at all. Now, there are transitional periods where we actually put people on cooked food because, psychologically and physiologically, it's an easier bridge for them—but there's no mandatory reason a person must eat cooked food. I think it's habitual. Even at the Institute, when we have people for whom going raw is a radical change, we give them a stepping stone of a little bit of cooked grain, a little bit of cooked something that of course, would be sprouted. We do this to make them a little more comfortable and secure, but in rapid order, we can get them on a 100% raw food diet.

35. WHAT ARE THE MOST IMPORTANT FOODS TO ELIMINATE FROM YOUR DIET?

FRED BISCI

That's a simple question. Eliminate all the processed food, 100%. The processed food is a killer and it's a modern-day curse. It won't kill you all at once, but sooner or later, it's going to get to you or it's going to get you on an operating table or on medication or into a nursing home.

BRIAN CLEMENT

Well, any animal flesh—from fish, right through pork—any dairy food. These are the most important foods to get out of your diet, and then, cooked foods. In my first volume of *Food is Medicine*, I have up-to-speed, up-to-date research on the acrylamides and cooked animal foods and how we now clearly show the chemical cooking link between diseases such as cancer. It's not only the raw food Elders and the research and clinical work that we're doing, but mainstream science is confirming, validating the work we've done for more than 200 years combined.

GABRIEL COUSENS

All junk food, white flour, white sugar, GMO food, should be eliminated immediately. Generally, minimize high-glycemic foods unless you're a particular body type (25% of the population) who genetically need a higher complex carbohydrate diet. In that case, I recommend sprouts, leafy greens and vegetables in general for carbohydrate needs.

VIKTORAS KULVINSKAS

Eliminate pasteurized dairy products.

36. SHOULD I STRIVE TO BE 100% PERFECT ON THIS DIET? OR IS IT OK TO "CHEAT" SOMETIMES? IF I CHEAT, WILL IT BE HARDER TO MAINTAIN THIS HEALTHY DIET?

VIKTORAS KULVINSKAS

Our research shows that the majority of people are not geared toward raw foods. They are emotionally toxic or, at least, hold so many memories associated with food and social experiences that they have a sort of addiction toward food. It makes it a perfectly natural thing for them to consider eating unhealthful food. The question is, will it make a difference in terms of long-term health? Yes it will. If you follow the Hippocrates approach, this is the approach that will give you the kind of results you want. We allow the individual to have berries and a little bit of fruit twice a week. We have cooked food served twice a week, which is better than having it on a daily basis. By taking enzymes with your meals, you will have no difficulty whatsoever in digesting them. Eventually you'll eat cooked food less frequently, and only on special occasions. Make sure you take extra enzymes when you consume that meal.

I don't think you should have any judgment about it. I mean, cheating, what a nasty word. There's no cheating here. You basically work at doing the best that you can as an individual. Don't place judgment on yourself, "I'm no good." Forget it. You're good. You're perfect. You're doing as perfectly as you can. Eventually you'll find that as you do emotional detoxification—through meditation, through spiritual practices—you'll find that cooked food has no allure. Right now, if you need it, go for it. Don't worry about it. Try to keep increasing your raw food and stop the judging mind. Following the Hippocrates program, you will find no difficulty in maintaining healthy standards and you will experience blissful and intellectual and above average aspirations and personal development. It will be easy to maintain such an approach. When you're ready, you'll do all raw.

GABRIEL COUSENS

It's not a good idea to cheat. It is wiser to create a cuisine and macronutrient balance that feels consistently comfortable and is sustainable day in and day out. One may move to that gradually. If people move to 100% live food too quickly, there may be emotional detoxification, because people use food to suppress emotions. Dead food suppresses dead and toxic emotions in our body. When we stop eating these foods, we create a situation where there is more release of those toxic emotions, and therefore, we can have some level of healing crisis. Best is the steady, gradual, persistent progress until one reaches 80%, (which was defined as being a live food cuisine at the gathering of live food leaders in January of 2006). One should hold there until feeling very balanced and stable, and then move up to 95-100%, if one so chooses. I describe this higher percentage as the Olympic cuisine, which helps one become a more active superconductor of the Divine. When one cheats or yo-yos, the body gets confused. It can't adjust as well, and it's harder to stay with the cuisine. It is better to move at a sustainable rate, whether it takes a day, a week, a month, or four months. In slow pacing, if one doesn't have any major diseases like cancer, heart disease, candida, or diabetes, first eliminate red meat; then eliminate poultry; then eliminate fish; and then eliminate grains and beans; and, finally, maintain a live food cuisine. We want to be gentle and loving with ourselves. An 80% live food cuisine is the basic ideal and 95-100% is more powerful. It's more about your cuisine comfort zone. The optimal macronutrient balance is the same for both levels and all cuisines.

BRIAN CLEMENT

Every time you cheat, it brings you a little bit closer to your addiction again and that pattern that you've created in the past life. I would strongly advise not to do it, but, you're going to do it. I did, I don't know an honest person who did not do that, and I think it's perfectly fine to admit that that may happen. It's more about getting back on the horse, dusting yourself off and continuing on, rather than going into that spiral of self-degradation where you say, "Oh, my God. See, I can't do it—it's hard for me to do. My aunt does this, and my friends do this." So, don't eat that first cookie, because you may end up eating the entire cookie jar. It's better to stay 100% raw for that reason, if nothing else. Is it the end of the world? Providing you're not sick—no, it's not the end of the world and expect that it's going to happen. I don't know anyone it hasn't happened to.

"I don't know anyone it hasn't happened to..." - Brian Clement

FRED BISCI

My philosophy in life is, don't cheat, no matter what you're doing. Don't cheat in what you're saying; don't cheat in a business deal; and I certainly don't advise you to cheat in your diet.

I do recommend that people design a food plan that starts with eliminating 100% of the processed food. You have to design a program that you can live with, that you can afford, that you can continue over your lifetime, and that will enable you to live with the social ramifications. A lot of people can't follow a 100% raw living food diet just because of the social ramifications. They won't even consider it. My wife is one of those people. She's very healthy, eats a good diet, but she's a very social person, so she has a different priority here.

37. WHAT ARE ALKALINE FOODS AND WHY ARE THEY IMPORTANT TO EAT?

BRIAN CLEMENT

There's a lot of misinformation and exaggeration and embellishment on the subject, but the bottom line is, on a proper raw living diet, you're on an alkaline-based diet. About 80% of your body chemistry and your food should be alkaline, 20% acid, and you don't have to be a chemist or a physicist to do any of this, you pretty much just eat the proper foods. They're the kind that the Elders will teach you about.

Our observation is that in early stages—we're talking about years not days or weeks—the acid or the pH can swing. So, don't think because some writer or purported expert tells you that we need a seven and if you don't have a seven you may die, that's going to happen. The vast majority, and we've done this testing with thousands of people over the decades, have not achieved that constant stable level. So, it takes years on a good diet for your body's biochemistry to regulate and to perpetuate numbers and it's not going to be exactly 7 for everyone.

The other thing I may have to say, don't be fanatical about this, the fact is that the body does function best at about 80 alkalinity, 20 acidity, and that keeps the organ systems in good order. If you don't have that, if you eat the diet that I grew up on (the Western diet), that many of you are either eating now or have eaten in the past—you're highly acidic, and that does break down the immunity, it also breaks down the organ systems and the chemistry of the body, making you more vulnerable to disease.

Statements like, "if you have an alkaline body, you will never get a disease," are absurd. Disease is created through emotional states and unpredictable environmental states, like radiation. So, could you live the way that the Elders are teaching, and, under certain circumstances, get a disease? But, is it going to be harder for this disease to seed itself or to create itself in your body if you're otherwise healthy? The answer is obviously yes, it's very hard to permeate a very strong and well-built wall where a weak wall is easy to negotiate. It's just common sense; eating well, living well, having a strong anatomy and strong chemistry creates an unfriendly place for disease.

FRED BISCI

Alkaline foods are foods that leave an alkaline ash in the human body. On a scale of 14, 7 or above is alkaline. 1 to 7 is acid. Fruits and vegetables, in general, leave an alkaline ash.

The most powerful alkaline foods are the green chlorophyll-rich foods, predominantly green vegetables and sprouts and green juices. Your blood pH is supposed to be between 7.3 and 7.4. Your own body chemistry is always trying to keep you within that range. A plant-based diet makes this process easier.

I recommend that you design a diet that you can stay with for the rest of your life. Give it a real chance to work. Exercise, drink clean water, maintain positive thoughts, be spiritually grounded, and get out in the fresh air. All these things increase your alkalinity, in addition to the foods you eat.

GABRIEL COUSENS

The discussion of alkalinity is a little confused because we have the alkalinity of our blood, the acid/alkalinity of our urine, and the acid/alkalinity of our saliva. All of them tell us different things. According to our constitution, our blood pH will vary significantly. For example, the blood pH will actually get more acid with protein if one is in the autonomic nervous system (parasympathetic), but if one is in the bio-oxidative system, the blood pH will actually get more alkaline with protein. This appears paradoxical. Saliva pH is related to digestive power, and urine pH is related to the body's overall cellular pH. Urine pH is ideally between 6.4 and 7.2. The body works optimally in those ranges.

In severe cancer, sometimes the body becomes very alkaline to compensate for its extreme acidity. While that seems paradoxical, the body activates different buffer systems to maintain equilibrium. Generally speaking, for optimum mental functioning research indicates a blood pH of 7.46 is optimal. This is higher than what the Germans recommend, which is 6.35. I find that 7.46 will give you optimum mental and brain function. For saliva, digestive ability is optimal between 6.4 and 6.8. Additionally, sometimes people can have bladder infections that will actually make the urine pH go higher. There are times one may need to acidify the body, particularly the urine, if one has a bladder infection. In this case there is a danger of over alkalinizing.

When I first began eating live foods, my urine pH was closer to 7.8-8.0, and it did create a little alkalosis, which expressed as muscle spasms and fasciculations. I had to monitor it and bring it into a normal range. Also, in fasting, my urine pH regularly will go to 8. This tells me that I don't have a lot of toxins in my body because often, during a fast, people will see their urine pH go down because they're detoxing. On the other hand, it can create some discomfort because I can have more muscle spasms and hyper-reactivity. If I'm at an 8 pH, I will take a teaspoon to a tablespoon of apple cider vinegar, and it will immediately bring my pH down into the low 7s, and hold it there for a while. I use apple cider vinegar to balance the excess of alkalinity in my body.

After a few years on a live food diet, people do get more alkaline. It takes a few years before your body is at a regular level of healthy alkalinity. I don't recommend tricks to create the illusion of alkalinity, like alkaline water or taking a lot of sodium bicarbonate. There are some reasons for doing that, but really, the best way to build alkalinity in the system is to take in high alkaline minerals, such as magnesium, calcium, and potassium. In other words, it is good to eat a high alkalizing, high mineral diet.

Generally speaking, foods that tend to be alkalinizing for the body tissues—not the urine, the saliva, or the blood—are vegetables. Our mainline alkalinizing foods are leafy greens, sea vegetables, and sprouts. They're important to eat because the body works best at a healthy slightly alkaline tissue pH, measured by a urine pH between 6.4 and 7.2.

VIKTORAS KULVINSKAS

Your human body is made up of 100 trillion cells, as well as 20 to 100 times more of friendly bacteria. The cells are tiny little batteries with a central nucleus being acidic and the cytoplasm that surrounds the nucleus being alkalinized. The body maintains different levels of alkalinity. The most extreme form of alkalinity is found in the internal organs such as the heart, liver, kidney and lungs. The reason for it is that you need the high alkalinity to be able to function without needing ongoing rest like muscles do, they have a very low alkalinity and need some down time. The heart, the liver, they do not take down time; they work 24/7. Their alkalinity is 10,000 times higher.

"All cooked foods are acid forming." - Viktoras Kulvinskas

The blood tries to be slightly under alkaline. Too high of an alkalinity will push you into alkalosis and too low will push you into acidosis. Alkalosis will make you feel completely wasted. That occurs, for example, when you're taking some of the alkaloids such as marijuana, and other drugs, in continued usage—especially on a raw vegan alkaline diet. Eventually, you won't be able to handle drugs of any sort. You need that alkaline balance.

Most people are consuming acid foods. There are only alkaline foods that are found in raw foods. There are no alkaline foods in cooked foods. All cooked foods are acid forming because the minerals have gone through disorganization and they're not bioactive and all they represent is a stress on the organism as it's trying to evacuate this cooked toxic chemistry.

Most alkaline foods are your greens, though there are some that have a lemony taste that are acidic in nature. However, your greens would be the best source of re-alkalizing, all your sprouts are alkalizing whereas the grains, especially all the cooked beans and legumes, are all acid forming. Your sweet fruits are alkaline. The melons are alkaline. All the other fruits are acidic with the exception of bananas. They represent hybrids. They're very high in sugars. They've been inbred to have such a high sugar content that they're going to put a stress on the organism and the sugar can make them acidic through the process of internal fermentation.

As a rule, fruits are picked unripe in order to accommodate the marketplace. If you have a sensitive system, you'll start noticing some aches and pains in the lower back associated with your kidney being overstressed by the acidic condition. That includes citrus and lemons. Lemons are good for pulling mucous out of your system and helping in many other ways but they are definitely acidic. Consume more and more alkaline foods, and also consume adequate amounts of water to spill out the acid waste products that are metabolic in nature. Water helps to alkalize in the sense that it leads to expelling the acid waste through the process of sweat and urination, plus exhalation.

38. DO OILS CONSTRICT THE ARTERIES? ARE THERE ANY "HEALTHY" OILS?

BRIAN CLEMENT

Oils and fats should be discussed. Do animal fats clog and constrict arteries? Yes. At some level, does even saturated coconut oil provoke your body to make cholesterol that can contribute to the arteries being clogged? The answer is yes. Are there oils that help to break that down? Yes. Omega-3 oils, from things such as sprouted chia seed, sprouted flax seed, and hemp seed, walnut oil, the algae, blue-green and green algae oils. Do they help to emulsify the fats in your arterial or ventricular areas? The answer is absolutely yes, but I think oils in any part should be eaten in a minute amount.

When one has had cardiovascular concerns, maybe the avoidance of oil and the consumption of seeds that are sprouted to get your omega oils should be recommended. I'm a major believer, as I think any serious nutritional scientist would be, that the essential fats are powerfully important agents in cellular health, and even neuron health, brain cells for thought, for memory, for a lot of the things that are concerning to us today in our culture and society.

FRED BISCI

Oils do not constrict your arteries. Certain oils will clog your arteries and contribute to hardening of the arteries. There are healthy oils. In fact, I think the right combination of flax seed oil and hemp seed oil is very, very important and it will take the place of fish oils. Fish oils, in my opinion, are not everything they're cracked up to be. I think that they're causing problems in some people and I don't encourage them. The best way to get your oil is from whole foods, such as nuts, avocados and seeds. Salad dressings are best made with whole foods. For those who wish to use olive oil, flax seed oil, hemp seed oil, sesame oil, they must be raw and cold pressed and used in moderation. All commercial processed oils should be avoided. The inflammation in our arteries, which is measured by CRP and homocysteine, is the main reason that we build up arterial plaque. I have never seen a person who is on the correct type of diet and omitted all processed food, who had clogged arteries. In spite of what some people say, not all oils are disastrous. Some of the healthiest people in the world, such as the Mediterraneans, use some oils. Occasionally, I use high quality olive oil for variety.

VIKTORAS KULVINSKAS

First of all, oils do not constrict the arteries unless they're heat processed oils, in which case, they'll deposit in the arteries and reduce the openings of the cardiovascular system. The problem with oils is that they create stickiness for the red blood cells and, as a result, lead to poor circulation, especially in the extremities. This reduces your ability as a thinker, as an intellectual, as well as an athletic performer, because metabolism is driven by oxygen, and you have a radical reduction of your circulatory oxygen for the brain as well as for the muscular system.

Are there any good oils? Yes, there are. They're found in real whole foods. You'll never get good oils in a bottle. Forget it. You will get great oils in blue-green algae. You'll get great oils in soaked seeds and nuts by means of soaking your seeds. Basically, you activate the lipase, the fat splitting enzyme, which reduces the accrued fat which is next to impossible to digest into essential fatty acids that are bioavailable, and yet have a high sources of omegas and all that your body needs.

The oily foods, such as the nut butters, including the raw sprouted nut butters, are fake, because they are not really made from sprouted nuts or seeds. If you sprouted the seeds and then made them into nut butter, you would not have that huge volume of oil in the containers. The commercial nut butter containers are filled with some sprouted nut that has gone through the milling process and added oil. Don't buy these. All oils, immediately upon being exposed to light and air, start going rancid. Rancid foods are carcinogenic. There's no benefit in consuming any of those nut butters.

GABRIEL COUSENS

Research done on olive oil eaten alone, showed a 36% constriction of the brachial artery. That does happen, and that is a problem, because it can disrupt the inner lining of the artery. That said, the rest of the research suggests that if you take your healthy olive oil with appropriate anti-oxidants, such as on a salad, it makes no difference in constriction. Are there any healthy oils? I really don't recommend fractured foods. Oils are fractionated food.

At the same time, I know that many people suffer from low cholesterol and/or Alzheimer's and need higher amounts of long-chain omega-3s. Coconut oil is a way to reverse brain insulin-resistant Alzheimer's disease. It also moves us from a conversion rate from short-chain to long-chain omega-3s of 1.5-3% to 6-10%. That's valuable! As I stated earlier, coconut oil converts to ketones in the liver, and these ketones give particular energy to the brain, supplying up to 90% of the brain's energy, and can help reverse the Alzheimer's process, connected to insulin resistance, that starves the brain of sugar. Ketones are a superfood for the brain. Coconut oil will raise your cholesterol. As I suggested earlier, the conclusion reads (viewing all the research with literally 1.25 million people and a huge amount of data) that cholesterol between 160-260 has literally zero effect on heart disease, while low cholesterol, and low omega-3s, clearly have a negative effect on emotional and mental states.

All aspects of brain and nervous system health are negatively impacted with low cholesterol and low omega-3s, with as much as six-fold increase in depression and increased suicide. Personally, I avoid all but a minimum of oils in my cuisine as they are a fractionated food, and they're easy to oxidize and go rancid (especially flax oil).

39. WHAT ARE THE BEST FOODS TO INCREASE ENERGY?

VIKTORAS KULVINSKAS

Energy foods can be defined by what I saw working with Olympic and other athletes; blue-green algae, enzymes, wheatgrass and probiotics. There are many other very powerful influential foods, but energy comes from alkalinity and increased oxygenation. If you want increased energy, then you will need to not be consuming any form of fat. As a matter of fact, increased energy comes from fasting on green juices, though you have to be prepared. If you are on a traditional diet, or even a cooked vegan diet, then you go on a green juice diet, all you're going to experience is a cleansing reaction and feeling wasted. If you are already on a raw food, green juice diet, and then you go on green juices and water—what you have done is now eliminated the stress associated with digestion and, all of a sudden, your energy just goes way up. If you want some stimulants through increased circulation, cayenne would be extremely beneficial. It is one of the primary well-known nerve tonics, without having any caffeine like derivatives or alkaloids. Taking two capsules of it you'll see a radical influence on your abilities.

There are other superfoods that will make a difference. Maca is a good example, and many of the Chinese herbs associated with the ginseng family. I would suggest moderation in this area, because now you're moving into alkaloids. The alkaloids can have an exhaustive effect, green juices will not. You're much better off working with green juices, the predigested proteins coming form microbial cultures and from soaked seeds and nuts.

Practicing de-stressing of your spine by lying down and doing yoga stretching and deeper relaxation will recharge your system. Doing breathing exercises will recharge your system. Alkalize, increase your oxygen levels and increase your circulation. These are going to give you tremendous increases in energy. See yourself as a winner. Have no negativity or doubts, and as a result, your powers will escalate physically, mentally and spiritually.

GABRIEL COUSENS

This depends on one's unique metabolic constitution. The energy producers in the body are the mitochondria, which are the factories within the cells. Mitochondria function is determined by the genetics of one's mother, and one needs to have the proper balance of carbohydrates, fat, and protein, depending upon those genetics. At least 60-70% of the population needs a higher protein, moderate fat, and moderately low complex carbohydrate diet; and 25% need a higher complex carbohydrate cuisine, with lower fat and lower protein. The less one eats, the longer one lives, but also the more energy one has, because, at least a third of energy goes to digesting food, and that creates limitations in overall function. Eating less is important. Eating according to constitution will give one that long sustained energy. Also beneficial is the use of a variety of herbs that can be helpful in protecting or increasing energy and longevity, as well as foods and herbs that particularly support adrenaline function.

"The less one eats, the longer one lives, but also the more energy one has..." - Gabriel Cousens

FRED BISCI

Here we're going back to the same issue. We're going back to, should you eat a lot of fruit or should you not eat a lot of fruit? Remember, the foods that create energy are the carbohydrates, the fats and the proteins. Carbohydrates are a very direct source of energy. When you have that direct source of energy, and you're still eating too much, then your body has to compensate. Your body has to secrete insulin, and if you're not exercising, that might not be the best thing. For half an hour to 45 minutes after you exercise, your body does not secrete insulin, so you can eat a lot of fruit and take in a lot of sugar, but that's not a good idea if you're not burning it up by exercising.

Animal proteins are not a good source of fuel. I always recommend the plant-based diet, preferably vegan. Eat a variety of different foods, based on your activity level and what you like.

At 84, I'm still exercising and have plenty of energy on a simple raw food diet. I exercise at least an hour and a half to two hours a day. I do a half hour to 45 minutes of Qigong martial arts exercises in the morning, and I walk or run through the hills, or take my dog to the beach and I walk for about an hour.

You've got to make sure you're getting enough calories and enough sleep. Incorporate juices, wheatgrass, and E3Live. Make sure you're getting some of the essential fatty acids from hemp seeds and some nuts. Once you get along far enough into the living raw foods diet, I'll be very shocked if you don't have unbelievable energy.

BRIAN CLEMENT

Protein foods increase energy and stabilize blood sugar, and the Hippocrates diet, as well as the general diets of the Elders, are high protein diets. With a stable blood sugar, you develop energy. Fresh water and salt water algae, sprouts, pollen—these are powerful agents for giving you energy.

Then of course, hydration. Hydration is one of the most overlooked areas of health. We see on a weekly basis, 52 weeks a year, people who come in to us from all corners of the globe and we insist they drink, drink, drink. We're handing them juices and water all day long from morning till night and by the third day the majority of them are saying "My God, I've not felt this good for years." Now, statistically, what we do know, from all the universal studies done on dehydration, is that about 6 out of 10 people in the Western world lack hydration. The majority of us are dehydrated. When you hydrate people, brain function, body function, immune function, all accelerate, they go up. That, in and of itself, is going to give you energy.

We also know from research that about 40% of the population somehow lack the mechanism in their brain to tell them to drink. So, there may be many of you that have to write down on a piece of paper, here's how much I'm drinking every day. Now, if you're not a competitive athlete, or living in a very dry and arid climate, you need approximately ½ of an ounce of pure fluid for every 1 pound of bodyweight. A 200-pound man would need 100 ounces of pure water or fresh raw juices, or a combination of those, every day just to maintain. If that man was an athlete in an arid climate, it could actually be double that amount. In my life as an example, seven days a week, no matter where I'm traveling in the world, I take a sauna and with that, I require more fluid than a person who would not do that. I'm also an exerciser. A lot of these things have to be taken into consideration for energy.

40. IF I CONSUME RAW LIVING ORGANIC FOOD, IS THAT ENOUGH? WILL IT BE NUTRITIOUS? WHAT IF IT HAS COUNTERPRODUCTIVE ELEMENTS OR INGREDIENTS? WILL IT GIVE ME LONG LASTING BENEFITS WITH LIFELONG CONSUMPTION?

VIKTORAS KULVINSKAS

First of all, the Hippocrates program is based on consuming meals six days a week and having one day of juices. It's based on the tradition of the Essenes, who lived on about an 85-90% sprouted, baby green oriented type of diet, as well as microbial cultures. They developed this agriculture within a desert community and they were noted for their extreme longevity. Their average age, according to the historian Joseph, was 124 years. You should have no problems with this kind of a dietary orientation.

However, all non-grain foods, (none blue-green algae foods) have undesirable components in them, according to a magazine entitled Natural Toxins in Food, put out by the Academy of Science. It's a monthly journal that researches foods in general. Basically, all foods contain something that is stressful on the organism. The human body sorts what is not acceptable and excretes it out of the system. This is done through the immune function. The immune system is driven by enzymatic support, according to Les Cobart. Within a matter of 20 minutes, orally administered enzymes, which also includes enzymes coming from food or from a supplement, empower the immune system function by 1100%. Our ability to have our enzyme levels rejuvenated not only by our sprouted foods, but also by the probiotics that we have along our gastro-intestinal tract, is unquestionable. Food in a raw form will always enable you to have strong immune function and to eliminate whatever side toxins you might have. If you go out eating other herbs, spices, eating randomly and excessively then yes, you will run into problems, which has been expressed by many of the herbalists. You have to be careful with strong tasting foods. Things that have a mild taste, they are agreeable and you can utilize them.

BRIAN CLEMENT

Well, the bottom line is yes, a diet of raw organic living food, properly combined and with a wide cross-section of foods, is not only enough—it's what we should aspire to, what we need to eat, it's how we were built to eat, and we have shown that empirically here at Hippocrates. Will it be nutritious? It's the most nutritious food on the planet. That one is a redundant question. Will it give long-lasting benefits? Of course, it's cumulative. It builds up like building brick by brick—a very sound building, that's what you're doing with this—building sound muscles and sound tissues of the body, etc. Providing that you constantly fuel your body with raw organic living food in great part, it doesn't have to be in total, you'll maintain lifelong benefits from this, as well as longevity.

GABRIEL COUSENS

A raw, living, organic, vegan cuisine is the best cuisine. It yields long lasting benefits. All foods have some ingredients that can negatively affect us. If we eat excessively and exclusively only certain foods, there may be negative benefits, but, the live food cuisine is good. In today's world, with the nutritional stresses, electromagnetic stresses, and the general stresses of life, is it enough? My answer is no. I think that everyone needs supplements. We'll be talking about that when we get to the supplement section. I, myself, take supplements. All my supplements are what we call food concentrates or herbal supplements, which definitely give me sustained energy throughout the day—that's a 9-10 hour workday consistently! I have sustained energy and a feeling of wellbeing at all times of the day. I don't know what the word tired means. I attribute this, for me, to a low glycemic and all natural, organic live vegan cuisine that helps maintain very steady energy all day long.

FRED BISCI

If you do it correctly, and you obey all the rules of nature, the answer to that question is yes. Drink water, get rest, and eat enough food to get enough calories to sustain your activity. If you do it incorrectly though, you could run into trouble. Some people may have to supplement with Vitamin B12 or a few other supplements.

41. WHAT ARE FALSE FOODS AND HOW CAN WE AVOID THEM?

FRED BISCI

The false foods are not whole foods; they are any food that's been processed. The whole foods in a plant-based diet are fruits, vegetables, nuts, seeds, avocados, sprouts, and their juices. All the other foods end up being false.

BRIAN CLEMENT

The latest trend is the term superfoods. Well, super unfortunately makes my mind immediately click into money because "superfoods" pretty much encapsulate the overconsumption mentality that Westerners have become trapped in. So, we're always looking for the quick fix, the one thing that will solve all the problems. There are some so-called false foods, and I wrote about this in a magazine. Go to the Hippocrates website, www. hippocratesinstitute.org, and look into our magazine archives, and you'll find that issue. We talk about things such as chocolate. Most of the "raw chocolate" is not raw. Most people that eat the chocolate add sugars into it. We talked about sugars already, sadly like the so-called raw agave, none of which is raw, as it's all heated at a minimum of 180 degrees Fahrenheit.

So, these unhealthy trends, for example, berries that are superfoods—it's almost taught to you like you could survive on these foods. Many of these are embellishments with stories such as, they come from the monks in the high Himalayas. When we really delve in and look closer at this, which we have, we find out the vast majority comes from China, and they are not organic, and God knows what's in it. Be cautious of this. I never use the word superfood. Are there superior foods? Yes, so we have our superior foods, and we've mentioned those previously.

GABRIEL COUSENS

The key foods to avoid include: white flour, all sweeteners (except stevia), all gluten and gliadin foods, all GMO foods, all foods with trans-fatty acids, foods higher up on the food chain (as they are 15-30 times higher in radiation, pesticides, and herbicides), and all synthetic foods.

VIKTORAS KULVINSKAS

First of all, is your visual—how attractive is the food? Your smell; does it smell bad? If it smells bad, there's a questionable condition. Sauerkraut smells good and it has a lemonish fragrance. When it's badly produced it will smell like poop. You wouldn't want to be eating it. Your smell is giving you an indication. Your taste buds are also giving you an indication of what is good for you, your normal senses. You can also utilize kinesiology in terms of as a way of establishing what is good for me? There are many different ways of establishing what is okay for you.

The Hippocrates program is based on the science of optimal health and our experience has been now over 50 years and we are thriving. So is Dr. Gabriel Cousens and other similar research centers. They support your digestive functions according to what is best for you and how you can avoid the "false food". The Hippocrates Health Institute as well as within my own personal health experience … part of the teaching, we take people to a health food store and offer them some shopping experiences.

False foods are saturating the health foods industry and are present in 99% of the regular marketplace. Overeating is a pathway to shorter life and also the method of madness and profit in the business of "food."

Seasonings are one of the biggest attempts to get you into an addictive mode. Both spices and seasonings encourage you to overeat. As a result, you end up buying more produce. Likewise, all processed foods encourage you to overeat. They are all dehydrated. Some of the strongest seasonings available are the false salt-based products such as what you may find in the soy liquids. Do not touch any of them unless it has sea salt and is fermented…otherwise it is dead.

Through kinesiology, the weakening effects confirm it's not acceptable as a food resource yet raw foodist are consuming it in volumes. As a further example, nut butters; even though from raw seeds these are false foods and you are better off not consuming them because of an overall rancidity though it's good enough for emergency and take plenty of enzymes and you'll be able to tolerate it.

Starches are the worst culprits in regards to food combining. Even more so, the processed lasagna, spaghetti and pasta contain 1000's of carcinogen derivatives created by the manufacturing, high pressure and heat to create the finished product. Minimize if not completely eliminate them from an optimal diet. However, when you do consume starches...never eat them within a meal that has anything acidic, like lime, lemon, vinegar or fruits...as it makes the starch indigestible and creates an uncomfortable fermentation within the digestive system.

Anything that comes in a can or a bottle or a plastic bag is questionable. Read the ingredient list. Very likely it's going to be containing some form of preservatives and toxins. That includes that ever so popular kinds of fruit juices or coconut water in a bottle, not fresh coconut water. Kombucha tea, oh it's a health drink; it's got over 400 different research papers showing that it's very beneficial and it is a traditional type of drink but at the same time not only is it acidic but also has alcohol in it and some of it has also caffeine. It might stimulate you and make you feel vital but the longer term benefits are undesirable.

All your wonderful chips, the raw foods that are prepared, they're good transition foods but food that is other than the one that you make at home and also grew the sprouts yourself, it's often a little bit questionable unless you know the source and it's fresh dated. When you end up purchasing greens or other packaged items, look at the label, see its expiration date. I would trust every kind of supplement you take with kinesiology. Even though it says on it raw, organic and all that kind of stuff I question it because it might have been at one time raw yet it has gone through degradation and muscle testing will tell you. The question you should always ask is it good for me and also try the different dosages; one capsule or a half a teaspoon, etc. Remember what destroys you is actually what you do on a continual daily habitual practice. If occasionally you have something that is out of sort such as a chip or other ingredients you will do okay but once you start you begin developing addictive habits this is an issue alone.

In the false food category I would include also black peas, even green peas, definitely coffee, all the milks that you can buy; the soy milk, the almond milk; they're all fake foods. You have to make it yourself if you want the real thing. Again, they're transitional foods look at them as indulging. Anything other than what is coming from your garden, from your sprouter or from local resources or at least from reputable organic growers is in question.

42. WHY DO SO MANY VEGETARIANS LOOK UNHEALTHY?

GABRIEL COUSENS

Many vegetarians and vegans look unhealthy because they're not taking a total approach, or they are following the non-scientific conventional teaching of a low fat, low protein, high complex carbohydrate, and/ or no supplement approach, which may only be appropriate for 25% of the population. Another infrequently discussed set of problems is hygiene and faulty food preparation. All walnuts and many nuts and seeds have fungus and some bacteria. At the Tree of Life Café, we soak all nuts and seeds in hydrogen peroxide. Foods that are in the dehydrator too long may become fermented or rotten. Uncontrolled fermentation, such as seed cheeses and rejuvelac, can grow pathogenic bacteria. Seeds and nuts should also be tested for rancidity. These are sources of low-grade infections, which may eventually lead to chronic disease.

Sometimes, failure comes from junk food vegetarian cuisine, or too much focus on their taste. Rather than eating according to their constitution, people eat according to a particular theory, and the going theory in the vegan world is a high complex carbohydrate, low-fat, moderately low-protein diet, which, as I made clear, really weakens one's condition, because they don't get adequate omega-3 oils and cholesterol. They may also be getting too much sugar. As I mentioned, genetically, 75% of people, according to the Stanford research, need to have a higher protein and lower complex carbohydrate diet, with moderate fat intake. There are a lot of problems like that. When one eats according to a theory from a book, that's when one gets into trouble. When one eats consciously, one will do what is necessary to create the optimum diet and cuisine for their unique physiological genetic program.

BRIAN CLEMENT

Because they become very cerebral; in their world, everything is food. They're not exercising enough. They're not taking the other areas of health into account, and they're not happy. Happy people who eat bad food look healthier than unhappy people who eat good food. The happy factor is a big part of this. You can't impose on yourself something in order to restrict yourself. What you have to do is understand why you're using the tool of good

"Exercise, get out in the sun, eat the proper foods and have a life, get a life. Get a life!" - Brian Clement

food. It's all about liking oneself and nourishing oneself. It's also important to be conscious enough to realize the repercussions of your actions—are you helping other people, helping the planet and, in general, the future of life as we know it.

Exercise, get out in the sun, eat the proper foods and get a life! You're going to be a productive, viable member of humanity, rather than this enigma out there, this oddball who feels odd themselves—that's why you look bad and are unhealthy.

FRED BISCI

That's a good question, and it's true. I remember many years ago, when I was a teenager, I was working out with weights and weighed 200 pounds. I would look at vegetarians and say, "Wow, they don't look very healthy at all." My friend Frank, who was a dedicated natural hygienist in the early days, looked pretty good, and he took me to a natural hygiene meeting. I have to say, it was frightening, because those people didn't look good. They were very thin. They didn't look healthy at all. I found out later that most of these people were going through detox. They were in the early stages. I got to know some of them later on and they started to do better with some improvising and making some changes, and they ended up doing well. Some of these people ran into serious problems later on in life, which included my friend Frank, who I believe died from a long term B12 deficiency. There was a large group of people from Rochester, New York, including a family who ran into serious problems after the third generation. I could write a whole book about this. Many vegetarians eat lots of processed food, thinking that leaving out the animal protein is enough to keep them healthy. This is not true.

VIKTORAS KULVINSKAS

Vegetarians not only tend to eat predominantly cooked food but, often, they are prone to overeating. Further, they're not necessarily organic or athletically inclined. They're not living a holistic lifestyle, so what they've done is eliminate meat and chicken and fish, but they still include dairy products, pasteurized dairy products. All of this basically adds up to non-healthy lifestyles. The studies that have been done by www.Mercola.com on vegetarianism are quite extensive, and they show that the longevity of vegetarians is no more than that of meat eaters. They have eliminated meat, but they haven't done much more to improve their overall lifestyle habits. It's good from the humanitarian point of view, so our planet is better off, as are the animals that are not being consumed by people.

Veganism is a good step upwards, as prescribed by www.PCRM.org. However, again, unless it's made up of raw foods, it's basically not going to be a very good diet in terms of long-term effects. Traditional aging might be reduced by as much as 20 years by following holistic lifestyles, and adding fasting will make a big difference.

43. I TAKE PSYCHOTROPIC DRUGS—CAN I GET OFF OF THESE WITH THE PROPER DIET?

GABRIEL COUSENS

As a psychiatrist, I have had extremely positive results taking people off psychotropic drugs. In my book *Depression Free for Life*, I show a 90% success rate in treating depression and getting people off all psychotropic drugs. With manic depression, I have had an 80% success rate—meaning "off all psychotropic drugs." Significant imbalances are created with psychotropic drug use. Contrary to what people think, the SSRIs, which supposedly increase serotonin, actually create serotonin depletion over time because, while they may temporarily increase the serotonin levels at the synaptic gaps, the serotonin is blocked from being reabsorbed at the synapses and gets urinated out over time. There are some serious troubles with these drugs. One of my mentors, Dr. Jonathan Cole, the head of National Institute of Mental Health, actually presented the fact that there is a four-fold increase in suicidal ideation on SSRIs. That isn't really what the FDA wants to hear, but suicidality is well documented on these drugs, as well as a variety of other difficulties. Entire books have been written on these side effects. One can take themselves off of them. Live foods, even without a variety of supplements, can build up the neurotransmitters and, in some cases, improve the neurotransmitter function enough to get free of psychotropics. Live foods themselves, in my observation, significantly stimulate the natural production of neurotransmitters and return function to a higher level. That is part of my program in helping people come off psychotropic drugs. One also needs to be aware that there can be serious withdrawal when coming off psychotropic medication.

VIKTORAS KULVINSKAS

Yes, we ran Dr. Gregory's substance abuse center and we had exceptional results. The best recommendation is, get on a cooked and raw vegan diet for a period of a week or so, and then take mild herbal laxatives at bedtime, and you should be taking them throughout the week. The next day, plan to fast.

Generally the reason why you have such an addiction towards psychotropic drugs is because you are acidic and psychotropic drugs are all alkaloid so they temporarily neutralize the acids making you feel fantastically vital and good because now you have become more alkaline by reducing the acids. They bring with them many cousins whether you're looking at cigarettes, you're looking at caffeine, you're looking at coffee or you're looking at cocaine, any of these things; they leave you more and more acidified and you excrete tremendous volumes of B complex, calcium, vitamin C and enzymes in the processing of using these drugs.

When coming off of psychotropic drugs and following it up with a vegan diet, I've seen consistent, continuous, no more cravings, good results. Get into spiritual practice. One of the great leaders in this movement was Yogi Bhajan. He was a proponent of the 3 Hs, which stands for healthy, happy, and holy. He published many papers on getting people off psychotropic drugs by putting them on a vegan diet. Get into yoga, practice meditation and you'll never go back to psychotropic drugs.

FRED BISCI

Again, I'm not a medical doctor or a psychiatrist. I see some people who come off their drugs and I see some who can't. We must remember, no matter what, you're better off eating a healthy diet. Even if, for some reason or other you can't come off all your drugs, there's a very good chance you can reduce them.

I remember one fellow in particular that I still see; he was very sick, emotionally and psychologically. He started to get interested in raw foods and someone told him that drugs were poison and that he should get off all his drugs and eat a raw food diet. He did—and he slashed his wrists and tried to commit suicide. He should've never come off his drugs like that. Whoever told him that must've been out of their mind themselves. Everybody's an individual and you just don't make blanket recommendations for people who have emotional or psychological disorders.

BRIAN CLEMENT

Well, diet is one part of that, of course. For 30 years, I've been using targeted supplementation and it has been helpful. Although the pharmaceutical industry is corrupted at its core, I am happy that they have made certain psychiatric drugs to help people who, decades ago, would have been institutionalized.

On the other hand, I have discovered, over the decades, that about 8 out of 10 people on psychiatric drugs can slowly, but surely and eventually, come off them under the supervision of a trained healthcare professional—a physician, psychiatrist, etc. Sadly today, the number one drug prescribed is an antidepressant. As I pointed out before, 80% of people do not need to be on that. Am I happy that there are drugs now that help schizophrenics? Yes. Manic depressants, which are bipolar disorders? Yes, I am.

The use of these medicines temporarily and, in some cases, long-term, is helpful for 20% of the sufferers. The other 80% of you wake up, change your life, get a Doctor you can trust, and an Institute that you come to so that you can work with them.

44. EVEN VERY HEALTHY PEOPLE GENERALLY WANT SOME FEEL GOOD FOOD. ANY YOU CAN RECOMMEND?

FRED BISCI

If you're talking about processed food like cake, candy, soda or ice cream, martinis, or anything like that, you're really speaking to the wrong guy. No, I don't recommend any compromise like that, because it just doesn't work well. If you want to have a feel good food, some of the raw food recipes are actually delicious. We have some raw restaurants in New York City that are absolutely fabulous. They make ice cream out of nuts and coconut, and some of the foods are just tremendous. They're 100% raw and the ingredients are good. The food combination might not be the best, but they're certainly edible. I go up there every once in a while with a fellow who works for me. We sit down and have something and I always come back alive, so I think anybody could do it. Everyone has personal preferences. Some people like avocados, some people like bananas and some people like mung bean sprouts. A large green salad with mung beans sprouts is a feel good meal for me. I also like bananas and dried apricots.

BRIAN CLEMENT

Again, when you really feel good, you don't need feel good food. You feel good by running, dancing, singing, having joy, working in a way you love, exercising—that's really where the feel good comes from. You should go back to the superior foods that I just mentioned and they can propel the body and the mind to pursue happiness. How do I become happy? Well, don't look at food as being the source of it.

If you need a sprouted bread to make you feel a little normal, or bring you back to the memories of your mom, or those nice days you had together eating as a child—we try to make a bridge at Hippocrates where we make food look like, feel like, and taste like familiar foods. If you don't make this realistic and just put people on algae and sprouts, 99% are going to fail in the early stages. I certainly would have. Sometimes, you may need to make raw cookies, cake, fruit-based ice creams, etc. with Stevia, and they are the ways that you make it over to this side of the road, where you're stable and not needing all of these perks and so-called feel good foods.

GABRIEL COUSENS

In the long run, a cuisine that one is happy with is all feel good food. In my 21-day program, I have a psycho-spiritual technique, called Zero Point Process, that I teach people, which helps them get away from their "feel good food" addictions, so that they are more addicted to *actually* feeling good than "feel good foods" that bring short term pleasure but leave them imbalanced afterwards. One understands, over time, what really brings sustainable wellness—and those are the foods that they gravitate toward, once they give up their food addictions. Unfortunately, food in our Western culture, where there's so much abundance, is a major way to help people suppress emotions. People tend to want their illusion of comfort with unhealthy comfort foods.

VIKTORAS KULVINSKAS

If you want to feel good, you should call a friend and have a conversation while you're not feeling good, do some writing, go for a long run, or enjoy any kind of activity that has given you pleasure in the past. Do some meditation, yoga; these are the real feel good activities, not stuffing your face with food. If you don't feel good, you probably need to be fasting from food, instead of looking for satisfaction by eating something. If your stomach is empty, have

"Get your body in motion, and you'll get out of that emotion which is making you feel lousy." - Viktoras Kulvinskas

some green tea; that will stimulate your brain a little bit. Have some blue-green algae. Or, if your energy is stuck, do some Qigong reflexology, or even simply massage yourself.

Food is the last area for feel good. For some it would be a cup of coffee and for others it would be too fast and meditate. I'm going to make one recommendation which would help—fast one day a week, of course you should have an empty stomach, add a couple ounces of celery juice and add a pinch or a quarter of a teaspoon of cayenne and/or ginger and drink it down. You will have a feel good experience. It might take about 5-10 minutes, you might not enjoy it during the drinking process but you will experience an altered state of consciousness.

45. HOW BIG OF A ROLE DOES CALORIC RESTRICTION PLAY IN ACHIEVING OUTSTANDING HEALTH?

BRIAN CLEMENT

An enormous role, but we have to be cautious here and point out to you that we cannot talk about caloric restriction with 100% of the population. There are some people who are so sad deep inside and so broken deep inside that bulimia, anorexia, or overeating to the point of morbid obesity is a real concern. Yes, ultimately all sane and healthy people should look at having a low caloric intake.

VIKTORAS KULVINSKAS

Studies have been done with animal subjects that show an increase of as much as 400% in longevity by having as much as 50% calorie restriction from what is considered the SAD diet. As far as human subjects, studies have shown that 1500 calories per day was the average of the long-lived individuals like the Equatorians. In John Robin's current book on longevity, folks over 100 years of age show that lifestyle habits play a central role in longevity. It's not only restricted calories, but also restricted protein, desirable levels of physical activity, quality of relationships, quality of joy and happiness; these are all important.

GABRIEL COUSENS

The less one eats, the longer one lives. The less one eats the healthier one generally feels, because one is using less energy to digest one's food. The less one eats, the less one needs to detox. In general, I consider it important, but I don't like to think about it as calorie restriction. I think about as a scientific approach to finding out the right amount of food one should eat at each meal, and eating that amount of food for optimal wellbeing. If one feels a little tired after eating, that means that they've either eaten the wrong food and they're allergic, or eaten too much. The concept from Ayurveda, and other systems is that the most important thing one can do is to learn how to push away from the table. We want to subtly under-eat. A guide to appropriate food intake is, "I want to eat so that when I get up from the table, I feel so good that I could walk a few miles." Rather than, "I have to lie down to sleep so that I can digest the food."

I don't see calorie restriction as a constriction. I see it as how we can be a nutritional and spiritual "nutrition athlete," and we're always eating to sense where we feel the highest energy before, during and after eating. In this way, we can call it calorie restriction, but for me, it's about eating for optimal wellbeing. How can one eat in a way that totally amplifies every part of one's life and, ultimately, create holiness by upgrading the planetary network of life? Chewing helps.

"A guide to appropriate food intake is, 'I want to eat so that when I get up from the table, I feel so good that I could walk a few miles." - Gabriel Cousens

Chewing one's food at least 50 times per bite stimulates a tremendous amount of energy and builds the saliva, which, in itself, is an important thing. Chewing naturally leads to under-eating, because one actually focuses on the food and eats the appropriate amount, feeling fuller sooner.

FRED BISCI

I believe it plays a big role. When done correctly, a 100% raw, living food diet is inevitably a calorically restricted diet. I remember the hardest thing for me when I was transitioning to a raw food diet was going from being a big guy to being a very slim guy—but you can be strong on this type of diet, especially if you're young and you know how to train. Caloric restriction makes a tremendous difference. If you are training for the Ironman, you do not want to follow a caloric restricted diet. But, I have seen many people eat small amounts of food and do very well.

Dr. Luigi Fontana is a medical doctor with a PhD from Washington Medical School and a world-renowned specialist in caloric restriction. He's done all kinds of research and he actually did a study with raw foodists. He found that people who were on a raw living food diet, across the board, had the arterial system of a 14-year-old kid. There was no build-up of arterial plaque. There was nothing wrong with their arteries or their heart, but he did see some younger people that had osteoporosis. I think that the issue could certainly be avoided by adding some Super Green Food, E3Live and wheatgrass in the diet. There are 100% raw vitamins and minerals out there, like the Innate. They're fabulous. Personally I do not believe in the accuracy of the bone density test. In my sixties, I had a bad car accident and did not break a bone, although I suffered some serious injuries.

I knew a gentleman, years ago, who had a little farm in Staten Island and he grew all his own vegetables. This man was really, really remarkable. He was working at a very advanced age. He had some goats and he raised a few chickens. He did eat a small amount of animal protein, but basically, he lived on vegetables and figs. He had a lot of fig trees there. He did not eat a lot. He didn't have a sophisticated education, but he was a very intelligent man. He was very musically inclined. He was fabulous with the mandolin and I remember him playing for us. One thing that made an amazing impression on me was that, when he was 100 years old, he drove to Florida all by himself. He got tired of winters in New York. He had two daughters who lived in Florida, and my brother was married to one of them. He died at 104.

Another gentleman, I met in my neighborhood. I live in a very hilly part of Staten Island and I used to see him walking through the neighborhood on a regular basis. One day I was out working in my front yard and he said "good day" in Italian, and we started a conversation. I got the impression that he was a little bit lonely, because he kept coming back. He lived with his great-granddaughter and he wasn't happy there because she used to pick on him, so he'd go out walking early in the morning, and he would walk all day and talk to people until it got dark. Then he would go home and have something to eat, wait a while, and go to bed early. He was talking about history and the parts of Italy he came from, and then I started to get an idea of how old this man really was. I said to him "Luigi, how old are you?" He says "*Cento quattro*," which, in Italian, is 104.

I was stunned. I dropped my rake on the lawn and just started talking to this guy. I asked him what he ate and he said, in Italian, "*Io non piace mangiare,*" which means, "I do not like to eat." He had this huge head of gray hair and he had all his teeth. I said, "Luigi, you've got beautiful teeth." He said, "Yeah." I asked him, did he brush his teeth? He said no. He said he cleaned his teeth with his fingers. I asked, "What do you eat?" He said "*Verdura, salata,*" which is—and also cooked vegetables, soup (*zuppa*), and "*Un piccolo bicchiere di vino,*" which is "a little glass of wine." I said "Luigi, how about meat? Do you eat meat?" He said "*Io non piace carne.*" He did not like meat. Sometimes he would eat beans, fagioli he'd call them. He said he really wasn't a pasta guy. He liked chestnuts and he liked nuts. That was it. I asked him the big question. "Luigi, how many times a day do you eat?" He said "*Uno*" which is "one." If anybody was on a calorically restricted diet, it was my friend, Luigi.

I've seen other people like this. My own mother lived to be 101. I put her on a vegan diet when she was in her 80s. She had a stroke and she lived to be 101. Her girlfriend, Valeria Barbera, lived to be 104. She ate like a bird. I don't think she weighed 100 pounds. I used to think she was starving when we were children because she hardly ate. I said, "Mama, what's wrong with Valeria? She hardly ever eats." She said, "Don't worry, Freddy, she knows what she's doing." It turns out that what she said was true.

I do not believe in the reductionist mentality that the food giants and nutraceutical and supplement businesses are creating. A plant-based, whole food lifestyle with small amounts of other freshly prepared foods is the best way to go. I am not dogmatic because of this. I believe the 100% raw diet is working well for me. My future will tell that story. I am well aware of that.

CLEANSING/DETOX/FASTING

"Fasting is a very essential feature of youthing, healing and life extension." - Viktoras Kulvinskas

*"Fasting is one of the most healing, beneficial processes we have. It has stood the test of time over thousands of years. It is one of the best ways to detoxify and rejuvenate the body."
- Gabriel Cousens*

"Eating a good diet, exercising, taking saunas and baths, getting body work, massage—all of this helps you cleanse the body, and rapidly." - Brian Clement

"There are many different ways to cleanse the body, but the most important way is to leave out all the things that intoxicate your body." - Fred Bisci

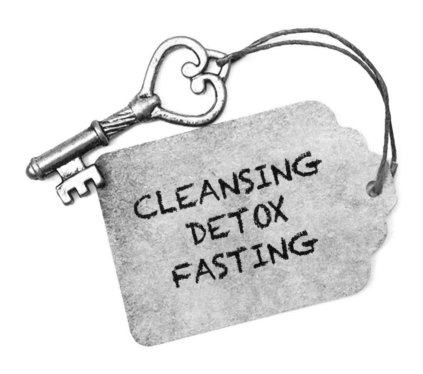

46. WHAT'S A HEALING CRISIS AND WHAT CAN I DO ABOUT IT?

BRIAN CLEMENT

Now, here's where we must be cautious. If you know that they have a serious disease and you're with an inexperienced person who purports to be an authority or an expert, they can easily mistake a detoxification - headaches, nausea, etc., with a real problem. Make sure that you're with somebody like an Elder in an institutional setting with extensive experience. Our medical team can differentiate between a crisis, and a healing and detoxification process.

What you also have to know is that the body will go through hell. You're paying for your sins of cumulative waste collecting. It's sort of like a house that you haven't cleaned in five years. Oh, my God, I'd hate to have to go into that house and clean it after five years; you'd have much greater problems than if you cleaned it on a daily basis. It's a very practical thing, but make sure you are not just doing this on your own, reading a book and having cheerleaders at your side. Do it under the auspices and realms of an institution such as Hippocrates.

VIKTORAS KULVINSKAS

A healing crisis is one or more symptoms associated with either improvement of lifestyle habits with the resulting increase of energy, or with having strong vitality, especially when you are still young and yet you have been backsliding for a duration of time, resulting in threatening the homeostasis of your body. Thus, it initiates a healing crisis. The symptoms can be a mild headache, diarrhea, increase in temperature, sweating, rashes or breakouts on the skin, continuous mucus discharge through the nasal passages or coughing it up. It might be exaggerated ongoing morning discharge of waste through the tear ducts.

What can you do about it? Go into cleansing mode. Go on a liquid program, herbal teas, warm water, as well as diluted veggie juices. Also recommended—mild herbal laxatives, enemas, colonics, taking a sauna or soaking in a tub of warm water with 3 pounds of salt, resting more, or just lying down, taking enzymes every hour or two. The symptoms usually don't last too long, though it could go on for days. What is important to know is that you are getting healthier and better, and more toxin free. It will be gone in most situations in three to five days.

GABRIEL COUSENS

A healing crisis occurs when more toxins are released from the body than the body has the ability to detoxify through normal channels. We can control the rate of detoxification. There is variation in detox physiology. Some people can fast, but they don't necessarily feel any detox symptoms. Other people go on fruits and vegetables and feel a variety of detox symptoms. We have genetic variation in how well we are able to detox. Ideally we can minimize detoxification and not push our bodies into detoxing faster than they can handle it.

I, personally, have worked out a variety of methods that seem to help. One of these is the use of high intensity proteolytic enzymes. They dissolve the amount of protein gunk in the basement membrane. As babies, we have big holes in our basement membranes, which separate our capillaries from our cells. On these basement membranes, food can go in, toxins can easily come out. With age, these holes get clogged up, and we aren't able to move toxins out of the body as easily. These high intensity proteolytic enzymes dissolve this excess protein residue in the system and allow an easier detox. When I measured it electronically, there was literally a 400% improvement in people's ability to detox, without going into healing crisis, with the use of proteolytic enzymes.

At our fasting retreats we support all avenues of detox. These include: 1) a colonic or an enema every day during the fast; 2) skin brushing (skin is the third kidney); 3) certain herbs and Bach flower remedies, which improve the ability of the kidneys and liver to detox; 4) flower essence and general essence elixir remedies to help us take energies into our system; 5) tongue scraping; 6) pranayama breathing exercise to blow out the excess CO_2 from the lungs; 7) mild exercise; 8) nude sunbathing, which gives the body a chance to outgas because there's a lot of toxins coming out of system that emerge as gases; 9) lymphatic massage; and 10) yoga. We do the Tri-Yoga, which is a flowing form of yoga that squeezes and presses the tissue to release toxins into the system and supports the lymph and blood flow. Those are the areas, again: lymph, blood flow, liver function, kidney function, skin function, bowel function, lung function, and also we use the tongue scraping to take the toxins coming off the tongue, as well as breathing exercises. These are all the avenues we support to maximize our ability to detox. With this total approach on the physical plane, we minimize the physical detox processes.

FRED BISCI

A healing crisis is when your body is going into a remedial process. When your body has the vital force to undo an unhealthy condition, you're going to experience some symptoms of discomfort as your body heals. There's a big difference between a healing crisis, during which a person is getting better, and a chronic ailment. When somebody has a chronic or an acute disease, the symptoms may seem almost the same as those of a healing crisis, but in this case the person is actually deteriorating; they're slipping into a more serious situation. A healing crisis, on the other hand, is when somebody has the chance to get ahead of the curve and go into a planned detox, to accelerate the cleansing so that their body can heal more rapidly.

It's extremely important that, if you're in a healing crisis, you get professional guidance and of course, rest is extremely important. I believe that rest is the ultimate healer. When you're resting, your body goes into an anabolic stage. It is replacing diseased or worn out cells to remedy whatever situation you have. Fasting, juice fasting, cleansing the lymphatic system and the GI tract, colonics, enemas, massage and oxygen therapy are all useful.

47. SHOULD I DETOX/CLENSE MY LIVER, GALLBLADDER OR KIDNEYS?

BRIAN CLEMENT

Well, there are many popular kidney and liver formulas, and we have to be cautious. There are some people with cirrhosis of the liver, hepatitis C, liver cancer, gallbladder problems, similar kidney problems, as well as other conditions, who should not go and do some abrupt natural method to cleanse themselves. This could actually create everything from kidney failure to breakdown of the liver and/or gallbladder. Again, people should do this under the auspices of a trained healthcare professional, a physician, an institution. I think that you systematically have to use some common sense in all of this detoxing.

I know, although many people are trained consumers, they should still make sure that whoever is guiding them knows what they are doing and has the experience. As I've often said, as we get older and deeper into the work that we do passionately, we've made enough mistakes in our early days to know now how to guide you. None of us really become brilliant somewhere along the way. The last time we were brilliant is at conception and birth. We Elders are seriously in love with the work we do. We've learned what works and what doesn't work from mistakes made early on. So, be in the hands of somebody who's mature, professional, secure and historically endowed with a lot of knowledge and a lot of experience.

VIKTORAS KULVINSKAS

Whenever you improve your lifestyle, you are cleansing the whole body. Your body is continuously regenerating all of its cells. The skin regenerates every 30 days, your mouth tissue regenerates every 3-6 days, your whole body is regenerated within a matter of 7 years, depending on the amount of cleansing and quality of lifestyle, hence cleansing of any single organ is not exactly doable. You cleanse the whole body. The body is a self-cleansing, self-rejuvenating organism.

We can accelerate the process with some herbal or enzyme choices, as well as certain lifestyle choices. For example, milk thistle, burdock root, dandelion leaf will all be helpful for detox of the liver, as well as other organs. All of the body's systems will benefit by systemic and regular enzyme usage for cleaning out incompletely metabolized protein, starches, and fats. For cleansing and detoxification of the kidney, plenty of liquid and herbal teas of nettle, uva ursi and diuretics like dandelion tea and parsley tea can be employed. Since cleansing also means cellular renewal, you will want to include a little bit of sea salt for the full spectrum of minerals, which will optimize the genetic materials of rebuilding cells. Take blue-green algae or the juice of sea veggies.

For a gallbladder flush, you can do a 3-5 day program of eating green apples with some garlic and drinking of plenty water throughout the day, as well as some green juices, especially made up of celery, cucumber, dandelion and kale. On the 4th, 5th or 6th day, drink liquids in the morning, then, in the afternoon, make a concoction of 3-4 cloves of garlic, a tablespoon of fresh ginger, half a teaspoon of cayenne, half a cup of cold pressed olive oil and a mixture of orange, lemon and grapefruit juice (predominately lemon) and half a teaspoon of salt. Drink that, and then 4 hours later, eat half a grapefruit and lie down on your left side. By evening, you will have a strong urge to evacuate. The following day, take green juices and green salads, and from then on, keep up with quality lifestyle practices. During this cleanse, it would be good to do some chi-gong liver exercises, which would involve putting your left hand on your liver area with your right hand over your left, and imagining that there is a clock on your body, move your hands in a clockwise direction 50 times, stroking up from the genital region to your head. Do this 2-3 times a day. When you are cleansing the kidneys do the same thing, except your hands are on your kidney area on the back and go counter-clockwise 50 times and stroke downwards instead of up. The gallbladder cleanse would be the same as the liver. This will increase your overall chi.

You will also benefit from doing reflexology on the liver, kidney and gallbladder spots on the soles of your feet and palms of your hands. For general toning massage your ears—rub, pull, twist—this will increase chi. And, of course, pray, meditate and ask for cosmic guidance to have the best of all possible experiences. Enemas are strongly suggested in order to eliminate waste ASAP and for preventing wastes from absorbing. Also suggested are saunas and plenty of rest. When you feel vital, exercise, and then rest again.

GABRIEL COUSENS

My advice on the liver gallbladder cleanses, which I do recommend, is to do it gradually, and not more than four times a year. When there are no more gallbladder stones coming out, then one really doesn't need to do very many continual gallbladder liver cleanses. People tend to overdo these cleanses and create minor stress on the liver. The kidney cleanses do really well with fasting, and these include the proteolytic enzymes which clean all levels of the kidney system.

FRED BISCI

I think a detox or cleanse should be under the care of a physician or some kind of a healthcare professional. Cleansing can be very beneficial, but it should be conducted in conjunction with colonics. Liver, gallbladder and kidney cleanses, done with supervision all can be very helpful.

48. IS THERE A TIME TO DO COLONICS AND IS THERE A TIME WHEN I SHOULD NOT? IS IT DANGEROUS IF YOU ARE VERY ILL?

BRIAN CLEMENT

Although everyone at Hippocrates gets at least one colonic as part of the program—we are big advocates of colonics to help cleanse out the waste so you don't go through as much pain, suffering, septicemia, toxic blood, etc., we give colonics—there are certain people who should not have colonics, for example, people who have had recent surgical procedures on the intestinal tracts. Certain impacts, certain tumor masses, already perforation or history of septicemia, you have to know the medical history of these people. A professional, well-experienced and licensed colonic therapist would be asking you all of these questions about your health.

In the early stages, it's like deconstructing a building that's been built poorly and is broken down, and then reconstructing a building, but again, this must be done in the hands of a health professional. Every time that you do an enema or a colonic, you follow it up with fresh juice and a wheatgrass implant. We have thousands and thousands of blood tests to show you the electrolytes improve when you do that, but I'll also show you that if you do a colonic or do an enema and do not follow it up with wheatgrass infusions, in many cases (not 100%), you can lose the electrolytes which are the batteries for your cells. You don't want to lose it.

The other thing I want to point out is that the goal is not for you to do colonics and enemas and implants of wheatgrass your whole life. The bottom line is that you're supposed to get to the point where you don't need these things. That you're living such a clean and healthy lifestyle, exercising, breathing fresh air, and drinking pure water, that you really don't need them.

VIKTORAS KULVINSKAS

I personally, have had a very limited background in the use of colonics. During the early years, over 45 years ago, even though the cost was only $5.00, it was $5.00 that I rarely had. Primarily, I relied on enemas. With an enema, you can do a very good job on cleaning the internal system while relying on your own feedback mechanism; that is, levels of discomfort, and whether you should be doing it or not. The pressure is very gentle and it will require at least a minimum of an hour to do a thorough enema. Utilizing approximately 4 to 5 quarts during this phase of cleansing, where the colon has been totally emptied. It involves some self-massage of the colon region. Colonics is an art and a skill and the amount of fluid that is taken in is both larger in volume, and creates more pressure internally, than an enema.

Listen, contraindications really means an indication or symptoms that make the execution of colonics inadvisable and so, absolute contraindications prohibit treatment of any particular disease. For example, colon hydrotherapy is absolutely contraindicated for patients with pronounced rectal bleeding. Those contraindications involve a risk benefit relationship. In the case of colon cancer, colon hydrotherapy's ability to eliminate poison toxins is evaluated against possibly making an already compromised colon wall weaker.

Following is a list of absolute contraindications for colon therapy. If you have any of these, colon hydrotherapy is not advised. Once these conditions have been eliminated, colon therapy maybe indicated.

Abortion less than 6 months, anal fissures or fistula, severe anemia, aneurysm, cirrhosis, colon cancer, colon surgery less than 6 months postoperative, tumor in the rectum or large intestine, colostomy, epilepsy, GI hemorrhage or perforation, heart disease, severe hypertension, severe hemorrhoids—minimum bleeding is okay—hernia, abdominal or inguinal, history of epileptic seizures, kidney dialysis, miscarriage less than 6 months, pregnancy up to 4 months, recent heart attack, rectal bleeding besides minor hemorrhoids, renal insufficiency and ulcerative colitis active or bleeding.

The following list is relative contraindications for colon therapy and usually a physician's prescription is necessary for somebody to get sessions of colon therapy.

Crohns disease, acute colitis, severe diverticulosis, acute diverticulosis, colon cancer, or colon surgery.

Something to remember is that insurance usually does not cover colon hydrotherapy treatments, even though I believe there are some companies now that are becoming conscious enough to take that into consideration. So, for anybody with a healthy colon, healthy digestion and desire to cleanse, colon therapy is usually done in sessions of 3 or 6, or even up to 20 sessions, depending on your needs. Then of course, one of the biggest problems that people ask about is washing out all the friendly bacteria in the colon. I don't believe that most people have any bacteria in their body anymore because of all the inorganic food that has been eaten and a lot of antibiotics that have been consumed. It is very difficult for healthy bacteria to live in a garbage can. Most people who eat the modern diet that is prevalent here in the United States, and in most of the world, probably don't have the kind of environment that is necessary in order to have a healthy bacterial content. What is required for healthy bacteria culture is fiber, especially green fiber.

There are a few other things that you might want to consider as well. People say that colonics can be addicting. I've never met anybody in my 40 years of practice who has ever been addicted to colonics. It's not the most pleasant treatment to receive. One of the things colonics do is, they help the body to relieve the toxic conditions that accumulate in the tissues and the cells of the body. A lot of the body will vibrate into a different frequency because there's less resistance, there's less toxic build-up and so, somebody wants to do some cleansing in order to change their lifestyle, their vehicle is colon therapy. It's advisable that you get an examination beforehand and see what kind of condition your colon is in. Or if you're a person who's pretty healthy, and you haven't had any acute kind of colitis or diverticulitis, or any of those types of diseases, I would be willing to say that you could receive a gentle cleansing of the colon.

If you're on a three week program at the Hippocrates Institute, you receive it three times. We also heavily promote detox through sweat, so we'll have you do a sauna. In the seven-day program, you may receive it five times. Some people may want more. In the twenty-one day program, you're probably going to get around twelve or thirteen in that period of time. Along with the herbs, and the juices, and the other things, watching the liver, testing the alkaline count, appealing to the body to see how much more alkalinity is coming in. There are a number of things we take into consideration. We also have three or four different kinds of waters, as well as making sure the metabolism is comfortable, to determine exactly how many colonics you're going to have to have.

What do people experience?

There are many stories. The stories that you always remember the most are about the people who have been having chronic constipation for years and they have a tremendous build up. The best stories are the ones about people that have had chronic colitis, chronic diverticulosis, chronic constipation, and their bodies start to eliminate that impacted cecum tar and gummed up mucous from dairy products and white flour. They relieve that stuff and experience a change immediately, because the fact is you're taking out resistance. Once that resistance is removed they celebrate their life again, in a way.

I decided to answer this question by referring to my long time friend of 35 years, who has been a colonic irrigationist, naturopath, and also went through nurse training. He has served a wide variety of people, like the President of Costa Rica, some of the Victoria's Secret's models, the less famous, as well as those who were considered the upper echelon of both the commercial and the celebrity world.

Theodore has operated spas in Hawaii as well as Mexico and many of the USA mainland states. During the last five years, he has been my neighbor in Costa Rica operating the Instituta Otrez. He can be reached via email at dharma250@yahoo.com.

A good follow up to colonic irrigation is retention enema wheatgrass and/or probiotics. Also, oral penetration probiotics.

GABRIEL COUSENS

Colonics and enemas are all part of the detox strategy. They support the overall detoxification flow. During a fast, I may even ask people to do two or three enemas in a day if they're suffering a detox symptom. If people are too weak, a gentle colonic can be very helpful for getting toxins out of the system. Generally speaking, because of protecting the overall *apana*, or downward flow, I don't recommend enemas outside of when one is doing a water or juice fast, because they're helpful in removing the toxins at that time and decreasing the healing crisis. For weak bowels and for serious constipation, I may recommend a series of colonics to get the bowel system working. I usually recommend a monthly colonic. Colonics provide stimulation to the smooth muscles of the colon that actually improves one's ability to have downward flowing energy and so may help with constipation. I recommend an enema or colonic at least daily when you're doing any serious detox protocol, particularly water or juice fasting.

FRED BISCI

Some people are so debilitated that they don't have the strength to sustain a colonic. Once again, everybody's an individual and should be guided by a professional. But most people that are reasonably healthy, under the care of a good colon hydrotherapist, should not have any kind of problems.

I've never seen anything that was really detrimental happen to anybody that had a colonic. Get advice from a professional if you have any doubt about what you're doing there. Make sure you're in the hands of a good colon hydrotherapist. Most of them are very knowledgeable and they can advise you about nutrition as well. Most of them are very honest and you can get good advice.

49. IS FASTING BENEFICIAL? WHAT TYPE OF FAST IS BEST? IS LONG TERM FASTING DANGEROUS?

BRIAN CLEMENT

Well, at Hippocrates, we fast on green juice one day a week. Decades ago, I was a big advocate of water fasting. I myself had done a 56-day water fast in Europe, as well as here in North America. At Hippocrates, I've fasted with hundreds of thousands of people, and had the opportunity to direct for one year the original living food center created by Dr. Kristine Nolfi, Humlegarden. This was in the mid-1970s, and what I found was that healthy people were fasting there. Now, my experience to that date was that, here in the United States, only very, very, very sick people, and a handful of very open-minded people, came to the Institute. My observation was, I didn't know what was happening with these people because most of them were so sick to begin with.

It was difficult, at that early stage of my career, to differentiate what was affecting them poorly or well, and putting healthy people on a water fast, I started to see a whole lot of disruption and concerns. I started to delve into it in the 1970s, and found out that most of the Western population, statistically, is more malnourished than per capita in third world countries. So, why take away all nutrients?

The other thing is that this whole idea of pain and suffering being good is strange. We have to suffer when we're fasting? Put that out the window. That comes from your religious fervor from which modern day fasting came; it came out of the nunnery and the monks, and suffering for your sins, and so water fasting fits right into that category. Now I know that, physically, you'll gain much more benefit by doing green juice fasting. Fresh green leafy vegetables, sprouts that have nutrients, that have proteins, that stabilize blood sugars—so you're not feeling like you're starving and swinging back and forth is the way to go. Remember, 6 out of 10 of us have blood sugar concerns—either we're low blood sugar, high blood sugar or close to it—and we want to stabilize the blood sugar. We also know that in fresh raw green juice we're actually getting a lot of peroxide benefits, a lot of sun energy, enzymatic benefits that emulsify and get rid of a lot of the waste. You get more waste out of the body by doing green juices, and without the big swing in emotional drama and feeling like you're starving that you get with water fasts. We're big advocates of green juice fasting, for the majority of people, one day a week. Are there exceptions?

Of course, people who have an emotional food eating disorder, people who are very toxic, people who have, in fact, become emaciated to the point where they need constant ongoing nourishment and sustenance, so that they can rebuild their system. You have to look at this individually. I, myself, for 40 years have fasted one to two days a week, consistently. I don't miss food anymore. No matter where I am in the world, I do fasting on juices and of course, pure water. Now, you may want to put organic, ripe lemon juice into the water. That helps, but it is not necessary. Those who are still into the taste area, you may want to put in a little Stevia to make it taste like lemonade, so you feel like you're okay during that period of time. I also have learned over the years, because I travel extensively, that when I'm on long air trips, I do not eat. I go on a fast because it's harder on airplanes to get good hydration. I drink a lot of juice and water before I get on the plane and then again as soon as I get off the plane. Even when not fasting, we dehydrate enormously on a plane.

That should be a practice that everyone undertakes. It's great on long trips, more than three hours or so. Try not to eat that day; make that your fast day versus the typical fast day. At Hippocrates, it's Wednesday. It could be Saturday for you. It could be Sunday. Whatever day is best and easiest for you, but get into that. I learned that from a great health advocate, Paul Bragg, one of my mentors back when I began this work.

VIKTORAS KULVINSKAS

Fasting is a very essential feature of youthing, healing and life extension. If you are interested in long, healthy quality of life, you will think in terms of fasting, at least several times a year, for a duration of one week or more. It's even more so advisable to fast one day a week. As an example of a weekend fast, starting at noon on Friday, have nothing but juices the rest of the day, stay on juices the following day, that would be Saturday, and on Sunday stay on juices in the morning, then break the fast with a noon meal. A different way of fasting is to have the last meal of the day at 5-6 pm, then abstaining from food for the rest of the evening and through the night,

"If you are interested in long, health quality life, you will think in terms of fasting."
- Viktoras Kulvinskas

just drinking liquids like warm water and herbal teas, and then extending it in the morning, drinking again lots of warm water with a little sea salt and cayenne, followed by wheatgrass juice, then green juices, not eating until 12. This is a very good form of personal lifestyle practice. That is, liquids only one day a week, and then also reducing your meal plan to two meals per day, noon and evening.

If you are a business or corporate individual, it would be best to stay on liquids all day, protein green smoothies and green juices. Have two thermos bottles that you take to work and drink from one, then a couple of hours later, drink from the other. In this way, you will maintain the highest level of proficiency, concentration, focus and productivity. When you get home in the evening, you will have your munching, with either a protein or starch oriented meal.

During the fasting, as well as in every day life, to regenerate the adrenals and other internal organs, you should be very sensitive to your body's signals. If your are starting to yawn, or feeling tired, you should not put it off for minutes or hours; immediately lie down on a couch or a bed or the ground, and rest for a while. Otherwise adrenaline will kick in, giving you booster shots of energy—the second wind. Having at least catnaps during the day, even when you are not motivated, will help to reconstitute the spinal energy and nerve regeneration. At least every other day, at bedtime, take a fiber product with a mild herbal laxative that includes cascara sagrata,

You could gain extra benefits by doing occasional enemas, soaking for many hours in a bathtub with 3 pounds of kosher salt, then taking a shower and resting. Above all, keep the mind quiet through prayers, confirmations, meditation, qigong, pranayama and or tapping.

How long should you fast? As long as you don't lose more than 15% of what is recommended for you according to your body, weight and height. For example, someone who is 6 feet tall, with strong bones and body mass at 170 lbs, wouldn't want to lose more than 30 lbs of body mass. You will find that when you consume predigested liquid superfoods, such as blue-green algae and all the greens and microbial cultures, juices from sauerkraut and kimchi, the bacteria will be manufacturing an average 10 to 30g of protein on a daily basis, as well as making tons of enzymes and creating the B complex. And if you're getting sunlight, you're going to get calories. Your skin is a solar battery and the more you consume greens, the higher your red cell count, the less you will be dependent on what is called a traditional nutritional program and calories.

Detoxification and cleansing is a wonderful time to connect with the creator, the source of us all, by concentrating, meditating, doing focus and consciousness work. You will not only connect to the source, you will become a sorcerer, creating abundance and all the resources you want in your life. Believe in it, have no doubts. Fasting is one of the most powerful tools you have. Love yourself.

GABRIEL COUSENS

Fasting is one of the most healing, beneficial processes we have. It has stood the test of time over thousands of years. It is one of the best ways to detoxify and rejuvenate the body. I recommend fasting for at least seven days at a time, twice a year. I do not recommend long term fasting, unless one really has some particular chronic disease where fasting may help. I don't recommend fasting if you're 20 pounds underweight.

"Twice a year, one-week fasting particularly clears the bowel toxins which are lodged throughout the whole body." - Gabriel Cousens

I have some hesitations if a person comes in with eating disorders and wishes to fast, because fasting can potentially aggravate eating disorders, but my experience is that it usually doesn't. The twice a year, one-week fasting particularly clears the bowel toxins which are lodged throughout the whole body. Research in 1917 by Satterlee and Eldridge with 517 people is helpful to appreciate fasting benefits. They did a bowel toxicity cleansing on these 517 people, and they had dramatic healing of a variety of mental diseases, paranoia, anxiety, neurosis, stupor, fear, and depression. Anthony Bassler's work in the 1930s with 5,000 people and found that fasting also helped many varieties of physical ailments, in addition to mental problems.

At the Tree of Life Center, we do a diluted green juice fast. I found that people on water fasts tend to get mineral depleted and often have heart palpitations. Eighty percent of people I've seen clinically are mineral deficient, which usually means they need supplementation with liquid magnesium during their fast. People fasting on water don't have energy to participate in meditation, yoga, or walking, and their sense of wellbeing is often depleted. I favor a 50% diluted green juice fast as the most effective. I find that it gives the advantage of maximally pulling out toxins, while minimizing the common problems of water fasting. Because of environmental toxicity, almost everybody benefits from a one-week fast twice each year for general upkeep of the body, emotions, mind, and spirit. Fasting not only detoxifies, but also activates the vital life force, which is the primary healing power. The fasts I lead at the Tree of Life Center, in the U.S. and Israel, are spiritual fasts, which emphasize healing on the physical, mental, emotional, and spiritual levels. They are organized to help people access their sacred design and to connect more deeply with their souls. Spiritual fasting is designed to help people awaken their spiritualizing force called the "kundalini", which happens in about 90% of the participants over the course of any given spiritual fast.

FRED BISCI

That's a controversial question. Years ago, water fasting was the big thing. Natural hygienists thought the only true fast was a water fast. A true fast, technically, is when you are abstaining from everything but water. From a practical point of view, that is not true. The thing about fasting is, when you leave out everything but water, you're not getting any nourishment, and though it does have benefits, it also has risks, especially if you're doing it on your own or you're under the care of somebody that is not a good fasting supervisor. I've seen a few disasters from people who were on a fast.

From my own personal experience in water fasting, I've seen what the benefits can be, but it can also be dangerous without the proper supervision. I recommend fasting under supervision, and I no longer recommend long water fasts. I like the way Doctor Bernard Zablac in California recommended fasting: shut down, close your eyes and rest as much as you possibly can. Don't do anything. I did some of my fasts that way. You're actually meditating while you're on your fast and you are just getting up to drink water and staying down as much as you can, maybe just stretching out a little bit. They were the best fasts I ever had.

John Taub, who was an old time natural hygienist, had cancer, and he would only recommend for a person to do one long water fast. He said that after that, you could really have trouble. I agree with him. I know some people who did some repeated long water fasts and ran into a lot of trouble. I did some long water fasting also, but I didn't run into trouble because I knew what to do. I did it because I wanted to have a complete experience about fasting. I didn't just want to go by what I read in a book. If you want to go on a water fast, go to a fasting retreat and get supervision from somebody reputable who's been doing it for a long time. Check them out, make sure they've done a lot of good for people.

The big controversy is between water fasting or juice fasting, which is really a juice diet. I have seen fabulous results from juice fasting, with no risk to speak of and no supervision really needed. Juice fasting is the rage all over the country now. I haven't seen any real problems. I have literally seen thousands of people do juice fasting and have never seen a problem if done correctly.

50. WHAT IS THE BEST WAY TO CLEANSE THE BODY? HOW LONG SHOULD MY CLEANSE LAST?

VIKTORAS KULVINSKAS

We are continuously building up environmental, as well as metabolic, waste. Minimal would be one day a week, 36 to 48 hours, where you are staying on water, green juices and herbal teas. A good idea is to do it during the change of seasons. This would be for a week or longer. This would be a regimen for a healthy individual.

During the detox and healing process, the cleansing program that is recommended is raw food juices, and liquid programs of juices, followed up by rebuilding programs, followed up by cleansing once again for a month or two months and never losing more than 15% of your ideal weight. Repeat it until what is considered your cleansing program is also the same as your rebuilding program.

BRIAN CLEMENT

Eating a good diet, exercising, taking saunas and baths, getting body work, massage—all of this helps you cleanse the body, and rapidly. Saunas are a big part of that, infrared being the best. If you do things like steam baths, for example, that helps the lungs, that helps the bladder, it helps the kidneys. Body work, lymphatic drainage, neuromuscular work all take the acidity out, push the lymphatic fluid, and help the cleansing process of the body.

Exercise, everyone should be doing that. That's our natural way to detoxify most of our body. How long should you do it? Throughout your life. Should you become a mono-focused fanatic zealot on detoxification? Again, no, the objective is to go through this initial process, detoxify, get on a lifestyle that maintains exceptional health, and the body will be doing what it always has historically, up until the last several generations. It's going to be through work, exercise, relaxation, eating the proper food, eating organic food on a normal cycle biochemically, detoxification, elimination and rebuilding.

GABRIEL COUSENS

Again, it depends. Are you talking about a person who's generally healthy? Are you talking about a person who has deep chronic disease? We want to cleanse the body until the fundamental deep toxicity and chronic disease is significantly reversed. Usually, within a week, two weeks at the most, you will see if you're on the right track and are generally healthy. If, after a few weeks, you're not seeing any improvement, you may want to question whether the toxicity is the main source of the problem. My experience with fasting is that it's the best and safest way to cleanse the body. After the fast, about 90% of people with high blood pressure have a genetic and epigenetic reset, where they come off their blood pressure medications and don't need to go back on them. It's very helpful in type 2 diabetes, although I do not recommend it for type 1 diabetics because there are a lot of other physiological imbalances. I will only fast type 2 diabetics. Generally, the best way to cleanse the body is to do this whole spectrum that I've been mentioning, which is focusing on all aspects of the cleansing. One of the things that I didn't mention before is hot and cold showers. I suggest between three and seven cycles—being in a hot shower, then a real cold shower for a minute or so, then a real hot shower, real cold shower, alternating. That stimulates lymphatic cleansing. Bouncing on a small rebounder is very good for lymphatics as well. As I say, fasting is probably the best overall tested process, as well as repeated liver gallbladder cleanses.

FRED BISCI

The best way to cleanse your body is by leaving out all the processed food. That's a tremendous cleanse to start with. Then you can progress to fasting, as we just discussed. You can also go into juice dieting or into just eating fruits and vegetables for a while. You can also do colonics, enemas, or lymphatic massage.

There are many different ways to cleanse the body, but the most important way is to leave out all the things that intoxicate your body. Liver and gallbladder flushes should be done under supervision or at a retreat under professional guidance. The length of time for most of these things really depends on the individual—but leaving out all processed food should be a lifelong commitment for everybody who wants to live a long, healthy life. A whole book could be written about this. But I think this is pretty common knowledge within the raw food community.

51. WHAT IS THE DIFFERENCE BETWEEN WATER FASTING AND JUICE FASTING? WHICH ONE SHOULD YOU DO? AND SHOULD YOU HAVE COLONICS AT THE SAME TIME?

GABRIEL COUSENS

I recommend colonics or enemas every single day of any fast. The bowel toxins are a major part of the detox, and when you do a colonic or an enema, you're literally pulling toxins out of the bowel, which pulls the toxins out of the blood, which is cleaning the blood as it pulls the toxins out of the cells. This is the law of diffusion, which is very helpful in fasting. I've done 21-day water fasts and 40-day juice fasts. They all have their advantages. In the bigger picture, having fasted thousands of people since 1988, I find that 50% dilution of the juices is optimal for both detoxing and maintaining a sense of well being and mineralization. So, this is somewhere between a water fast and a juice fast; perhaps getting the best elements of both. With water fasts, which I generally don't recommend, I see so many people get exhausted, not have much fun, and worse, go into a variety of mineral deficiencies, particularly magnesium, which often leads to heart palpitations. I find that juice fasting with the 50% diluted juice is by far a safer and preferable way to do that. Again, I strongly recommend at least one colonic or one to two or three enemas each day of the fast.

BRIAN CLEMENT

Which one should you do? We're big advocates of juice fasting, not of water fasting. Should you have colonics at the same time? For a highly toxic person that's a candidate for fasting, we suggest colonics right after you break the fast, the morning after. Everything accumulates, the body does as much detoxification and elimination as it can and then at that point, you help it out by purging it with an enema and an implant of wheatgrass juice. We hold it in for 15 to 30 minutes. It absorbs, at some level, helping to coagulate the waste and microbes and pull that waste out of the body.

FRED BISCI

On a water fast, you're only drinking water and you're going to have a more profound detox. Juice fasting really isn't a true fast; it's more of a diet where everything is juiced. You're just drinking juices and leaving out all solid food. The juices are very alkalizing, so a lot of the endogenous material that's coming out of your system—and could otherwise cause a lot of discomfort—will be neutralized.

It's not a good idea to do colonics on a water fast. If you want to do enemas, you can, but if you do too many, you're squandering your energy. Sometimes, with water fasting, people do not move their bowels, so they build up a lot of vital force while they're fasting, and then afterward they could have a huge bowel movement.

"Do not do anything based on some philosophy or hearsay. Check it out before you try something new and make sure that you're being guided by somebody who has experience." – Fred Bisci

I had one girl on an 18-day water fast. She had fasted, the first time, for 12 days and she didn't go to the bathroom. Then, she went back to eating. She decided to do a second fast. She did 18 days and she had the most unusual bowel movement I've ever seen. It had to weigh at least 6 pounds and she had to break it up in the toilet bowl with a wooden stick. Enemas done in moderation with a water fast can prevent that sort of discomfort.

With juice dieting, it's not really risky unless a person is on a lot of medications. In NYC, there are a lot of juice bars showing people how to do 15-30 day juice cleanses and I haven't heard of anybody having any problems.

Remember, nothing is absolute and there's no panacea. Do your homework. Consult with experienced people before you do anything that could be a problem. Always err on the side of caution. That is critically important. Do not do anything based on some philosophy or hearsay. Check it out before you try something new and make sure that you're being guided by somebody who has experience.

VIKTORAS KULVINSKAS

Water fasting, you stay on water. Juice fasting, you stay on juices, green vegetable juices. The green juice program is going to be most beneficial for those on the S.A.D. diet or for individuals who have been on raw foods on a long-term basis. The reason for it is, when you are doing the green juice fast, you get enzymized, you get re-alkalinized and you get re-mineralized. On a water fast, you move into more depletion. We recommend a juice program, green juice. It should be practiced with any liquid program and certainly colonics would be beneficial, though not essential.

PREVENTING AND UNDERSTANDING DISEASES AND CONDITIONS

"Disease is chaos in the field. Health is order in the field."
- Gabriel Cousens

"Most people are kicked out of their body because of poor housekeeping, that is, accumulation of toxins, waste products and incompletely metabolized foods. They have become garbage cans. Eventually, life is not sustainable within such an environment."
- Viktoras Kulvinskas

"I'm a firm believer that just about all diseases begin in our bowels and our brain." - Fred Bisci

"Disease is disorder. It's pretty simple to think about it in this way. When you have order, you are healthy." - Brian Clement

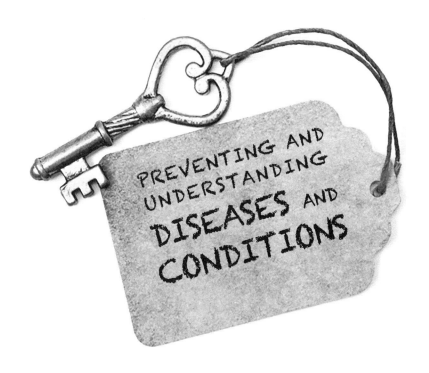

52. HOW WOULD YOU DEFINE DISEASE OR DIS-EASE?

BRIAN CLEMENT

Disease is disorder. It's pretty simple to think about it in this way. When you have order, you are healthy. The body is working in an orderly fashion—anatomically, chemically, psychologically and spiritually on the path and the rhythm of the universe. Everything is working the way that it ought to. Disorder or disease is an abnormality in one, or many, of these areas. Certainly, if we have a deep-seated abnormality, it affects the physical, the spiritual, the emotional, and the psychological state, and vice versa. The psychological affects the biological state.

VIKTORAS KULVINSKAS

Disease is lack of ease, needing to reach out for comfort foods and having an addictive, behavioral life style. It means that you have accumulated blockage in the physical, mental and emotional plane. Your homeostasis, a place of balance, is off-kilter. You are retaining waste products in a physical plane. You are out of the state of love and peace in the emotional and mental plane.

GABRIEL COUSENS

Disease is chaos in the field. Health is order in the field.

FRED BISCI

Disease is when the body is not functioning under normal healthy conditions and a person starts to feel ill at ease. Disease is very common today in the average person and they're taking medication to palliate some of the obvious symptoms. Because they're not addressing the cause of the problems, their diseases progress to become chronic and acute, and often terminal. The early stage of disease is really your body trying to give you a warning that something is not functioning properly. Unfortunately, many people wait until the symptoms are really debilitating.

A lot of people start to have joint pain and in most cases it's coming from eating a terrible diet that's acid forming. That causes stress and inflammation, and eventually wears out their joints. That's a state of disease—but when they're taking medications and painkillers, they're not dealing with the underlying inflammation. They end up getting knee, shoulder, hip replacements—or developing other, more serious conditions.

People were forewarned about all these different problems by their body. But, it's being ignored because most doctors just treat the symptoms, and the underlying cause is ignored until a person has to get surgery or some kind of major medical intervention.

53. THERE ARE DIFFERENT STAGES OF DISEASE. IS THIS A ONE-SIZE-FITS-ALL PROTOCOL? OR DO YOU SUGGEST A TAILORED PROGRAM DEPENDING ON THE SEVERITY OF THE DISEASE?

BRIAN CLEMENT

Well, we certainly are known and renowned internationally for tailoring and personalizing programs via our medical team at Hippocrates, and the different bio frequency testing and research that we do helps to personalize the guidance. We use state of the art technologies to deeply understand what's going on in an individual; not to predict or diagnose, but to see the lay of the land, see the large picture, and, this way, we can individualize and tweak things and change things. Remember, what we tell you today may not apply 6 months, a year, 2 years, and 10 years down the road. It will not, if you keep on your path of getting healthy. There are things that you will not need to do anymore and things that you may want to do at that point to even accelerate that enrichment and strengthening process.

VIKTORAS KULVINSKAS

We cover this in great detail in *Survival in the 21st Century*. Most individuals are out of control and would benefit from an instructive, well-researched, informative environment, where they can be supported and guided in their transition into a healthier lifestyle through a holistic approach. Usually when a condition has gone chronic or even acute, being in the presence of a place like Hippocrates Health Institute, which supports overall recovery, is the best thing.

Most people can handle the transition and lifestyle improvements on their own, as well as learning from books, DVDs and other informed individuals. Continued experimentation with one's body will lead to continuous improvement.

The idea is to overcome malnutrition, to begin re-enzymizing, re-mineralizing, re-alkalizing, re-oxygenating your system, while at the same time removing the toxins from the body through all of the cleansing techniques that are available. It is going to be a long-term process. You will learn from many different teachers. In the long run, your biggest instructor will be meditation, contemplation and observing your body as it goes through the changes.

GABRIEL COUSENS

There are different stages of disease. The more chronically ill a person is, the slower and more careful one has to be in detoxing. The stage of disease must be assessed carefully, because if an individual starts to detox too quickly, they can have a healing crisis and move into serious life-threatening difficulty. We have to be very careful and thoughtful about how fast we detox somebody. I do not fast type 1 diabetics. I just do mild detoxing. Again, the severity of the disease is important. People coming in with chronic fatigue or fibromyalgia often do exceptionally well on a fast. I've seen a great many people with fibromyalgia clear up on a fast because it is so related to toxins that are embedded in the tissues.

FRED BISCI

There are two major states of disease. There's acute disease and there's chronic disease. Acute disease is life threatening. People need surgery or they fall into some other medical protocol that's probably not going to help them in the long run. With chronic disease, there's a great variation in the stages of disease.

As I stated previously, some people get minor pain or they're having headaches or constipation. These are all stages of disease that most people ignore. I see people in my practice who tell me that they haven't moved their bowels in two weeks and were told by their physician that it was normal. I can't understand how a doctor could tell a person that. It's not like putting money in the bank; saving up waste material in your system definitely doesn't make you better off. That's actually the precursor to most disease.

Most people who walk into my office are not prepared for what I'm going to tell them. They're not ready to go into a raw diet or to give up processed food. I used to try to help everybody, but I don't do that anymore because I don't want to take somebody's money if I know they're not going to help themselves. If somebody's not ready to give up the processed food and they're very sick, I politely tell them I'm not really the person for them.

My personal belief from my experience is that all chronic disease is remedied by lifestyle change.

54. WHY DOES OUR BODY GET CANCER OR OTHER DISEASE?

VIKTORAS KULVINSKAS

Other diseases are signs that you are not living according to the laws of nature. The human body is divinely made and heals itself and never loses it to degenerative conditions. Due to faulty lifestyles, it eventually wears out and dies.

Most people are kicked out of their body because of poor housekeeping, that is, accumulation of toxins, waste products and incompletely metabolized foods. They have become garbage cans. Eventually, life is not sustainable within such an environment. There are those who have ascended to perfect lifestyles and they, too, leave this body, but they leave it by their own personal choice. They have finished this incarnation. Cancer is the result of unresolved emotional lifestyle behavior, usually associated with anger. You keep reaching for comfort food. They are all enzyme-less and dead. Dr. Max Gerson showed that all forms of cancer are preceded by pancreatic insufficiency in producing the protease enzymes.

"Other diseases are signs that you are not living according to the laws of nature." - Viktoras Kulvinskas

In the Science section of the May 23, 2002 issue of the *New York Times,* a study from Harvard Medical School showed that all forms of cancer are due to the consumption of enzyme depleted proteins, which leads to inflammatory conditions, which interfere with oxygen transport and normal reproductive cancer. Cells mutate to cancer cells and they act like vacuum cleaners, sucking up circulatory protein and putting our system out of circulation, so that normal oxygen transport can be continued. This procedure can go on indefinitely, for five, 10 or 20 years before the volume of malignant cancer cells and tumors interfere with the normal metabolic process. You have increased the garbage having effects beyond your ability to sustain and maintain life.

The medical procedures do not offer any hope. They, as a matter of fact, shorten your life. The true answer is to return to natural laws and regenerate your enzyme reserves, and you will find that you can eventually recover from cancer and every degenerative disease. Cleansing and detoxification, upgrading your lifestyle habits through improved positivity, settling your emotional storms, the process of forgiveness, living in the eternal now, all these are a part of the procedures, in conjunction with good dietary habits, adequate exercise, rest and living in a clean environment.

BRIAN CLEMENT

Well, cancer is a disease in which your immune system has allowed a mutagenic cell to occur. A very figurative way I can describe it is, all healthy cells move in a clockwise manner. If you put Mozart concertos on and watch this, we have microscopically felt they all move to the rhythm of Mozart's beautiful music. If you look at a cancer cell, it's like putting on hard rock music—the cell is radically moving in the opposite direction and coagulating. It's called antigenic. What's interesting is, the cell of cancer goes out and searches for stem cells, little baby, innocent cells. Stem cells come out and say, "Oh, what should I become? Should I become a liver or a kidney?" And the big spider-like cancer cell, with its long legs, tentacles, the antigenic effect, comes out and seduces the little innocent stem cell that comes up the tentacle and swims in the opposite direction becoming part of the tumor mass or the leukemia, whatever the abnormality is with cancer.

It all is happening because the immune system, the white blood cells and the eosinophils, neutrophils, granulocytes, lymphocytes—the armed services that you have—are not strong because you have not been thinking right, eating right, exercising right, environmental degradation has occurred. All of these things allow that army to sit back, and now these mutagenic disorders like cancer, and microbial like viruses, bacteria, molds or fungus or yeast come into the body. All of these nemesis can be fought by the immune system, or not, if the immune system is sluggish, weak and not functional at that point. That's how you get cancer and other diseases.

The major cause of cancer today, noxious absorption, similar to Autism, Alzheimer's disease, MS, Parkinson's disease, and ALS—is the toxemia factor. Those heavy metal and chemical toxins, have a lot to do with the diseases I've just mentioned. Every single year, as I've reported in much of my writing, 2,000 brand new chemicals, which none have really been tested in any way at all, are put into the marketplace. Those chemicals get into our environment and mix with the other tens of thousands of chemicals that have been put there to make hundreds of thousands, and millions and billions of different chemicals, this happens when chemicals meet, they morph into different chemicals.

These chemicals, which our body doesn't know how to deal with, and our immune system doesn't know how to have a defense against, go deep into the cell and of course the organs of the body, the bones of the body, or the tissue mass of the body, and that's where a lot of these cancers come from. These other diseases are directly linked with that, too. Other diseases like microbial diseases, viral diseases, and bacterial diseases are organism life forms that come into the body, and they create another form of infection. Many people today believe, as I do, that viral diseases either directly, like in cervical cancer, or indirectly, with all other form of cancer, contribute to cancer, but in great part it's the chemicals, heavy metals and lack of immunity that create most disease.

GABRIEL COUSENS

Many conditions, in addition to fructose and glucose intake, contribute to cancer. The cancer cells feed off fructose and glucose as much as 10-50 times more than other nutrients. Radiation exposure from Chernobyl and Fukushima is definitely a contributing factor. Those with cancer may have a variety of mental imbalances that reflect in psychosomatic issues that ultimately manifest as physical diseases. We're exposed to heavy environmental toxins. Another aspect is karma. Certain people come in the world with certain karmas, and the diseases are sometimes necessary to burn these karmas. This is separate from all their other physical or mental reasons. Sometimes people have a disease, and no matter what they do, they are unable to reverse it. These are things from past lives.

The great sage, Shankaracharya, was visited by a king. The king said, "You're a great sage! What is going on? Why do you have malaria?" The sage said, "It's my karma, but for our interview I'm going to put that malaria on this chair." The chair began to vibrate. Shankaracharya had a calm interview and said, "Now we're done." Shankaracharya took the malaria back and began trembling again from his malaria. In other words, sometimes there's a role for these, but the more we work on our health on the physical, emotional, mental planes, with a holistic approach, the more the outcome, although we may be destined to have it, is minimized and has a minimal effect on us. We have to be careful about making judgments about why somebody has a disease. We should be humble, because there's a mystery, and more is going on than meets the eye.

FRED BISCI

I'm a firm believer that just about all diseases begin in our bowels and our brain. Our brain chemistry is largely influenced by our diet and our lifestyle, which can lead to many emotional and psychological disorders.

"Eating late at night or too early in the morning upsets your body clock, which controls our circadian rhythm."
- Fred Bisci

The choices we make, based on our spiritual beliefs and the thoughts we entertain, can influence our health in many different ways. In preventing cancer, my focus is always on cleansing the lymphatic system, the lower and upper GI tract. The upper GI tract, in spite of what some people think, is most important. I've seen it over and over. My focus is to get a person well by cleaning out their digestive system. I help them get their metabolism to work optimally. The body has a God-given capability to overcome disease.

Most people are abusing their bodies by the way they eat. They're living on junk food and this is getting to be the standard way of eating in our country today. They're eating all day. They're being told to snack because snacking is good for you and that it stabilizes your blood sugar. It doesn't work that way. Many people are eating way too much animal protein and they're being told that you can't be a healthy vegetarian, which as we know is definitely not true. Many people are eating late at night, which doesn't contribute to a healthy GI tract. Partying has come to mean eating and drinking to excess and it's definitely a precursor to our diseases, including cancer. Eating late at night or too early in the morning upsets your body clock, which controls our circadian rhythm   I believe this is extremely important and is a factor in itself in the course of many different diseases. It leads to indigestion, fermentation, off-gassing from the upper GI tract, which is the precursor to cellular inflammation and all diseases.

When you're living that way and your GI tract is not functioning correctly, the indirect response is that your body is just not breathing properly on a cellular level. Most people are in agreement now with Otto Warburg that a cancer cell is a cell that's not getting enough oxygen and tries to survive on fermentation.

The human body produces approximately 3,000 metabolic enzymes. They are catalysts, and every function in your body requires them. Without metabolic enzymes, you will not absorb your vitamins. One of the most important metabolic enzymes is the respiratory enzyme. Without respiratory enzymes, your cells will not absorb oxygen. When you're eating a junk food diet, which is very acid forming, eventually you will impair your metabolic enzymes and your body will start to utilize non-oxidative fermentation. When a cell gets to the point where it is below 30% in its utilization of oxygen, it will switch to non-oxidative respiration. When it is thriving on non-oxidative respiration, then you've got a rapidly growing cancer cell.

New scientific evidence finds that many diseases which begin in our bowels cause fermentation, which leads to inflammation and on to other diseases. Some doctors are now treating colitis and Crohn's disease successfully with antibiotics. It has been known for quite a while that these 2 diseases going untreated could lead to cancer. I believe what happens, to keep it simple, is that when people are eating processed food, high animal protein, eating too frequently and eating late at night, they are actually living with chronic indigestion. This leads to a bacteria overgrowth, which off-gasses into your system. This bacteria overgrowth coming from the indigestion, putrefaction and fermentation, in my way of thinking, is the source of the problem. I believe this is at the root cause of most of our problems, inclusive of all the processed foods, chemicals and everything else that is being added to our foods, which is destroying the quality of our lives. I could write a whole book on this subject.

55. IS THERE A NATURAL WAY TO CURE THYROID DISEASE?

BRIAN CLEMENT

Well, I hate the word cure because cure takes away your responsibilities. Is there a way that people can control, manage and even eliminate the symptomatology of thyroid disease? The answer is yes, for the most part. The use of pharmaceutical drugs (there are many different names, depending upon where you are in the world), involves chemicals that go in and impose T4 on the body. T4 is what's lacking in the thyroid and what the chemical form of T4 does, is go and superimpose on top of that and get it to semi-function. Sadly, this doesn't really have any ability to help restore the thyroid. Even the pharmaceutical industry will grant that they have pharmaceutical drugs that are free of T4 that are more biocompatible, that work better with the human anatomy and body.

That would be one way to look at it, but look at the morality of taking glandular drugs like that. We have found, hands down, that the best way to help thyroid function with plant-based derivatives are the Chinese medicines. Wherever you are in the world, find a master Chinese herbal doctor and have that woman or man help you. If you've been on long-term Synthroid and other thyroid medicines, work with your doctors and slowly but surely get off of them and increase the herbal medicine. Yes, we've seen many cases get to the point where they didn't need any medication, but there are 20 to 30% of the population that are going to need some form of medicine throughout their life.

VIKTORAS KULVINSKAS

A natural way to improve the functioning of the thyroid, whether it is hypo- or hyper-thyroid, is to stop all pasteurized dairy consumption. Get on a cleansing detox program. Use the Melt Away supplement of Hippocrates with meals and in between meals. Then do the neck exercises that are found in yoga books. In conjunction, do the plow as well as shoulder stand. Consume sea vegetables. The thyroid is one of the ductless glands and it has no plumbing to go into it. It ingests through the skin, it gets nutrients and excretes hormones through the skin.

When the skin ends up being coated with mucal phlegm, it ends up being not able to absorb nutrients or excrete adequate volume of needed hormones. Through detoxification and cleansing, the organ function is returned to normalcy. Through optimal nutrition, you will be able to produce optimal levels of hormonal production.

GABRIEL COUSENS

There is a natural cure for thyroid disease. Incidentally, thyroid disease is really the only thing I've seen that seems to increase on a live food diet. Having deeply considered this, I see that a live food cuisine greatly increases the amount of oxygen in the system, and oxygen and iodine work very closely together. The result is that it begins, at least temporarily, pulling iodine away from the thyroid function to help the iodine and oxygen get into the cells. Iodine is needed for all aspects of bodily function. Iodine plays a role in skin and brain functions in apoptosis, the breakdown of dying cells, dead cells, and cancer cells. Iodine deficiency is also associated with fibrocystic breast and cancer of the breast, as well as prostate, colon, rectum, and a variety of different cancers. Iodine deficiency is associated with hypo-adrenalism and a variety of mental problems. Iodine deficiency is the leading cause of mental retardation in the world, and beyond this is cretinism. When the body begins to work more effectively and returns to health, iodine is pulled all over the body for healing.

My approach to healing the thyroid is to have people supplement with a nascent form of iodine, called Illumodine, that significantly improves iodine sufficiency. Keep in mind that 95% of Americans are indeed iodine deficient. In healing hypothyroidism, it's important to have a healthy replacement of iodine. A great deal of blood flow goes to the thyroid, so a great many toxins may be built up in the thyroid that need to be pulled out in a variety of ways. Specific clay packs are very helpful for pulling these toxins out.

Additionally, because water is often fluoridated and bread is prepared with bromine instead of iodine, as was the case years ago, and because bromine may be in swimming pools and hot tubs, there is a build up of bromine and fluoride in the thyroid and other bodily systems. This build up of bromine is reversed when the body is given adequate iodine. Within even a day or two, we will see as much as a 60% increase of fluoride or bromine in the urine, because the iodine is displacing and replacing it through competitive inhibition. We can reverse hypothyroidism by increasing iodine supplementation and taking herbs that increase the thyroid function and pull out the toxins from the thyroid that have been blocking the function. I also suggest avoiding foods that block iodine uptake, such as soy products.

FRED BISCI

Thyroid disease is like any other kind of disease. If you get to it soon enough, and you get a person to cleanse and take the burden off their body, and if the thyroid hasn't atrophied, there is a chance that natural methods can work. If a person has been on medication for a long time, there's a chance that they will not be able to come off their medications. If somebody has an overactive thyroid, there is a chance that if a person goes into a clean diet they will be able to reduce the activity of the thyroid down to a normal level. It's possible, but every case is individualized. There are certain supplements and herbal preparations that can help. Every case is individual and has to be personally evaluated.

56. DO HEAVY METALS CAUSE DISEASE? HOW SHOULD THEY BE TESTED? (URINE CHALLENGE TEST? BLOOD TEST?) WHAT CAN YOU DO TO ELIMINATE THEM?

VIKTORAS KULVINSKAS

Urinalysis and other procedures are available for establishing the presence of heavy metals. It can be eliminated through a detoxification cleansing program in conjunction with the consumption of super green foods, such as wheatgrass and algae, especially blue-green algae.

The body provides all elements, but it needs some heavy metals. We are getting way too much of it in our industrial age.

BRIAN CLEMENT

Absolutely, no doubt about it. How should they be tested? Urine is one way to test it and I think that's a more than adequate way. Blood does it at some level, but urine testing is the state of art in this case.

What can we do to eliminate them? Besides eating properly—not putting more into you, making sure you are wearing natural fiber clothe are a few important steps. Make sure your environment is clear of heavy metals and toxic chemicals—even making sure the bedding that you're on is organic, etc. Making sure that the water you drink, the air you breathe, are not riddled with heavy metals. That's where most of these come from. Making sure you take saunas, exercise, heat the body up and perspire profusely—all of these are the natural, normal way to detox and we have never seen them not work. We've been testing people on an ongoing basis for more than half a century. We actually see that, when people employ these lifestyle methodologies, with the inclusion of saunas, that they purge these heavy metals and chemical toxins from the body.

GABRIEL COUSENS

Doubtless, heavy metals, particularly mercury, cause disease. Mercury is associated with Alzheimer's, as are aluminum and lead. Lead is also associated with mental retardation, slower thinking, and poor memory. Cadmium is associated with kidney difficulties. All the heavy metals are associated with disease, one way or another. Perhaps the most accurate way to test for these toxic heavy metals is a hair test, because it gives you the accumulated amount of heavy metals over four months.

What can one do to eliminate them? Live foods certainly help. I use a zeolite called Natural Cellular Defense (NCD) that I find extremely helpful. In testing 40 people during a fast, I found that 38% of them clearly had some sort of heavy metal toxicity, and, after one week on our 50% diluted juice fast, 87% of all these metals were taken out. After two weeks, 100% of the heavy metals and pesticides were taken out. This is important because part of my work is to help prepare men and women for pregnancy, so that they have a viable cellular system. All these toxins are very detrimental to the functioning of the germ cell and proper reproduction. In that context, I get steady positive results with Natural Cellular Defense. It's been tested at the university level, with published reports showing that it pulls heavy metals from the body. I also find that NCD pulls out pesticides and herbicides. I personally take it on a regular basis.

FRED BISCI

Heavy metals are a real problem, no two ways about it. That's been proven over and over again. Too much mercury in your system can lead to neurological damage. Lead and cadmium can also cause problems.

According to the latest information, the blood test is not sufficient because a lot of these heavy metals are stored up in your fat cells, and that's why the urine challenge test is really important. You give a person a DMSA, which pulls the metals out into the urine where it can be measured.

There are a number of products and things that you can do to help get rid of the heavy metals. There are all kinds of magnetic clays, French green clay, DMSA, even Himalayan Sea Salt or Celtic Sea Salt can do it at a slower pace. The Sonne #7 and #9 is also an effective product. Medical doctors all recommend chelation, but I think a lot of people are being over chelated. It's definitely not necessary.

57. IS THERE A NATURAL WAY TO CURE DIABETES?

BRIAN CLEMENT

The answer is yes. I've never seen a type 2 diabetic not be able to bring about their own recovery. Type 2 diabetes is not a disease. It's a lifestyle choice and it's sad. There's an institution created around type 2 diabetes, and it's called a chronic disease and lifelong problem that you can only control. Well, again, I've never seen a type 2 diabetic who did what she or he was supposed to do, the inclusion of everything we've discussed, that was not able to reverse it.

Type 1 diabetes, on the other hand, is not statistically the same. In recent research that came out, it is clear now that many people who were either born with, or got shortly after birth, type 1 diabetes, had a mother with a celiac or wheat allergy during that time. That's one big part of this equation. You have to look at your diet if you're type 1 diabetic. You have to employ the same kind of Hippocrates lifestyle that we've been helping type 1 diabetics with, and certainly type 2 diabetics over the decades. You're going to actually have a much better state of health with type 1 diabetes and there are going to be a percentage of people who are able to reverse type 1 diabetes. I don't think we can be bold enough, or silly enough, to say that type 1 diabetes is as easy to control and reverse as type 2 diabetes, because that's just not what we have found.

VIKTORAS KULVINSKAS

All of the studies associated with type 1 diabetes have shown that the only nutritional factor that correlates to its development is consumption of pasteurized dairy products by the mother and/or infant. The mucus coats the Isle of Langerhans, the source of insulin production, reducing nutrient absorption and the ability on the part of the body to excrete adequate volumes of insulin.

By cleansing and detoxification, within two to four weeks, you will be able to clean out the mucus levels and produce an adequate amount of insulin. I have seen many, many cases of type-1 diabetes reversed. There might be some genetic origin, but I have great doubts.

Type 2 diabetes is where the individual has normal or way above normal insulin levels. They say that in type 2 diabetes, the insulin is resistant. What happens is the situation where the cardiovascular systems are coated with mucus phlegm, incompletely metabolized proteins along the blood vessels, thus disabling and creating a resistance to the movement of insulin, carrying sugar across the blood vessels into the interior for storage and conversion.

The answer is to clean out the blood vessels. The blood vessel detoxification is accelerated by consuming a totally mucus-less diet of plant-based raw foods, free of dairy products and all forms of animal protein. Taking enzymes with meals, as well as enzymes between meals, will accelerate the whole process. In a matter of a few days to a week, you can find yourself totally returning to normalcy.

GABRIEL COUSENS

In the revised edition of my book *There Is a Cure for Diabetes,* released in April of 2013, the results for healing diabetes are straightforward. Sixty-one percent of non-insulin dependent diabetics are healed in 3 weeks. Twenty-four percent of insulin dependent type 2 diabetics are healed in 3 weeks. Ninety-seven percent are off all medication in 3 weeks, and as for type 1 diabetics, 21% are healed in 3 weeks. Healing means that they have a fasting blood sugar less than 100 and are on no insulin or medications. Thirty-one percent of type 1 diabetics are off all insulin in 3 weeks, but their fasting blood sugar has not yet come down below 100.

How do we do this? The answer is with a relatively low-glycemic 100% live-food cuisine. By low-glycemic, I mean 25% to 35% carbohydrates. These carbohydrates are only sprouts, leafy greens, and green vegetables. No beets or carrots. This is the Phase 1 Diet.

My program also includes fasting on 50% water-diluted green juice for 1 week, which greatly accelerates the healing. I do not fast type 1 diabetics. I put them on blended foods, because of a variety of metabolic imbalances occurring within type 1 physiology as distinct from type 2.

"Sixty-one percent of non-insulin dependent diabetics are healed in 3 weeks." - Gabriel Cousens

There are supporting herbs for healing, but truly, the primary way to heal is with a Phase 1 Cuisine—which is nuts and seeds, all the leaves, all the greens, and sprouts. One week of fasting on diluted juices, many sea vegetables, and a certain amount of Illumodine (iodine) —because all diabetics are deficient in iodine and it is connected somehow with insulin production and enhanced pancreas functions which has an excellent therapeutic effect.

The results are very good with diabetes after three weeks, and for those who stay with it, even more people heal over time. People in our program are highly inspired because they get such good results in such a short time.

I'm going to mention fructose because fructose can no longer be considered a diabetic-friendly food. It's directly associated with causing diabetes, and high fructose corn syrup is particularly implicated. It isn't safer than glucose. In fact, cancer cells require 10 to 50 times more glucose than fructose in order to thrive.

FRED BISCI

I don't like the word cure. I don't use that word because it could end up leading to complacency, but I'll put it this way: I have never seen a person who had type 2 diabetes who followed the correct lifestyle and didn't go into remission. They essentially were not diabetic any longer unless they went back to their old lifestyle.

Type 1 diabetes is something else. In some cases a person with type 1 diabetes can be helped. I treated a young man who was a type 1 diabetic and now doesn't need to use insulin. A lot of people make claims for type 1 diabetes, but the question is, can a person do what has to be done, and is it a long-term remission? If people are willing to drink green juices, eat lots of greens, and go on a very low calorie type of a diet, they are likely to recover from their condition, but it's very questionable how many people would stay with that for a lifetime.

In the very near future, type 1 diabetes will be treated very effectively with stem cells. They're right on the verge of doing that now, but you can also definitely improve your condition by changing your diet. There are people with type 1 diabetes who will not be able to come off of their medication. I believe it is ridiculous to say that type 1 diabetes can always be cured by lifestyle.

58. I HAVE TROUBLE SLEEPING WHAT SHOULD I DO?

VIKTORAS KULVINSKAS

If you have a very busy mind, take notes and write, to quiet your mind. Do self-massage, in particular, the eyebrows, pinching and squeezing. Massage the earlobes and the ears completely, inside and out. Massage your shoulders by crossing your arms in front of you and digging into the shoulder area. Then massage the fleshy portion between the thumb and index finger, massage the toes.

Take digestive enzymes, especially HHIzymes, which will help to overcome digestive problems, often the foundation for keeping you awake. The major issue for not being able to sleep is systemic acidity. This is irritating your neurological system. The HHIzymes are also very alkaline, so it will address the acidic condition, which is further also aggravating the neurological stimulation. I would suggest five to ten enzymes at bedtime. You might also take five HTP, 1-300 units also at bedtime, preferably on an empty stomach, of course.

You can get excellent results by not eating for at least three hours before bedtime. Drink some warm chamomile tea. If that does not work, then take a salt bath. Put three pounds of salt in the bath and soak for at least an hour. Take a shower, then go to bed. You will sleep like a baby. This can overcome the worst case of insomnia.

As you improve your lifestyle habits, you will be able to sleep normally. Your sleep needs will be a function of the level of exercise you get, as well as of your state of emotional poise, which can be established through meditation. If you still cannot fall asleep, just practice a deep level of relaxation.

Once you master the corpse pose, or Savasana, you will be able to find that just by merely doing 20 minutes of deep relaxation, you'll have the equivalent of about four hours of sleep. Most people find this one of the most difficult postures to master. I have done it and I have found it extremely successful as an alternative to sleep.

As long as you are eating, you will need to rest. As long as you are exercising, you are going to need sleep.

BRIAN CLEMENT

Well, the most important thing is contemplation, meditation, and prayer—that is at the top of the list. There are some more effective herbal medicines. On and off, periodic use of melatonin is fine. I'm not a fan of its consistent use. It somehow throws off the liver and gallbladder function. Why, we haven't discovered this yet, but we're clear on it's happening. If none of this works, if you have a real problem, we even submit to temporary use of psychiatric or sleeping meds, but the key word there is temporary. Retrain the brain chemistry to go to sleep and then get off that med, go on to an herbal medicine and ultimately to the point where we don't need the medicine in any way.

GABRIEL COUSENS

Sleep disturbance can reflect a variety of imbalances, and it happens at a variety of ages for a variety of reasons. We have to be very careful. This happens for different reasons at different times. However, going to bed by 10:00 p.m., and sleeping at least through the hours of 10:00 p.m. to 2:00 a.m., gives a tremendous boost to the endocrine system, to serotonin levels, and to the immune system in terms of repair and energy.

The average person needs somewhere between seven and eight hours of sleep each night. There are 100 million sleep deficient people in the U.S. Sleep deprived people have 40 times more depression and a lot more endocrine imbalances. Even fasting blood sugar in the morning is higher if one does not get sufficient sleep.

The treatment for insomnia is complicated. Whole books are written on it. As you eat more live foods, there is a drop of insomnia rates by 400%, according to the research of one of our Spiritual Nutrition Masters students who took a survey. When people go on live foods, there is a dramatic decrease in insomnia. Simply eating live foods starts to create a rebalancing in the sleep cycle.

There are certain herbs and supplements that may help, as well. Sleep disturbance represent a vata imbalance, and one can best improve their sleep by calming vata with an emphasis on slightly sweet, salty, and sour foods, creating a calmer environment, and avoiding TV or computer use for about three hours before going to bed.

A gentle abhyanga massage or oil related massage on your body is recommended. Oil is very good rubbed on the body at least twice a day for insomnia. Also taking oileated enemas is very calming to the vata and calming to the bowel where vata is stored. These are general suggestions. Stay out of the wind as much as possible. I once cured a person of chronic insomnia in India by simply telling her to turn her fan off at night, because even a fan at night can create a vata imbalance.

FRED BISCI

It's not just a question of taking sleeping pills or melatonin or valerian or any of those herbs, because people have to try to get to the root cause of their problem. I have seen many people who did not sleep well. Once they get into a right diet and clean up their GI tract, a lot of the problems improve. Colonics and Epsom salt baths are helpful. Epsom salts can also be taken internally, as a salt flush to help clean out your GI tract.

Again, I take each person as an individual. Warm baths and exercise help a lot of people. Many people are very sedentary and they're eating a lot, so they go to bed and they can't sleep because they just ate. Then they're tired all the time during the daytime. Circadian rhythm and your body clock are a factor. On a side note, I have found medical hypnosis to be a powerful tool to help people with lifestyle changes. With the help of medical hypnosis, poor sleep always improves.

59. WHAT IS THE BEST WAY TO BOOST MY IMMUNE SYSTEM?

VIKTORAS KULVINSKAS

Dr. Leskovar published results showing that, within 20 minutes of orally-administered enzymes, the natural fillers activity increases by 1100%, macrophages by 700%. Enzymes are one thing, the consumption of probiotics is another thing, then of course a raw food program—all of these empower your immune system

BRIAN CLEMENT

Number 1—the sun, early morning sun, 9 o'clock and before and two hours before sunset, 12 months a year. If you're living in cold climates, wear natural fiber clothes. Go out and get a minimum of 30 minutes, five days a week.

Number 2—attitude. With my former colleague, Dr. Carl Simonton, and my current colleague, Dr. Janet Hranicky, we work together globally, with visualization, and the effect it has on the immune system, it is spectacular. The diet that we're speaking about, a raw living organic diet, and exercise—a wonderful work that was just published called Spark by Dr. Ratey from Harvard University, shows that you literally can change the mind to use the vehicle of looking at everything from immune function to sleep disorders. So, exercise is scientifically validated as a great way to boost the immune system today.

GABRIEL COUSENS

The best way to boost the immune system is to get adequate sleep. There are also a variety of herbs that can help; however, adequate sleep, moderate exercise, lymphatic massage, and hot-cold showers, consisting of three to seven cycles of hot and cold alterations, can all boost the lymphatic system, which supports the immune system.

FRED BISCI

Change your lifestyle. Do a juice fast or water fast under supervision. Start exercising. Clean out your digestive system. Get plenty of fresh air and sunshine. Drink clean water. It's the same situation as for recovering from any disease.

A lot of people don't realize that when you're eating a bad diet, your body is kind of like a garbage disposal system. The endogenous material is a perfect nesting place for bacteria. Everybody sneezes on you, and you're probably going to pick up a cold and find you have a weak immune system. If your system is clean, you exercise, you're not overeating, and you're eating the right food, people could sneeze on you all they want and you're unlikely to get sick. The host is a factor for contagion. I only recommend supplements as a last resort.

I deal with all kinds of sick people. I don't remember the last time I had a cold. Keep your system clean, and make sure you're moving your bowels once for every meal you eat. If you do that, and drink plenty of water, get plenty of fresh air and exercise, and try to maintain a tranquil state of mind, you're going to have a very powerful immune system, there's no two ways about it.

It goes without saying that we should be drinking pure water, trying to avoid environmental toxins, leaving out all the processed food, eliminating GMOs and dairy products. Cell phones are a disaster. They are doing far more damage than the average person realizes. I have seen demonstrations that are frightening. I personally do not put my cell phone to my head for the heat that it creates and the head ache that it gives me. A woman doctor told me there was a 40% increase in brain cancers in the last 10 years due to technology. The best way to boost your immune system to the point where you will almost be immune to disease is a total lifestyle change. I do not recommend magic bullets to improve your immune system. I think that is false information based on reductionism type science.

60. HOW CAN I FORTIFY MYSELF TO COMBAT RADIATION EXPOSURE?

BRIAN CLEMENT

When we were given the privilege to visit Moscow, shortly after the Chernobyl incident, Dr. Anna Maria and I helped people by giving them copious amounts of algae and soaking them in very hot baths with kelp in the water. In a 14-day period, on an average, the reduction of uranium radiation from their body was 29%. We showed and validated this under scientific constraint all the way.

"..be more concerned about your cell phones and your laptop computers, and all of the electronics surrounding you." - Brian Clement

Green leafy vegetables and sprouts are part of the diet of the Hippocrates lifestyle and also that of all of the Elders—because we are very similar in this. After we do enough work for long enough, we all come up with truth. That's why what you're hearing resonates in this book and is very similar, because everyone gets to the truth if you do this with an open heart and mind.

Just the diets that we're proposing for you will, in fact, help to protect you from radioactivity, which is not just a recent phenomenon. The same radiation that was here during Hiroshima is still on this planet, it did not leave. During older wars, where they were using radioactivity in warheads and during the Gulf wars and current wars that are going on, the radiation is still on this planet. But I'd be more concerned about your cell phones and your laptop computers, and all of the electronics surrounding you, than I am of the far away threats. You don't have the far away ones stuck to your head or sitting on top of your genitalia on a daily basis. Medical scans in 1980 gave the average person 15% of their radiation. Now it's 50%.

VIKTORAS KULVINSKAS

I quote in my book, *Survival*, the study that was done by the Army and the Navy and published in radiation reviews, animals that consume green foods were able to be subjected to lethal dosages of radiation and survive it. The other experience has been the consumption of fermented foods, in the form of miso, sauerkraut, and kimchi.

GABRIEL COUSENS

We have developed a remedy called Radiation Neutralization that, at the time of this writing, provides 100% positive results in neutralizing radiation in people. It's got over 100 radio nucleotides and special oxygen. Additionally, by taking Illumodine you can protect yourself from radioactive iodine via competitive inhibition.

FRED BISCI

Greens and green sprouts, wheatgrass, E3Live, and all live foods combat radiation exposure. There's a product called BioSuperFood, which is a concentrated greens formula developed by a Russian scientist for people who were exposed to radiation in Chernobyl. It works very, very well. But if you've been exposed to radiation, you should consult a professional. Have somebody evaluate you and prescribe the proper products.

61. DOES APHANIZOMENON FLOS-AQUAE (AFA BLUE-GREEN ALGAE) HELP PEOPLE WITH DISEASE, OR EVEN WITH NEUROLOGICAL CHALLENGES?

GABRIEL COUSENS

Absolutely. I published research on *Aphanizomenon flos-aquae* in the Journal of *Orthomolecular Medicine*. In one case, it actually reversed Alzheimer's disease. This person with Alzheimer's disease couldn't walk or even watch TV, and after six months, was walking, watching TV, able to follow her husband around the track, and able to dress herself. Another case was a lawyer with a rapid degeneration of Alzheimer's, which the E3Live stopped completely in its tracks. This was a case of a very intelligent lawyer whose IQ had dropped to 90 in his degeneration process. This is different than spirulina or chlorella, which do not have the same kind of neurological affects. I've taken *Aphanizomenon flos-aquae* since 1982 and observed a variety of improvements in regard to my own clarity of mind, thinking processes, memory, creativity, and overall brain function.

Research done in Nicaragua, in which kids were given a teaspoon or a half a teaspoon of E3Live daily, had dramatic improvement in their grades. Their conduct in school improved significantly, and, in general, their brain function, memory, mental acuity, clarity, and social behavior significantly improved.

Other research has been done in applying a skin preparation of blue-green algae to leprosy, with very dramatic healing results as well.

I once had a child who wasn't speaking at all. The child had been diagnosed as autistic. After just three months on the *Aphanizomenon flos-aquae* the child began to speak fluently. It can work on a variety of levels.

People have also used it to heal certain cancers, particularly of the brain and also of the seventh and eighth nerves. It generally supports every aspect of our physical and mental functioning, although it is a far more specific for improved mental functioning on every level.

BRIAN CLEMENT

For more than 30 years, we've been using blue-green algae, AFA algae, to help people. In my family, we take several varieties of algae every single day, and there's no doubt that this is a superior food that helps to restore every part of the body, cell by cell. It helps everything, from improving depression to endowing athletes who need extra energy. We have trained Olympic level athletes, and this is one of the foods we give them. I cannot emphasize enough the importance of consuming this supplement. It is a spectacular addition to one's diet, hands down. I can't say anything but good things about it and have decades of clinical research to support what I'm saying to you.

Before we accepted algae, we actually did an 18-month study and differentiated a group, with a control group. We put half the group on algae, half off and saw vast differences in the groups. That's why, about three decades ago, we adopted this as part of the Hippocrates program. We don't jump into things blindly and I never ever put money first. I don't care if we lose money on something. If it's not good, I'm not going to tell you that it is. If it is good, I'm going to support it 100% and constantly challenge it to make sure that we're at the state of the art in our level of knowledge.

VIKTORAS KULVINSKAS

Some years ago, a study was submitted to the University of Illinois Medical School, entitled *Two Hundred Cases of Incurables Treated Successfully with Superfoods*. One of the superfoods was AFA. The areas with the most dramatic response were in respiratory complications ranging from bronchial asthma to emphysema. Significant results have also been seen with ADD, ADHD and also intellectual development.

My own grandmother recovered from Alzheimer's disease. It should be done in conjunction with enzymes, probiotics and a mild herbal laxative, in conjunction with taking an adequate amount of hydration and taking high enough dosages of blue-green algae.

Most individuals will do well on four AFA capsules, up to a maximum of eight, twice a day between meals.

FRED BISCI

Yes, E3Live is a great supplement that I encourage people to use because I know it works. It has no side effects. E3Live BrainON helps a lot of people, and I use it myself. It is very energizing. People who suffer from depression often feel better when they use it. But there is no one specific thing that is a magic bullet. You have to try for yourself to see if it works for you. I found it to be a great help for people withdrawing from a chemical dependency and other forms of addiction.

62. WHAT WOULD YOU RECOMMEND FOR SOMEONE WHO IS A PAST OR CURRENT DRUG ADDICT AND HAS A BIOLOGICALLY ALTERED BRAIN?

GABRIEL COUSENS

This is a particular specialty of mine. It can be healed. Drug addiction, including the use of psychedelic drugs such as Ayahuasca, is associated with varying degrees of serious brain degeneration.

The research in Jamaica on cannabis alone showed that after 20 years, the people using it on a regular basis often develop serious brain deterioration. There's a book out now called *The Marijuana Syndrome*, and there are about 100 different syndromes in regard to ingesting marijuana alone. We've seen significant brain alteration and deterioration from all the psychedelics because they create a serotonergic oxidation, from excess serotonin, and then the oxidation of that excess serotonin destroys brain cells.

I've also seen this with Ayahuasca, which is an MAO inhibitor. It seems to cause different problems, and in the last three years, as people are using it more and more, the glowing reports of how safe it is really don't hold up. The only people I've seen recently for drug imbalances and drug psychosis crisis have been those who have taken Ayahuasca. It can severely alter the brain functioning in a variety of people. I see a lot of people who have these troubles.

For alcoholism, there is a tenfold better success rate when we put people on live food and on proper supplementation. For example, the usual rate of success for alcoholics at four years is 7% with AA. On a nutritionally balanced, supplemental approach, including *Aphanizomenon flos-aquae*, and an all live food diet, I see significant neurological regeneration and sustainable success rates of 75%. That's a 10-fold increase.

I also use certain supplements that help support the neurotransmitters for the repair of the brain. These supplements are neurotransmitter precursors to reinitiate the flow of energy. However, even in people who can't afford all the neurotransmitter precursors, when they go on live foods, there is a gradual and steady rebuilding of the neurotransmitters circuitry.

But the important thing is that if people are serious, they indeed can repair the biologically altered brain, and I've seen a very high success rate in my own practice. It may take up to 2 years, but with the right support, the brain is highly likely to repair itself. As a holistic psychiatrist and holistic physician, these are things that, over the last 40 years, I've seen to be consistently successful. The biologically altered brain can be repaired, and one must have the willingness to stop all psychedelic and other drugs—including alcohol.

VIKTORAS KULVINSKAS

Besides a plant-based diet, place emphasis on raw foods and greens, in conjunction with blue-green algae and enzymes, and plenty of exercise and meditation. Everyone can benefit from these practices.

FRED BISCI

I don't like blanket diagnoses. I take each person as an individual and prescribe a reasonable diet, starting from the premise of leaving out all the processed food. Processed food is addictive, so it exacerbates the need to medicate with either food or pharmaceuticals or recreational drugs. I would get a patient into the best diet that they would be willing to follow, preferably a diet that is vegan and at least 60-70% raw foods. If they won't follow that, some clean animal protein, free of chemicals, hormones, pesticides and antibiotics would be acceptable, but no more than three times a week.

A lot of physicians feed people a high protein diet and leave out all the carbs because on an immediate level, they seem to respond better, but in the long run, that's a real problem. I would design a diet that the person could follow and then gradually improve it to get them to their optimal diet that they can sustain for their lifetime. I have found BrainOn to be particularly helpful in these cases. Of course, like in everything else, detox is extremely important. We have to cleanse the lymphatic system, the GI tract, detox on a cellular level so a person can utilize oxygen completely and improve their brain chemistry.

I've worked with some people addicted to methadone and heroin, and I try to offer guidance and help them detox gradually and systematically. Especially with methadone, people can have convulsions, so I use a hyperbaric chamber and infrared sauna. Fresh air and exercise are also extremely important, and I design an individualized supplement program, often including the E3Live BrainOn and the bio superfoods. B vitamins in a good raw mineral formula help to ground the person.

My individualized treatment plans also usually include things like warm baths with Epsom salts, food-grade hydrogen peroxide, colonics, enemas, colon cleanses, systemic enzymes, anti-inflammatory enzymes and lots of probiotics. The probiotics with high CFU counts (over a trillion) work very well for people with emotional or psychological disorders.

BRIAN CLEMENT

Well, it's good that a person's alert and awakened and off medicines, drugs, whatever they may have been on. The core of any addictive pattern being changed and shifted is self-esteem. If you develop self-respect, understand you have a purpose, a reason, understand your whole job is to fulfill your life, to contribute, to give, you're going to permanently remove the addictive substances. Food is the most common addiction; 100% of the population has a food addiction. There are two kinds of us reading or listening today, current food addicts who are actively pursuing food addiction and then those of us who are recovering food addicts. But we are food addicts, every one of us. So, self-love, self-respect is at the top of the list.

Number two: by giving your body high protein, high mineral foods, we have seen thousands of people removing addiction. Just two days ago, I spoke to a man who, for 45 years had been an alcoholic; and a couple of years ago he adopted the diet after going through about 10 rehab programs, none of which succeeded. The diet in and of itself helped, because of the nutrient load it has and benefit of essential fats for the brain, was ultimately what reversed his addictive patterns. Now, the bottom line is, you're not going to have just food alone be enough. You're going to have to combine this, as we do, with psychotherapy. Every single guest who comes to Hippocrates receives psychotherapy, like it or not, that's the most important thing. We have to get to why you don't like yourself before you can like yourself enough to get rid of the disease.

63. WHAT IS THE BEST THING TO DO TO BOOST THE IMMUNE SYSTEM FOR PROTECTION AGAINST COLDS AND INFECTIONS?

VIKTORAS KULVINSKAS

Adequately hydrating is number one, taking extra enzymes with meals and in between meals, and consuming probiotics. The studies are extensive.

BRIAN CLEMENT

What we've learned in recent years is that the number one nutrient to protect you from colds and flu is zinc. Boy, can you get a lot of zinc in sprouted pumpkin seeds and mung bean sprouts, the white Chinese bean sprouts, but taking a liquid ionic form of these minerals if you have a lot of colds and flus would be terrific. Again, not taking dairy food, too many cooked foods, not taking bakery or flour products and other grain products, meats of any type, all of that is part of it, but really, the zinc is at the top of the list hands down.

Statistically now on several occasions in different research studies globally, they have shown that if you contract a cold or flu, you reduce it by one-third by taking zinc. If you have a 6-day cold or flu, it would be a 4-day one, just by consuming an adequate amount of the proper zinc. If you are feeling a cold come on, and you take enough zinc, the likelihood is that you're not going to contract that cold or, if you do, it's going to be a minor cold at that point. I'm a major fan of zinc, it does work and its organic whole food form is by far the best or if you're taking a supplement, again the ionic form.

GABRIEL COUSENS

Support the immune system with adequate sleep. One of the biggest causes of illness I've seen is not getting adequate sleep or being overstressed in one's life situation. Getting adequate sleep, minimizing stress, and eating at least an 80% live food diet for 2 years has been shown by one of my Live Food Masters students to improve immune function by 92%. Many supplements, like vitamin D and medicinal mushroom are also great protectors.

FRED BISCI

I think that's a misunderstanding. If your system is toxic, you're loaded with all kinds of garbage. Taking vitamin C or zinc is only going to be a temporary adjunct. The best thing to do is clean out your system. Detoxify; get to the point where you're moving your bowels regularly; eat a good plant-based diet; reduce stress in your life; and get all the chemicals out of your system. Then you're going to have strong protection against colds and infection. It's all about if you are a good host for bacteria proliferation. If you are a toxic waste dump, you are going to be picking up infections often because you are a good host for them. You are providing a fertile environment for the bacteria to proliferate. If you are clean from a healthy lifestyle, your so-called immune system will be strong. What this means is, you will not be a good host for bacteria proliferation.

64. I CONTACTED HEPATITIS C, A SO-CALLED "INCURABLE DISEASE. DO YOU HAVE ANY TIPS TO HELP ME LIVE WITH MY DISEASE?

VIKTORAS KULVINSKAS

There are no incurable diseases, only incurable personalities. I have seen dozens of cases of individuals overcoming hepatitis C and living superlative lives without any limitations, rejuvenated, looking healthier and younger than they ever did before. Get on the programs that are being advocated at Hippocrates and the other individuals within our community.

The thing that will help most is going to be the nutritional program, which includes the consumption of green juices, blue-green algae and bitter greens for liver regeneration, combined with the exercises, the holistic lifestyle. These will make you feel especially strong, as well as taking enzymes for immune system function and regeneration. If you do all of those things with the use of probiotics, you will have a stronger liver. Within a year, you may not have any of the symptoms of hepatitis C.

BRIAN CLEMENT

We have seen many people with certain types of hepatitis C. With our lifestyle, the Hippocrates lifestyle, combined with the intravenous use of substances like Argentyn from the Sovereign Silver Company, they may be able to reverse it. The good news is that allopathic mainstream medicine today has a whole new way to look at this and they're getting a very high success rate with modern technology, not the olden interferon technology that was failing in the majority of cases. I would go to an expert in your part of the world and delve into the state-of-the-art modalities. That and the lifestyle changes together can almost assure you of reversal in seven to eight cases out of ten.

GABRIEL COUSENS

The most important thing I've seen with hepatitis C, which I've definitely seen with my patients, is either a halting of the disease or a reduction of the titer to either close to zero or zero. A live food cuisine and the green juice fasting, as well as herbs for healing the liver, are all key.

Adequate sleep is important, and I would recommend a 100% live food diet, with the inclusion of fasting for one week 2-4 times yearly on 50%-diluted green juices and particular herbs for the liver.

FRED BISCI

Absolutely. I've seen plenty of people drop their viral load down to zero with hepatitis C. You've got to clean up your body to give your liver a chance to unburden itself of the hepatitis C. Seventy percent of our population has a fatty liver from eating a terrible diet. The average liver should weigh about 3-1/4 pounds. There are people that have 5-pound livers. It's a perfect nesting place for viruses and then the liver is not going to work correctly. Go on a juice fasting retreat, under supervision. Leave out all the processed food, and take systemic enzymes, probiotics, and digestive enzymes. In my experience, some of the supposedly incurable diseases have ended up being the easiest to overcome, believe it or not. You can get better. Your body is a miraculous healer. Leave out the causes of disease, give your body free reign and watch the miracles.

65. I HEARD THAT EATING RAW LIVING FOODS CURES CANCER—IS THIS TRUE?

BRIAN CLEMENT

Again, the word cure is an ominous word, it should be called remission. What the raw living food lifestyle does, along with exercise and all of the other things we continually mention, is to boost and support the immune system and the immune system can heal cancer and put it into remission as it does other diseases.

VIKTORAS KULVINSKAS

No, it does not. Though cancer does disappear in a high enzymatic nutritional program that includes an abundant amount of raw foods, live foods and, in particular, fermented foods and enzymatic supplementations. It is a lifestyle habit change that causes symptoms to disappear.

GABRIEL COUSENS

We certainly get a higher percentage of healing cancer with people. I am not a cancer specialist, but occasionally people come to me and will refuse to go to other places, for whatever reason. These have a high percentage of healing.

Usually I refer them to Hippocrates in Florida, which has a high percentage of healing using 100% live foods and juice fasting, as well as particular herbs that are helpful, along with NCD. Live food cuisine is particularly good for healing cancer. These diets that I put people on require absolutely no fruit at all and really no sweeteners at all except stevia and a little xylitol. The other thing that generally helps is the use of iodine, such as Illumodine, which has a strong anticancer effect. I have also found Natural Cellular Defense (NCD) to be helpful.

Cancer is very tricky and I feel people should go to a live food cancer healing center as their first choice.

FRED BISCI

This is an inaccurate statement. I'm not saying you can't get better. I just don't like the word "cure" and a lot of people are making ridiculous statements, as if the raw living food diet is a panacea. It's not. It is definitely the best way to go, and it can do miraculous things. But people on a raw food diet can still get cancer. I've known a few, so there definitely have to be other factors. The raw living food diet is the best way to go, but it will not resolve all cases of cancer. There are many other factors, which would require extensive conversation.

66. MY AUNT HAS STAGE 4 BREAST CANCER AND HAS BEEN GIVEN 6 MONTHS TO LIVE. IS THERE ANY HOPE FOR HER?

VIKTORAS KULVINSKAS

Hippocrates Health Institute is doing a study where this irreversible degenerative condition is healed by the body through lifestyle improvement in a matter of less than six months, where one becomes totally cancer-free. Yes, there is hope. It means doing the whole program.

We anticipate the results will be published in 2016 or later in medical journals. The study is being done in conjunction with the University of California School of Medicine. My own personal experience has been dozens of cases of stage 4 breast cancer of ages between 30-60 completely reversed in a matter of 5-6 months by following the Hippocrates Health Institute program.

BRIAN CLEMENT

Well, this is the kind of individual we deal with on a daily basis, and we have seen numbers of people reverse advanced breast cancer and others. Now, in the archive mainstream medicine what we do know is that they tell you in writing that they fail with stage 4 breast cancer. They also have recently, slowly but surely, globally published some real current data and information on how chemotherapy and radiation can actually create cancer. You may want to look into the Hippocrates website magazine archives; we refer to some of these medical research studies that are coming out in medical journals. You may want to also look at an extraordinary documentary called *Healing Cancer from the Inside* by Michael Anderson, a very poignant and very clear portrayal of the truth surrounding cancer. You may also want to consider coming to Hippocrates to support your body in its healing process.

GABRIEL COUSENS

There is always hope. A 100% live food approach significantly increases the chances of healing. There is always hope, and it's surprising how many times we've seen things turn around.

FRED BISCI

Yes, there is always hope. I've seen a number of people with stage 4 cancer who changed their lifestyle, did the right thing as best as they possibly could and they bought a lot of time, and some of them actually went into remission. I've seen one person who had six months to live with pancreatic cancer, which is rare—and he lived 16 or 17 years before he succumbed to his cancer. Every case is different.

There's always hope, but you have to be very aggressive. You have to do a complete program. If you have an advanced cancer, you can't go on a raw food diet and not do the cleanses like colonics, because you need to get rid of the endogenous material you're releasing into your system. The cancer could actually get worse if you're not doing the cleanses. You need guidance. You have to go to a retreat or work with an experienced professional.

67. WHY DO SO MANY PEOPLE HAVE B12 DEFICIENCIES? HOW CAN I PREVENT THIS?

GABRIEL COUSENS

Meat eaters and vegan live fooders do get B12 deficiencies. Our bodies don't synthesize B12, so it must be supplemented. There are some people who can get away without taking supplementation for up to 30 years, because of variations in enterohepatic circulation.

B12 bacteria grows in our colon, and if an individual has particularly good enterohepatic circulation in recycling it back to the liver, they may move into a deficient stage a lot slower. About 40% of meat eaters and about 80% of vegan live food people are deficient in general at 200 nanograms, which is a low normal value. At the optimum level of B12, which is closer to 400 to 450 nanograms, we're looking at probably 90% of the population of meat eaters and vegan live fooders will eventually get deficient. The best way to avoid this is to take a live food living B12 supplement. That's the easy way to go about it.

FRED BISCI

Undiagnosed B12 deficiency is a big problem in our society today. The lower normal ranges are too low. Many people are told that they are in a safe lower normal range when in actuality this is not true. Misdiagnosed B12 deficiency is being manifested in many different disorders. People who eat animal protein are also having problems with B12 deficiency. There is more than one factor in falling into a B12 deficiency. Most B12 is bound to animal protein. The B12 must be split and separated from the protein. We need hydrochloric acid and pepsin. If that metabolism is faulty you can fall into a B12 deficiency. If you are not producing the intrinsic factor, you can fall into a deficiency. You need other proteins, called R-binders, to carry the B12 into the small intestines. The small amount of B12 that is produced

"I believe that every raw foodist or vegan should be monitoring their B12 on a regular basis." - Fred Bisci

in the small intestines might not be absorbed if it is not coming from your diet. Transcobalamin 2 carries the vitamin B12 to the various cells and the excess to the liver for storage. As you can see, this is a complicated process where there could be some problems. The human body and its chemistry are miraculous and can do this easily.

The big question, "Is it possible for people on a long term raw food diet or vegan diet to have a good chance of running into a B12 deficiency?" The answer is "Yes". I have seen it happen plenty of times over the last 40 years. It could be a factor in other diseases and is misdiagnosed. The lower normal ranges are too low. There are people who are having problems that are in the lower normal ranges and when they supplement and come into the right range, they show dramatic improvement. I believe that every raw foodist or vegan should be monitoring their B12 on a regular basis. I know one case in particular where the person was a friend of mine, who I am sure succumbed to a long term undiagnosed B12 deficiency. One of the best books I have read on this topic is *Could It Be B12* by Sally Pacholok.

BRIAN CLEMENT

Some 20 years ago, my colleagues, Dr. Cousens and George Malcolm, brought to my attention a study done in Framingham that showed that blood testing of B12 was inadequate. When they were doing this testing, people that showed they had B12, in half the cases, did not. We then went on subsequent studies and found the Framingham study to be absolutely correct and we started to do deeper testing with SpectraCell, etc., and found out that approximately 70% of the population has a B12 deficiency. If they eat meat, if they eat dairy food, none of it matters. In general, about equal amounts of B12 deficiency are in every population of food consumers.

I really became a missionary in trying to discover why, and I went into the archives of medical schools and looked at anatomical sketches, charts and photographs, and discovered that our anatomy, our large intestine,

"Neurological disorders including dementia are the result of B12 deficiency." - Brian Clement

our colon radically changed its shape and functionality as hundreds of years passed. Over the last 300 years, and certainly into the last 150 years or so, we are lacking and missing a part of the lower part of our intestinal track where food would come out of the Ileocecal Valve after

coming from the small intestine, fall into this pocket that looked like an empty front of a boot. This part of our anatomy is now missing.

B12 is a soil based microorganism. Historically human anatomy maintained an elongated, large intestine, whereas at the bottom, collected this B12 bacteria and culturing it in the cellulose and other nutrient factors remaining after the digestion process. Somehow there has been a de-evolution where this section of the colon is now replaced by a shriveled up appendix. This mandates consistent consumption of an appropriate and living B12 supplement. Our research over the last two decades has established that 70% of the worldwide population lacks this essential nutrient. Neurological disorders including dementia are the result of B12 deficiency. Framingham researchers published a study in the late '90's that exposed the fact that B12 measurements in standard blood tests were flawed. Our conclusion has been harvested from efficient and effective B12 testing on thousands of people for nearly a generation.

Now we all need a daily intake of B12. The one supplement that we are absolutely definitive on that everyone must take, every day, for the rest of their lives, is the bacterial form of B12. We make ours through a culture, there are very few that do. Many use chemicals, like an alcohol fermenting process. Most methyls, though not all, are not really a good choice for you. They show higher B12 in the blood, but they really don't supply higher B12 in the cell. B12 deficiencies become dementia, neurological disorders, so not something anyone wants. B12 every day for the rest of your life. Thank you, Gabriel for tipping me off on that, and thank you for all the research scientists globally that have given us the understanding and ability to tell you that you need B12 and it's not something that's going to change anytime soon.

VIKTORAS KULVINSKAS

It is due to the prevalence of antibiotics and other ways of destroying the friendly bacteria cultures. The main source of vitamin B12 is your friendly gastrointestinal bacteria.

The lack of B12 leads to pernicious anemia, which is a form of wasting away disease. In *Survival in the Twenty-First Century,* I have quotes from medical studies. All forms of anemia, including pernicious anemia, were treated successfully with chlorophyll greens.

The greens supply nutrition for vitamin B12 manufacturing probiotics proliferation within the gastrointestinal tract. There are many causes for B12 deficiency. One is the destruction of friendly bacteria through gas and flatulence. Two is harsh herbs. Three is inadequate presence of B12 manufacturing probiotics.

A reason why the intrinsic factor is not absorbed within the stomach areas is that the stomach, for most people, is coated with mucal phlegm and it is not absorbing it. Within a matter of five years, it becomes severely chronic and you develop pernicious anemia symptoms.

If you do cleansing and detoxification, you will have all the vitamin B12 complex components absorbed and you will be functioning healthy and normal. As a preventative, as an antidote to this phlegm and mucal coating in the stomach, which is not going to absorb the vitamin B12, use sublingual delivery of vitamin B12 by purchasing quality B12 as available from Tree of Life and Hippocrates Health Institute. Chew it up and absorb it through the mouth cavity.

It enables you to act in a preventative way. Eventually you will not have a need for vitamin B12 supplementation.

68. SO MANY PEOPLE ARE LOSING THEIR MINDS WITH ALZHEIMER'S AND DEMENTIA. IS THERE ANYTHING THEY CAN DO TO PREVENT THIS FROM HAPPENING?

BRIAN CLEMENT

Well, B12 deficiencies are the number one cause of this. Essential fatty acid deficiencies, and going back to something I said early on in this book, is lack of brain use. Crossword puzzles, Luminosity, checkers, reading, interaction with other people, intellectual pursuits—even people who have the classic Alzheimer's gene, when they use the brain and live in a healthy way, they do not have Alzheimer's, even at 100 years old. Brain use, nutrition, that's what you need to do, you don't need heavy metals in your brain. You don't need chemicals in your brain, it will cross circuit and that's one of the problems.

VIKTORAS KULVINSKAS

Yes. Many years ago, Victor Coleman did some preliminary research with blue-green algae, *Aphanizomenon flos-aquae*, and he claimed that it provided a cure. It is much more complicated than that. We have seen results with all levels of introduction of blue-green algae, whereby when it is consumed initially one, then two, then up to ten capsules twice a day between meals, then some degree of reversal was taking place.

Dr. Gabriel Cousens noted in some of his published studies with stabilizing the Alzheimer's disease. I use the holistic approach, though I was not able to get dietary changes initiated. I made sure that they were not being poisoned by their dietary habits.

What I did was, with my own grandmother and several other individuals who had Alzheimer's disease, is put them on enzymes, in conjunction with a mild herbal laxative at bedtime, one capsule of cayenne a couple of times a day for circulation, and then I gradually increased the blue-green algae usage from two capsules, then three capsules every few days then four capsules, then six capsules, eight capsules twice a day. Then I let them stay on eight capsules twice a day for the duration of about two to three weeks, then cut back gradually to four capsules twice a day as a maintenance dosage.

I have seen consistently, within five to eight weeks, complete reversal of the Alzheimer's disease. Of course, this will have a favorable effect on dementia. Other individuals have had some good improvement with the consumption of Chia seeds.

In the studies that have been published in Time magazine, as well as in Newsweek, they said all individuals across the board that had Alzheimer's disease showed their brain was saturated with rubberized proteins. In other words, enzyme exhaustion, brains are becoming storage warehouse with protein, not amino acids or polypeptides, which are precursors to neurotransmitters. We are talking about incompletely metabolized proteins that are clogging up the brains, interfering with normal functioning.

Stop eating dairy products. That is the number one culprit. Then cut out animal proteins and get on a raw food program or vegan program, and you find that it is correctable.

FRED BISCI

Absolutely. Prevention is the answer, just as with cancer. We could reduce these problems in our society dramatically if we could convince people that we are the cause of our own problems. Don't stop detoxing. I don't care whether you're 60, 70, or 100, it's still going on, and the cleaner you are, the less vulnerable you are to these things. We've got to be aware that detox is just as important when you're older as when you first get into this. Long term Vitamin B12 deficiency could be a factor in dementia and Alzheimer's.

GABRIEL COUSENS

The answer is absolutely yes. But one of the things to understand is that the mental functioning is compromised with excess sugar intake. As I pointed out earlier, there is a decrease in the mental function with glucose and fructose. People who had the highest intake of carbohydrates were 1.9 times more likely to develop cognitive impairment as compared with those with the lowest, as shown in some recent research.

Sugar fuels the brain, and when people eat a diet high in sugar, they often go into insulin resistance, as we see with Alzheimer's. The blood sugar then cannot enter brain centers such as the hippocampus. The ensuing glucose deficiency affects the memory centers, bringing on senility. As I mentioned earlier, consuming coconut oil converts ketones very quickly and supplies a great deal of energy for the brain. This is a way to get around it. The brain must also be relieved of heavy metals, aluminum, mercury, and lead, for all of which, the gentle use of NCD is helpful. Gluten and gliadin grains have been shown to contribute to senility and Alzheimer's, if one is sensitive. Forty percent of the population is estimated to carry this sensitivity.

"There are many things we can do to prevent brain shrinkage."
- Gabriel Cousens

Aerobic exercise for 30 minutes, 4-5 times a week, can have a dramatically positive effect in prevention and treatment of Alzheimer's disease. Additionally, adequate hydration and nutrition is key. Vitamin B12 supplementation is especially vital, and many herbs can also help protect against Alzheimer's.

Brain shrinkage can be mitigated with adequate B12 supplementation, and prayer has even been shown to prevent brain shrinkage. High blood pressure, diabetes, and smoking all negatively impact brain function. Low hormone function also affects brain function, and a high stress environment will also shrink brain size. There are many things we can do to prevent brain shrinkage, as well as a whole variety of nutrients that can be used to protect against it. A moderate vegan ketogenic diet is very important for protecting against Alzheimer's disease and dementia.

69. I HAVE ARTHRITIS, WHAT SHOULD I DO?

VIKTORAS KULVINSKAS

Ana Schwartz, of the King Gustav Institute in Scandinavia, published that 85% of it is caused by the consumption of pasteurized dairy products. Then, the other components are animal protein and cooked foods in general.

The answer is, basically, get on true plant-based alkalinity, not acidic pasteurized dairy products, and start drinking celery juice. Minimum would be one quart per day. Get on a vegan program and start taking enzymes. You will find that the condition will get better every year. You can become pain-free within a matter of a month.

The other thing that will help is soaking in a saltwater bath, three pounds of salt, soaking for one to two hours, and allowing your feet to soak in hot water, where you add one cup of salt.

GABRIEL COUSENS

About 95% of osteoarthritis is healed with juice fasting for one to two weeks. Avoiding a cuisine high in sugar, processed food, GMOs, and other junk food, and eliminating meat, fish, chicken, and dairy from the cuisine really helps tremendously in the overall curing and maintaining relief from arthritis.

"Arthritis is relatively easy to heal when one eats a healthy diet. I also recommend the avoidance of all grains—of course if one is eating 100% live food that's not a problem. It's important to note that a variety of food allergies can cause arthritis." – Gabriel Cousens

Gentle yoga is very good for supporting the healing of osteoarthritis. One patient, a lady who was 92 years old with diabetes, hypertension, and wheelchair-bound due to debilitating osteoarthritis, came for my Diabetes Recovery Program. In three weeks, on a 100% live food cuisine and a little fasting, she was free from her wheelchair and has not been back in the wheelchair since. That's at 92. She also healed her diabetes and her high blood pressure.

Arthritis is relatively easy to heal when one eats a healthy diet. I also recommend the avoidance of all grains—of course if one is eating 100% live food that's not a problem. It's important to note that a variety of food allergies can cause arthritis.

BRIAN CLEMENT

Dr. Anna Maria, when I met her back in the late 1970s in Stockholm, Sweden, was directing Europe's most famous center on reversing arthritis naturally. Unlike North America, the Swedish government supported millions of dollars worth of research. They went in and showed them why what they were doing worked, and advocated the use of a raw plant-based diet to reverse arthritis. Research showed that and sent people there. We have been using not only what Hippocrates developed over the last 60 years, but what Dr. Anna Maria developed at the Brandal Center in Stockholm, Sweden over the decades with Alma Nissen, the founder of that center. Rheumatoid arthritis is something that is always correctable—osteoarthritis is correctable in almost all cases. We use electromagnetic cold laser therapy, and movement, and physical therapy, depending upon the state of the arthritic person.

FRED BISCI

Change your lifestyle. Change your diet. No two ways about it. I see people who are bone-on-bone, walking around pain-free because they're on the right diet. After my car accident, three specialists all said I needed shoulder replacement surgery on both shoulders. I didn't do that and I have no pain. I exercise very strenuously. If I weren't on this diet, I'm absolutely positive that I would be in a lot of pain. If you have arthritis, get into a plant-based diet. Detoxify your body. Reduce or eliminate animal protein. Get all the unnecessary hormones, chemicals, and pesticides out of your system. Drink plenty of clean water. Investigate Qigong. Drink plenty of juices and detoxify, detoxify.

70. CAN DIET HELP WITH HORMONE BALANCE?

GABRIEL COUSENS

Yes. A plant-source live food cuisine, properly applied, will help with all levels of hormone balance.

BRIAN CLEMENT

Can diet help to correct hormone balance? No doubt. Is it enough, on its own, all of the time? The answer is no. This is why, at times, we use bio-identical hormones prescribed by a physician who's an expert and well-seasoned in this. Bio-identical hormones became popular because of the implosion, thank goodness, of mainstream pharmaceutical hormones that were directly and clearly linked to cancer. On the other hand, you need to have a well-seasoned person who was doing this far before it became popular, having a lot of experience. Again, as any honest Elder will say, we made enough mistakes early on to now know what not to do, and as mentioned, that's the type of woman or man you want to work with.

VIKTORAS KULVINSKAS

Yes, on the most obvious level in reference to the fact that over 60% of our couples of reproductive age are sterile. You can rejuvenate reproductive function, which is hormonal, by adding sprouted grains. Within a matter of 6 months of eating sprouted grains at least once a day as a cereal, you will regain your fertility and libido.

On a more serious level, whereby the hormone system continues to deteriorate, lets look at why. It's a combination of toxemia and malnutrition. Toxemia especially, the kind that is mucus-forming incompletely metabolized proteins, as well as dairy products, coat these ductless glands which are hormone producers, reducing the absorption of nutrients—while at the same time reducing the excretion hormones necessary for regulating body function and an optimal life. So, the combination of cleansing and detoxification is of the highest priority for regaining the function of the organs, the functioning of the hormone system.

Then of course, overcoming the malnutrition. The best type of foods would be the sprouted seeds—which would include lentils and mung beans, as well as baby greens—wheatgrass, sea veggies and blue-green algae. Fasting and detoxifying herbs, especially cayenne, play a big part. Furthermore, you would do well to get involved in yoga and Qigong practices.

For instances for thyroid issues, you would want to consume sea veggies, do shoulder stands, plow position, neck exercises, all of which would be extremely helpful. You can rejuvenate and regenerate your system through the use of adult stem cell accelerators that are becoming popular, these are nutritionally based, as well as some of the human hormone nutraceuticals. By improving your sleep patterns, you will be regenerating the whole body, including the hormonal systems. I have found some very good natural herbal products that help in having long, deep and restful sleep, which you can find at www.viktorasconsultations.com.

FRED BISCI

Yes, it can. Many women on a plant-based whole food diet, devoid of processed food, go into menopause with no symptoms; no hot flashes, no irritability, no problems. Menopause is supposed to be a beautiful time in a woman's life. Estrogen production doesn't stop completely, it just goes down to non-reproductive levels. A poor diet causes even less estrogen production, along with disturbance in the hypothalamus, which controls our body's temperature, leading to the hot flashes.

Bio-identical hormones are not the answer. It's a total misinterpretation of what we're supposed to be like. A lot of men think that if they don't have the libido of a lion they're losing their manhood. You never were supposed to be that way in the first place. Sexuality is supposed to be the fulfillment of a bonding, loving relationship between a man and a woman. You could be 90 or 100, and if you've been living a healthy lifestyle, if you and your partner want to be sexually active at that point, you should be more than capable.

71. FOR INJURIES, WHAT IS THE BEST WAY TO DIAGNOSE? SHOULD WE AVOID X-RAYS, CT SCANS AND MRIs?

VIKTORAS KULVINSKAS

X-rays, CAT scans and thermographs. First of all, at the time of injury, the immediate reaction should be—especially if you break something or injure it through blows—to do the laying on of hands, putting the left hand on the area of trauma and the right hand diagonally opposite. If that is impossible try to use just even the polarity of thumb and index finger. That would be number one.

Secondly, get a diagnosis by whatever methods are being recommended by your physician. I would not worry about radiation associated with hopefully infrequent accident occurrence. The consumption of green things, green foods and blue-green algae will protect you from the radiation.

FRED BISCI

Yes, try to avoid these things if you can, but if you have a severe injury, or if you have something wrong and you're not sure and it could be life threatening, you have to weigh the benefits against the side effects. You have to determine the cause of the problem. The radiation in CAT scans is probably 100 times more than in X-rays. With X-rays, the effect of radiation is cumulative, so you definitely want to avoid it where possible, like at the dentist's office. They may say, "Oh, you're getting as much radiation as if you're out in the sun," but since it is cumulative, it can be a factor in developing diseases down the road. MRIs are safer, but you've still got to be careful. Consult with somebody who understands this and is going to give you an objective evaluation based on what's best for you and not what's best for their pocketbook. Remember, with a live plant-based whole food diet, you might rarely need this kind of evaluation.

BRIAN CLEMENT

Sadly, today the state-of-the-art in diagnosis all have side effects. X-rays, CT scans and MRIs, all of these give radiation to the body. It's easy to find on the Internet research that shows exactly how bad scans are and that the more often you take them, the more cumulative the radiation is in the body. But on the other hand, we are resigned to the fact that some of these must be used or we can't really get a true understanding of what's going on in the person. You can't walk around and just make believe an injury hasn't occurred, because injuries can become permanent abnormalities if they're not corrected properly. You can reduce the effect of radiation by just living on the Hippocrates or similar lifestyle, and by taking large amounts of fresh water and saltwater algae before, during, and after this period of time. Reduce or avoid as many of these scans as you can, but use common sense to determine when you actually need them.

GABRIEL COUSENS

It is best to make a clinical diagnosis if possible.

I had a torn cartilage in my left knee from playing football. I could reach in and feel the complete cartilage torn. No X-rays were taken. Treatment was very simple: 100% live food cuisine and yoga. After a period of time I was able to sit in full lotus for three hours, and I haven't had any further trouble with this for the last 50 years.

However, it would be foolish, if an X-ray, a CT scan or MRI were really needed, to avoid such a thing. There are times these may be appropriate. One must really ask the doctor how necessary it is. That's the key idea here. They shouldn't be used frivolously. They shouldn't be used as preventative screening, because all that radiation builds up over a lifetime. For example, the more that breast tissue is exposed to radiation, the more likely a woman is to get breast cancer. For breast screening it is best to use infrared.

72. IF I TOOK A LOT OF ANTIBIOTICS AS A CHILD, IS THIS GOING TO AFFECT ME AND HOW DO I REPAIR MY BODY FROM THE DAMAGE DONE, IF ANY?

FRED BISCI

If you took a lot of antibiotics as a child it could possibly affect you as an adult. It could affect your immune system and your intestinal flora, allowing the trillions of bacteria that are in our digestive tract (pathogenic) to cause us problems. You can reverse the effects of long term antibiotics with probiotics, enzymes, colon cleansing, a plant-based diet and detox. Proper elimination is critical.

GABRIEL COUSENS

Any good rancher knows that if you give antibiotics to animals, particularly as babies, they gain weight. Indeed, children who've had a lot of antibiotics tend to be overweight.

Adequate probiotics are extremely important for our health, our immune system, and our overall wellbeing. Surprisingly, they are actually part of our biochemistry and are needed for certain biochemical reactions that maintain health. The best thing one can do is take probiotics on a regular basis. Breastfeeding plants a health-producing lifelong culture. Taking antibiotics as a child can seriously damage our basic lifelong culture. Most children's health issues are better handled with homeopathy and other natural remedies.

Sauerkraut and kimchi deliver as much as ten times higher amounts healthy probiotics into the system as do probiotic supplements. If one must take antibiotics, it is important to at least double probiotic import for several months.

BRIAN CLEMENT

Yes, of course it will affect you, because antibiotics weaken the immune system. How do I repair my body of the damage? The good news is, the body is constantly morphing and regenerating. Every seven years, you have a totally brand new body. Parts of your body and your brain take 2 ½ days to regenerate, the stomach lining five days, the heart 30 days, the lungs 70 days—and all of these are constantly getting brand new cells. If they were not, we probably all would have died at a very, very young age because our bodies become irreparable without change. And when change happens, moving from bad to good, we're renewing and cleaning up and healing the damage we've done. Yes, you're going to eventually be able to get rid of that, the only concern would be, you may have created scar tissue, and even healthy cells morph into scar tissue. The healthier you become, the less scar tissue you have.

VIKTORAS KULVINSKAS

Primarily, everything is capable of being rejuvenated. Enzyme deficiency, B complex deficiencies, especially B12 and all of those sorts of things can be corrected through nutritional means. Mainly through a high volume of enzyme usage with meals and in between meals, in conjunction with the consumption of sauerkraut, probiotics and good sources of the vitamin B complex, found in sprouted grains and legumes can help. Everything is reversible. Do not worry. Be happy.

73. CAN MENTAL HEALTH DISORDERS BE CONTROLLED OR ELIMINATED BY DIET? WHAT FOODS CAN COMBAT DEPRESSION AND ANXIETY?

BRIAN CLEMENT

Well, we do know a lot about that today and I would say in light of mental disorders, depression, etc., diet may be enough—avoid the sugars, take the proteins, take the essential fats, etc. In moderate to strong disorders, the inclusion of proteins have been very effective, everything from GABA protein to lysine and right down to targeted herbal supplementation can be used.

At Hippocrates, we use electromagnetic stimulant therapy, neuron therapy that's been proven effective. Even in light cases of depression and in sleep deprivation, this has been spectacular in helping people reverse those problems. The kind of foods that help to combat these, again, are high essential fats, the seeds, sprouted chia seeds and flax seeds, or, the easy to digest, highly usable algae that goes right through the blood brain barrier. We get 50 times more benefit from sprouted hemp seeds than just eating it in its shelled raw state is also helpful. At some level, walnut oil is good.

VIKTORAS KULVINSKAS

I will address the question on four different levels. First, what can be almost an immediate solution is a distraction strategy. Tapping on your scalp or any kind of motion to get you out of connecting with your thoughts. Instead, you end up paying attention to the external world instead of the internal world. Keep this going continuously through dance, song, breathing exercises as well as any physical activity including tapping.

Meditation works wonders and has been studied as such. Within a matter of minutes, the person who is depressed, their brain patterns go through quick immediate change as soon as they start engaging in this mind exercise. So, it's a simple and immediate solution that shifts your focus from what is going on internally by externalizing your attention, thus forgetting all about the irritable thought patterns which are registered as organic protein complexes created by your hypothalamus, as well as your pituitary and other glandular systems.

"Blue-green algae contains small chain amino acids and polypeptides which are the precursors to neurotransmitters that facilitate clear thinking." - Viktoras Kulvinskas

For over 70 years a Moscow Psychiatric Institute has successfully treated all forms of mental disorders with exercise and fasting, following it up with a vegan diet. All of it was essential and a five year follow-up showed full regression of these conditions. Besides activity and motion on a biochemical level what will help you is blue-green algae.

It will have further impact if you chew a few of the algae. If you do, it will give you a very holistic new feeding of your brain so that, even though you are in an acid depressed state, the alkalinity of the blue-green algae will increase electrovoltage operating the brain and you will be operating with a much larger brain capacity. Secondly the blue-green algae contains small chain amino acids and polypeptides which are the precursors to neurotransmitters that facilitate clear thinking. Also, it has five times more chlorophyll than wheatgrass, and as a result, it quickly starts increasing the red blood cell production, which will mean more oxygen throughout your whole system.

Other foods that will make a difference include green tea, which will put you into an improved state of activity and functionality. Chew on gotu cola. In Florida, you can go in the fields, it's one of the most common weeds that you could possibly find—it's everywhere. Just chew on a few leaves and you will change your whole outlook. You've heard that expression "gut brain?" Well, if your energy is stuck in your stomach due to indigestion—and most people are suffering from indigestion as well as malfunctioning immune systems due an inadequate amount of enzymes—the immune system will aggressively attack these protein molecules of negativity, gobbling them up. So taking enzymes with meals, as well as in between meals, you'll see a great clean up of the blood, which will provide increased energy availability out of the gastrointestinal tract.

The best food is no food just alkaline juices. That is celery, cucumber, wheatgrass, blue-green algae, sprout juices, etc. All of these will help you to start functioning on a higher level of consciousness, with increased energy available for your brain activity. Start fasting on liquids, get into an exercise routine, get plenty of rest, engage in holistic living and every day you will be experiencing improvements in your state of consciousness and how you feel about yourself.

In yoga, they teach you how to change your states of consciousness through the practice of breathing. That's pretty much what you get in cardiovascular exercise, as well as in any other physical activity. The more you engage in physical activity, the less you will be likely to be depressed, anxious. It will even increase your energy and vitality and you'll overcome fatigue.

I know many of you are on medication. You're taking one of hundreds of prescribed psychotropic drugs, and many of you are self-medicated. You are using the most popular antidepressant called coffee and cigarettes. Many of you are doing marijuana. Some of you are doing cocaine. The majority of you are doing socially accepted drugs, which are far worse. Is there a way of getting out of this vicious cycle? There is.

I have been there. I have been there with you. By seventeen, I had a bleeding ulcer. I had emotional disorders for which I started seeing a psychiatrist intermittently in my teenage years. Eventually, when I got to graduate school I had four years of psychotherapy included, also studying, part time, theories on personality, ego. Very superficial, but it did help me to start taking more and more personal responsibilitiy. The greatest help for me throughout all this has been fasting and meditation.

Eventually, I started working more and more with the real issues, which have to do with developing healthy relationships. A loving relationship with yourself, defining and getting to understand yourself as an entity, a human being. Giving birth to yourself. Nurturing yourself in ways that no one else could. No lover, no mother or father. You just have to do the whole thing yourself. Ask yourself what would a loving person do for this human body? The temple within which you live. That means taking it for walks, giving it loving thoughts, keeping negativity out. There are so many excellent techniques and books available in the market place. Find your style. Exercise, rest, fasting, meditation, etc.

By the time I was in my twenties, I was on medication, as well as drinking fifteen to twenty cups of coffee a day. So I know what it feels like to give up and to move into personal responsibility moving those demons, those toxic CDs that we just love to keep replaying in our life so now, we're only creating the new CDs, the new future, by working on our self on an ongoing way, moment to moment. You can notice when you're playing a negative CD. It's when you feel uncomfortable, anxious, depressed. Just check your head for what is going on inside of your brain and quickly, before even bothering to watch what's going on in the brain, start tapping. Start singing. Move your head, left, right. Move your eyes. Blow your nose. Take a deep inhalation. Tap dancing—move your body and immediately these negative thoughts disappear. Just keep on doing this, eventually, after many months of continued vigilance, they just don't visit you on a regular basis. Whenever they do visit or some new beasts start being creative, just keep doing the same things. Keep them out through activity. Namely, always invite messengers about what is going on externally in the real physical environment, and stop paying attention to the illusions of delusional CDs that were created in childhood and sometimes in adulthood.

Most of the things in our society are false. They're results of lies that have been inculcated in us and we make believe they are true. Whether it is religion, our parents, our teachers, politicians, military leaders and great teachers. Scientists who go around expounding truths, which are their own personal opinions, is a big part of it. And it's simple, even a child can understand it, your body will tell you that when you avoid taking responsibility for any kind of pain and hide away from the symptoms instead of treating and addressing the symptoms, and moving on, you end up becoming entrapped by these bogus CDs of illusion, disillusionment and depression.

Nutrition will make a big difference. Why the Russians had them use a vegan diet is because in the meat oriented diet, you are taking in the fear, pain and suffering of the slaughterhouse animals that are watching their brothers and sisters being killed. They register all of this through the actions of pituitary, pineal and hypothalamus as well as sensory matter and it becomes part of their flesh, part of their blood, and when you eat those corpses, you end up taking on the same fearful energetic vibration. Namely, you are in a slaughterhouse and you better be scared, you better be depressed and that's the way most people feel. You can numb yourself with alcohol and psychotropic drugs or you can start working on yourself. Gradually, as you get stronger and stronger physically, you can cut down gradually on the medications you're taking. Eventually, you may not need any of the medications that are being administered.

You need to get stronger continuously. Get in to lifestyle habits that are not going to be benefited by the psychotropic drugs. I will give you a simple example, which has to do with one of the alkaloids, which is marijuana. In their early history, individuals on a totally acid cooked food diet—which is pretty much what everyone eats—when they did marijuana, they felt improvements. They got strong alkaline rushes and their brain started working at a higher capacity. They started understanding that killing was wrong. They started understanding that living in cities was not a good idea. They started to understand that a vegan diet was an exceptional alternative, that relationships mattered. There were all kinds of wonderful discoveries.

But, as they started eating more vegan and lived in communities where they grew their own foods and ate food in a raw state, they became more and more alkaline and that marijuana, which temporarily neutralized acidity, was now moving the blood towards the alkaloid state, and they got into alkalosis which was experienced as a bum trip. Individuals that were sane gave up the use of marijuana. The ones that indulged in an acid vegan diet, which is a cooked vegan diet, continued to enjoy the temporary wonders of the usage of marijuana, which gave them a good trip, as one would say, because it temporarily still neutralized acidity without pushing them into alkalosis.

A much better approach, is to stay high all the time by being on an alkaline diet so you won't need the alkaloids—whether it's cocaine, marijuana, coffee or cigarettes—to feel blissful, which is your natural state. For more experience in all of this, join me at *viktorasretreats.com*, where we study blissology in nature, an experience which will transform your lives. I am in Costa Rica, we have year-round access. The whole idea is hydration, so that you sweat and you keep that gastrointestinal tract also in an alkaline condition so you don't develop pain and spasms as it's excreting these acids into the GI tract. If you keep your body hydrated, you'll feel comfortable, and end up sleeping better and coming out of this severe extreme acidosis. Indulge involvement in reflexology, acupressure—these will help speed the process of recovery because you open up the electromagnetic acupuncture meridian channels and electrical energy flows much more freely.

GABRIEL COUSENS

This is a particular specialty of mine, as a holistic psychiatrist. I describe in my book *Depression Free for Life*, healing over 90% of depression without medication. A nutritionally balanced, live food cuisine plays a big role in healing depression naturally, but it is only one of 5 components to an optimal approach.

For 80% of people with manic depression, cuisine can play a positive role in healing. One of the biggest pathological elements in any diet is high sugar, because it imbalances the blood sugar and depletes neurotransmitters. Imbalanced blood sugar disorganizes the brain function. There is a center called the locus coeruleus. When blood sugar gets too low, that center, which controls anxiety and depression, stops working properly. This results in increased anxiety and depression. The sugar blues are a real phenomenon.

A healthy, low glycemic, 100% live food cuisine can play a major role in healing this. Almost everybody who comes in with depression will have some sort of endocrine imbalance and so I focus on balancing the hypothalamic and pituitary adrenal axis. The thyroid, which is connected to depression, often needs to be healed, as well as the liver and pancreas.

Third, there are certain allergies that swell the brain. Gluten and gliadin allergies, which are now being found in 30-40% of the U.S. population, are big causal players in many forms of depression. About 40 years ago, when I was in training as a psychiatrist, I witnessed an injection of wheat extract into a perfectly calm person that brought that person into acute schizophrenic psychosis in about three minutes.

Certain foods create brain swelling and create serious mental imbalances, so one needs to be screened for all possible allergies in the bigger picture, to foods, as well as for paint and gasoline and other common environmental factors that one may be reacting to.

Another causal aspect of depression I often see is low omega-3s and low cholesterols. These contribute very much to anxiety, depression, and suicide. People low in long chain omega-3s and cholesterol will have two to six times more depression and/or rates of suicide. It is well documented that being low in long chain omega-3s and cholesterol often results in serious health consequences. I have discussed that all women with postpartum depression respond well to DHA. To prevent this, it is good to have cholesterol above 159.

One also needs to have a cuisine that's going to supply a great deal of vitamin B, vitamin C, and magnesium, as fundamentals, as well as vitamin E, and particularly B3, B6, and B12. Those are important factors for a properly functioning brain and mind. Cuisine plays a major role in mental and emotional equilibrium.

FRED BISCI

That's a good question, because every case is individual. I've had clients with paranoid schizophrenia who were able to live without medication by following a raw diet or a very healthy diet. Other people are not so successful, so you've got to be very careful. I don't want to say things that are not realistic and I don't want to make people think that they can't be helped. I believe that a good diet can help everybody to one degree or another, but you can't say how much good it's going to do to that person until they try it, because there are other factors involved.

Many mental health disorders are just a manifestation of toxemia. Fruits and vegetables and a plant-based diet are the basis of helping both physical and mental disorders. I cannot mention enough the importance of leaving out the processed food. I have seen many people, who by the elimination of processed food, have recovered good health

74. WHAT IS THE RELATIONSHIP BETWEEN SKIN CANCER AND SUNLIGHT?

VIKTORAS KULVINSKAS

With the rise of individuals moving from outdoor life to life within the office environment, skin cancer has increased radically. Skin cancer was practically unknown during the days when people lived under the sun, now we have toxic individuals going out to the sun, which causes an elimination of waste through the process of perspiration and the skin.

The toxins from the internal part of the body accumulate in the skin area, especially where perspiration is stopped by the greasy sun blockers, and the consequence is cancer. The sun is your friend. You are a solar battery. You need sunlight. Cleanse, detoxify and gradually increase the usage of sun.

Initially, get exposure for as many hours or minutes as possible before the 10:00 am sun and afternoon sun after 3 or 4:00 pm. Eventually, you can tolerate the sun at all stages of the day. However, you don't want to lie around, burning yourself and destroying your skin. Ageing can be accelerated through addictive sun baking.

BRIAN CLEMENT

What's ironic is, many years ago I started to get caught up in all of the research and data that was coming out saying that skin cancer is caused by the sun. Then, I took a step back and looked at the data coming out of Africa and South America looking at the indigenous people who are out in the sun seven days a week, close to the equator, which showed that they didn't have any higher incidents of skin cancer today than they had 50 years before.

This made me question what differentiated the Western white cultures from these indigenous people—

they certainly got far more sun than we do (it was their lifestyle). After the Second World War, we radically began an experiment where we poured into the body massive amounts of animal fat. Remember, people ate moderate amounts, or little to none, before that. As affluence grew, as the middle class grew, we aspired for more—and we aspired to be like the wealthy who overate, and became obese. The only really sick people in those days, in the 19th century and before the early 20th century, were the very elite and wealthy. We all became like them and we haven't stopped. Ironically now, the things that people aspired to eat that only the rich could eat 60 years ago, are what the poorest people eat the most of because they've been commodities that had been controlled and manipulated by governmental and industrial forces.

The poorest people eat the most sugar and the most fat. These used to be delicacies at one time. And to that, we now add heavy metals and chemicals. To go back, the number one way to boost the immune system is the sun. You asked that question earlier. Get out into the sun the immune system is being boosted, the immune system cells, the army, pushes the waste out—not out of your buttocks or your urinary track but out of your skin. The average person eliminates up to 2lbs of waste out of our skin, our largest organ, every single day. Guess what? Now we have heavy metals and fats and chemicals mixed together. Your skin becomes like a frying pan surface! You can now develop skin cancer. Once you've cleansed the body, the chance of getting skin cancer is very, very small. This is why we say, go out early in the morning, and two hours before sunset year round, no matter where you live and you can get sun. It's the number one way to get vitamin D, and we'll talk about that later. Make sure that you're getting that sunlight with natural fiber clothes on.

GABRIEL COUSENS

What is the role of sunlight and skin cancer?

I find that people eating a live food cuisine can be in the sunlight four times longer than other people. Joanna Budwig, with her use of flaxseed oil in the curing of cancer, also found this to be true.

I first noticed this for myself, as a Native American Sun Dancer having fair skin relative to my Native American brothers and the other dancers there. I was not sunburned, and at the same time I was the only one to complete four days without food and water. I also completed the Eagle Dance where I stood from sunrise to sunset hooked and tied to the Sundance tree. I was not sunburned from this sun exposure, where others, including Native Americans, did get sunburned.

One eating live foods takes in so much green sunlight energy that they literally resonate with the sunlight. It becomes food for them so that they don't get burned. Nevertheless, in general, people who put a lot of junk on their skin and eat a lot of junk food tend to have a lot of toxins accumulating in their skin as the skin's trying to eliminate them. That interplay between those toxins and junk sunscreens creates conditions conducive to skin cancer.

Research has shown that people living in nature, without necessarily eating a non-junk food cuisine, yet maintaining ample outdoor activity, had less skin cancer than people living in the city environment and consequently spending more time indoors.

FRED BISCI

If you're a very toxic person living on all kinds of garbage and you're a sun worshipper, there's a very good chance that you could develop skin cancer. Sunlight is actually very healthy, as long as you don't get a burn, and it draws all those endotoxins out to the surface of your body. That's why a lot of people who don't eat a good diet and are out in the sun a lot have brown spots on them. A person on a good diet can sunbathe in moderation and get the benefits of the sun as long as they don't burn their skin. Skin cancers *"Vitamin D deficiency is a factor in cancer and that includes skin cancer." - Fred Bisci* are not coming from the sun; they are coming from burning from the sun, which draws out endogenous materials onto the skin. A recent study shows that there is a large Vitamin D deficiency in Florida and Hawaii.

153

How can that be? It is commonly believed by people in the health field that this is caused by the extensive use of sun block. It is a proven fact that Vitamin D deficiency is a factor in cancer and that includes skin cancer.

75. SO MANY PEOPLE SEEM TO BE GETTING AUTOIMMUNE DISEASES. WHY IS IT BECOMING SO PREVALENT AND HOW CAN I PREVENT IT?

VIKTORAS KULVINSKAS

The answer is, go back to a plant-based diet, enzymatic nutrition support of probiotics and you will overcome immune system dysfunction.

FRED BISCI

I have my doubts about the term autoimmune disease. I personally don't believe that there is such a thing. I have seen plenty of people with so-called autoimmune diseases change their lifestyle, get into a good diet, do very heavy detox and go into remission, so I don't believe in labels any more. I try to focus on the bottom line, results. I believe autoimmune disease is just another manifestation of toxemia like many other illnesses. Change your lifestyle. Experience the truth.

BRIAN CLEMENT

When you hear the word autoimmune diseases coming from the mainstream medical field, it usually really means, "We don't know what this is, we're going to call it an autoimmune disease." They reduce it down to a staggering embellishment and they say to people, to the patient "Your immune system is attacking you." This is not correct. A better way to describe it is, when you've done enough wrong for long enough, not slept enough, not eat right, being under an enormous amount of stress—pollutants come into your body, etc. Your immune army becomes weak, they become like drunken soldiers, and the drunken soldiers can no longer protect you.

"How do you correct it? By doing everything that we've even talking about throughout this entire book." - Brian Clement

Now, the way to place this in the minds of people is that you have an inadequate, drunken immune system that's incapable of keeping everything in order. Remember, disease is disorder, out of order. That's how you have these so called "diseases." How do you correct it? By doing everything that we've been talking about throughout this entire book. Think right, eat right, exercise, develop a spiritual value base, a virtue-based life, and develop passion and fulfillment. This is what we've seen 100% of these people able to correct their so called autoimmunity diseases with personal responsibility.

GABRIEL COUSENS

The autoimmune disease represents a disorder of the immune system where the body is so disordered it gets confused, and then goes against its own tissue because it can't identify the tissue.

Disease is chaos in the system. Health is order in the system. These autoimmune diseases are disorder in the system. The amount of radiation, chemical exposure, pesticides and herbicides, and junk food eating all contribute to this. With the use of 100% live food cuisine, high intensity proteolytic enzymes, and specific immune-boosting supplements, I have been successful in minimizing or eliminating these autoimmune diseases.

76. HEART ATTACKS ARE THE NUMBER ONE KILLER IN THE UNITED STATES. CAN A LIVING FOOD DIET HELP REPAIR DAMAGE DONE TO MY HEART?

BRIAN CLEMENT

Very soon, cancer will supersede heart attacks and strokes as the number one killer. Canada, in 2008, was the very first country ever to have cancer be the number one killer, even superseding heart attacks and strokes. Now, heart attacks and strokes, 97% to 98%, are not diseases. These are, like type 2 diabetes, lifestyle choices and the prescription is the same. Get up and start to move and exercise, eat proper food and get rid of stress in your life. It's the other 3% or so mechanical problems that are actually disorders or diseases.

The solution is to exercise, have a happy life, reduce stress and eat plant-based diets. Go back to Dr. Esselstyn's work out of the Cleveland Clinic. Nobody can doubt that, I mean, he has photographed the scans and shown how the arteries reverse the so-called, "plaques" and "diseases", through the methods I've just mentioned.

GABRIEL COUSENS

Absolutely. The main causes of heart attacks and cardiovascular disease has nothing to do with cholesterol. It's been well established by research that inflammation is the driving cause behind chronic disease. Trans-fatty acids and a high carbohydrate diet have been causally related to increasing rates of heart attacks and cardiovascular disease in general. The evidence of the biochemical pathways explaining this is well documented. I present some of these in my revised edition of *There Is a Cure for Diabetes*.

The research by Dr. Spindler showed that there is a 400% decrease in inflammatory gene activation with live foods. While we must acknowledge that genetics also play a role, research shows after the age of 40, genetics only play about 25% of the role.

All the men on my mother's side of my family died of heart attacks before age 50. On my father's side, most everybody died at a very early age before 60, the average age being 57. This is really about inflammatory diets and genetics. A live food cuisine can minimize the amount of inflammation and therefore significantly decrease the rate of heart attack. We are not bound by our genetics, and we can be elevated into enduring, radiant health by a properly applied 80-100% live food cuisine.

VIKTORAS KULVINSKAS

Enzymes are the flagship nutrient of the raw and live food movement. Enzymes are highly concentrated in sprouts and fermented foods.

Dr. Max Wolf of Fordham University created healing of all forms of cardiovascular diseases with enzyme saturation.

Dr. Gordon, a 30 year medical cardiologist MD, claims, "Doctors are doing a great disservice to their clients by not recommending enzymes. I have not lost a single patient in 30 years by having patients taking enzymes before and between meals."

By going on an enzymatically rich, nutritional program, which consists of alkaline juices, sprouts and fermented foods, you will not only rejuvenate your enzyme levels...but also end up cleaning out your blood vessels and returning your system back to a totally normal cardiovascular health. Personally, I've seen hundreds of people achieve those results. Getting off all medications in a short period of time, like 3-5 weeks and coming back into full function, be it simple daily life, mental and spiritual rejuvenation or even competitive athletics.

Cardiovascular health, just like any other condition, is reversible. The body heals itself, all you have to do is remove the causes. Heat treated animal protein, pasteurized dairy products and to a smaller extent, sedimantary lifestyles, sugar, white flour products and all the heat treated oils all have a less-than-optimal effect on the human body. Everything improves physically when you address your dietary choices and get on a predominantly raw, living foods program. For example, for breakfast have a green juice, half hour later a green protein smoothie with soaked seeds or nuts with dried fruit, a capsule of probiotics, blue-green algae and other favorite herbs. You can also add other greens such as kale or cilantro, then blend it all with water to a cream. Lunch can be a simple green salad with an emphasis on sprouts, especially fenugreek, alfalfa, mung bean, lentil with some buckwheat lettuce and/or sunflower greens.

Your evening meal can consist of a big green salad. For dressing you can blend 1/2 avocado with cup of cucumber, 1 clove garlic, 1/4 tablespoon of sea salt and the juice of 1 lemon with half cup of water and cayenne pepper to taste. You can also include some steamed kale, califlower or baked squash.

For extra, rapid rejuvenation of depleted enzyme reserves, take enzymes with all your meals. Enzymes between meals is very important, especially systemic enzymes or strong potency enzymes like "Meltaway" or "Astraextra" between meals to clean out the cardiovascular system. They should always be taken on an empty stomach. If bowel management is an issue, use "Internal Cleanse" and take 4 capsules at bedtime. Make sure you're very well hydrated by drinking not only additional green juices but also adequate amounts of water that is appropriate for your body weight. Go out daily for walks...enjoy your life. Don't do anything that leads to discomfort or pain. If the cleansing reactions are to hard to manage...add more steamed vegetables to your diet.

FRED BISCI

Most heart attacks are caused by coronary artery disease, which is where your coronary arteries or the other arteries in your body are blocked, and that's coming directly from your diet and your lifestyle.

I've even seen the benefits of a living food diet in my dog. He stepped on a hypodermic needle and got septicemia that damaged his heart muscle and he had a couple of weeks to live. I had him on a raw food diet with raw animal protein, but I switched his diet to blended salads and raw egg yolks and he lived a year and a half, which the veterinarians couldn't believe.

Coronary artery disease is correctable. I believe that is pretty common knowledge that it can take place on a vegan diet. To answer the question, "Can I repair damage to my heart?" That requires a different answer. Of course, there is positive help. Sometimes there is damage to the heart muscle itself, where the pathways to cellular regeneration of the heart tissue might be irreversible. Nobody knows where that point is. The human body is remarkable. This can work sometimes where all else fails.

77. HOW DO YOU DEFINE CONSTIPATION? WHAT DISEASES CAN RESULT FROM CONSTIPATION?

VIKTORAS KULVINSKAS

An exceptional article with over 300 documentations can be found in my book Life in the 21st Century, written many years ago. Every form of disease has its origin in toxemia and toxemia is generated by constipation, which comes from acidic dietary lifestyle choices. Normal evacuation will take place easily on a plant-based diet with high amounts of fiber and the consumption of friendly bacteria.

GABRIEL COUSENS

At the causal level of constipation is a lack of apana, which is the downward force. I found in the live-food study by one of my Spiritual Nutrition Masters students, that constipation dramatically decreased on a live food diet. It was more than a fourfold decrease.

Constipation is, obviously, inadequate bowel function. In our study of over 525 people on at least an 80% live food cuisine—there was a significant decrease in constipation. But, part of the definition of constipation also has to do with your constitution. If you are a kapha, you're more likely to be going once a day, but pittas and vatas really need to be going two to three times a day.

Now, when people went on a live food diet, there was a significant improvement in their constipation tendency. In the study with 525 people, the percentage of people reporting two or more bowel movements daily increased from 25% to 78%—a threefold increase in bowel function.

Those complaining of constipation decreased from 73% to 30% on a live food cuisine. Live food, being well hydrated, and the fiber in live food all contribute to a more normal physiology. All manner of chronic disease is related to constipation because all the un-eliminated toxins are re-circulated back into the system affecting physical, emotional, and mental states. Dr. Bassler's study in 1933, about autointoxication with 5,000 people, showed that almost every disease imaginable was associated with constipation and could be reversed by detoxing the bowel.

BRIAN CLEMENT

Constipation means that you're not evacuating fecal matter at least once a day. Now, ideally in the healthiest people I know, and I haven't quite achieved this yet, two to four hours after they've eaten a solid meal, it's evacuated. If you are evacuating minimally once a day, and you're evacuating the majority or all of the waste out of your body, that is fine. If that's not happening at least on a daily basis, you're constipated. Now, I grew up in a household where my mother prided herself on not going to the bathroom for a week at a time when she would be on a holiday. I thought that was normal. Of course as a child, you watch your parents and the people around you, and that's how you learn what is normal or not.

If you have waste inside of your body, it seeps through and gets into the blood stream, you become septic, that means poisoned, and as you become poisoned, you become more acid, and that leads to becoming more vulnerable to diseases. It's that simple. What type of disease? Every known disease, more headaches, more nausea, more mental illness—all of these things are resulting effects of inflammation constipation.

FRED BISCI

Constipation is improper elimination of what is in your bowels. Constipation is a problem that should not be ignored. Just because you're moving your bowels every day doesn't mean you're not constipated. If what you ate three or four, or even six or seven days ago is coming out of you today, even if you're moving your bowels twice a day, you're constipated. It's not moving through you fast enough. What you eat today, if you're clean, should be coming out of you tomorrow and if it's not, you're constipated. If you're constipated, you have a perfect nesting place for bacteria. You're overworking your intestinal flora. It might be losing the battle there.

"Constipation is a problem that should not be ignored." - Fred Bisci

I believe that just about any disease can evolve from constipation because most of our diseases originate in the GI tract. When you're constipated, sooner or later, your body is going to stop breathing on a cellular level. You're not going to get the oxygen you really need, and you're going to be getting a lot of other stuff delivered to your cells from your GI tract that don't belong there. This is a factor in all diseases, especially cancer.

78. DO GENETICS AFFECT YOU? I HAVE RELATIVES WHO EAT HORRIBLE DIETS, DRINK AND SMOKE—YET ARE STILL GOING STRONG INTO THEIR 80s. DO I ASSUME I INHERITED THEIR GOOD GENES? OR SHOULD I TAKE PRECAUTIONS?

GABRIEL COUSENS

Everybody has a certain destiny. Everybody has a certain genetic play, but again, after the age of 40, genes only play 25% of the role.

What I'm saying is, those people not living in a healthy way into their 80s are seriously compromising their ability to live longer and with vitality. Remember the quote about Moses—he lost none of his natural health and vitality. At age 120 "his eyes were not dim nor his natural force abated." (Deuteronomy 34:7) In other words, maybe these people are living into their 80s, but could actually have the potential to live much longer. However, their health is compromised because they're not living at their potential. The idea is not to live long, but to live up to your energetic potential at every moment.

FRED BISCI

Everybody should take precautions. Let's take a good look at the people doing everything wrong and living into their 80s. Most likely, they're on medication. Most likely, they had some type of surgery. A lot of people are living in nursing homes with dementia or Alzheimer's disease, or they're in wheelchairs, on oxygen. The quality of life isn't there, no two ways about it. People following a raw living food diet or a vegan diet or a diet with minimal animal protein, generally have a high quality life when they live to an advanced age.

Just because you know somebody who is 80 years old and doing all the wrong things doesn't negate the fact that, for most people to make it to 80 years old and beyond still running around, dancing, putting in full days, with all their faculties, they need to make healthy choices because it's what we do that affects the expression of our genes. A bad diet takes its toll on everyone. Don't look for excuses to do the wrong thing because it might not pan out for you.

Another thing to think about is that 80 years ago (1934 and on) the general population ate fresh foods and very little processed foods. They learned to eat small portions and there were no fast food and take-out places. They ate less animal protein because of financial reasons and really focused on a plant-based diet. I know this first hand because I was a product of this era.

BRIAN CLEMENT

We'll try to answer this in an easy way. Before the Second World War, all food was organic. Television did not exist, radio was relatively new, stress loads were low, pollutants were minimal, and corporations were not creating massive heavy metals and harmful chemicals and putting them in the environment. The population of the world was less than half of what it is today - more people equals more problems and more waste—all of these things radically changed after the Second World War and now have gathered together to create a perfect storm.

Your 80 year old relative was built in a much more solid and strong way anatomically, and had an inheritance of a genetic system that was stronger. The degradation of human structure DNA and genetics over the last three or four generations has been catastrophic. There's no easier way to say that, so you are not the same person as your relative.

In the Caucasian cultures, the only remnant—and I mean Remnants with a big R—that we see with strong genetics come out of the Polish and Russian populations. There's no other culture generally that has strong genetics in any way. That is going away because they have been corrupted by the media and fast food world.

What you have to know is that people got away with a lot because they had a good foundation, a good beginning. You did not have a good foundation and beginning.

If you look at the *Okinawan* studies, one of the populations of the world that lived long lives, yes, most or all of what they eat is a plant-based diet, they exercise, they have great attitudes, and a wonderful cultural structure. Even those who smoke cigarettes and drink, because they have a genetic reserve, live the way their ancestors did hundreds of years ago, they don't get cancers and heart disease and strokes the way we do, but they are not you. Don't rely on fantasy, rely on common sense and reality, and then you'll be participating in protecting your health.

VIKTORAS KULVINSKAS

In my book *Physiognomy*, I show the visual science of genetic degeneration. It's shown by the nose structure when the nose is flat with wide nostrils. It's an indication of strong heart and lungs. The longer are your ear lobes, the stronger is your detoxifying ability of the kidney and liver. Most kids nowadays in their 30s and 40s and younger have no ear lobes, indicate that they are not going to last too long, unless they change to vegan live food.

Over 25% of the clients at Hippocrates suffering with old-age degenerative disease are being brought to the institutes by their mothers and fathers—parents are bringing in their children! We are living at a time when the parents will outlive the children, unless the parents and the children switch to a live food diet.

If you get on the live food program, you will not only greatly reduce the potential experience of any of those diseases, but also your longevity will be totally increased far beyond your grandparents who might have lived to their 80s and 90s.

MIND/BODY CONNECTION

"The more you become alkalized, the more you do liquid programs, the increased intuition, psychic abilities, all this will become natural phenomena." - Viktoras Kulvinskas

"Without a doubt, the live food cuisine greatly enhances our ability to become superconductors for the Divine. It balances mind-body-spirit in a way that makes it a wonderful connection."
- Gabriel Cousens

"Absolutely, especially if you're on a 100% raw living food diet, you're not eating a lot, you're doing periodic cleanses four times a year for each season, and you're meditating and praying. You're going to become a totally different person." - Fred Bisci

"The diet, in spite of my own staggered and stagnant negative attitude, provoked change." - Brian Clement

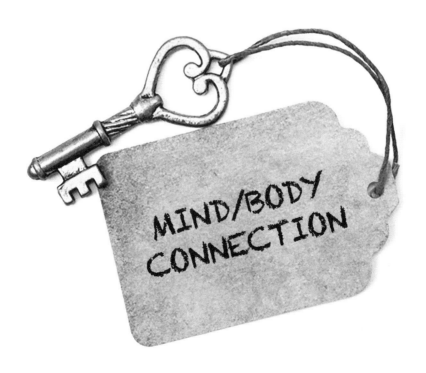

79. WHEN INCORPORATING MORE RAW LIVING FOOD INTO MY DIET, WILL I NOTICE A DIFFERENCE IN MY MIND BODY SPIRIT CONNECTION—POSSIBLY HEIGHTENED AWARENESS?

GABRIEL COUSENS

It is highly likely. That is why I became interested in live food. I was specifically searching for a cuisine that could enhance the mind-body-spirit connection and help people become superconductors of the Divine. Without a doubt, the live food cuisine greatly enhances our ability to become superconductors for the Divine. It balances mind-body-spirit in a way that makes it a wonderful connection. In our Masters study, 87% experienced an enhanced body-mind-spirit connection.

VIKTORAS KULVINSKAS

Your meditation will start becoming deeper. You cannot be a meditator and be successful at it on a meat-oriented diet. You have a scattered mind with a lot of suffering associated with the animals that you have consumed. Spirituality is impossible without ahimsa, that is, "do no harm." That means, don't go out killing other animals. You will see clarity of mind, sharpness of mind, cleverness, your intuition will increase. The more you become alkalized, the more you do liquid programs, the increased intuition, psychic abilities, all this will become a natural phenomena. If you are a meditator, you'll start increasing your mental maturity and sharpness. Instead of having an Einstein potential of functioning with 10% brain capacity you'll be operating at 20, 30, 50, even a 100% if you have mastered Samadhi, and have gone into the deepest levels of meditation.

For more information on this, read *Survival in the 21st Century*, Gabriel Cousens' book, *Spiritual Nutrition* and the many books on consciousness found at Hippocrates Health Institute.

BRIAN CLEMENT

This is going to happen. I mean, I was the most nasty, negative person you could ever imagine when I started this and one of the things that surprised me the most is how I started to have compassion, see things differently, love more, that's all I can say. The diet, in spite of my own staggered and stagnant negative attitude, provoked change. And then slowly but surely, I started to cultivate that and still aspire to become better, more open, happier, more loving and every day, I get a little bit better at doing that. Ultimately, life provokes life, and life is consciousness and awareness. We don't have to work hard on becoming conscious, that's a misnomer. Consciousness is omnipresent. It exists all of the time. We just have to allow consciousness to be—and it's right there for us to grasp.

I'm currently in a writing project that started with my colleague, Dr. Valerie Hunt, who recently passed in her late 90s. My objective is writing the new biology called *Quantum Human Biology*. I hope to publish that in the next two years and we speak mostly about what we're discussing right now and we can scientifically validate the biological effect of energetics in changing consciousness, awareness, etc. We don't want to start an elitist ideology, we just want to get back to our origin of consciousness and awareness. We've lost it, and it's not that we're going to become better at it. We're just going to become the way we're meant to be to begin with.

FRED BISCI

Absolutely, especially if you're on a 100% raw living food diet, you're not eating a lot, you're doing periodic cleanses four times a year for each season, and you're meditating and praying. You're going to become a totally different person.

That was my experience. I started out in life with difficulty learning to read. I didn't realize I was dyslexic.

It led to a problem with my self-esteem. I didn't want to go to school because it was embarrassing, and I really didn't think I had much of a future. Lo and behold, when I started paying attention to my nutrition, I started to see changes. Then I went into a vegetarian diet. I fasted for over 40 days twice and did other shorter juice fasts, and I transformed completely. My priorities and my spiritual beliefs changed dramatically and my consciousness opened up. When you make these changes you're going to develop a mentality that you can trust the logic in your mind, and you'll be able to apply that logic and use your intuition to vastly improve your life.

80. WILL THIS DIET/LIFESTYLE CREATE THE POTENTIAL FOR GREATER CONSCIOUSNESS AND SPIRITUAL CONNECTION?

BRIAN CLEMENT

Once again, absolutely, if you just use it correctly. It doesn't guarantee that you're going to become conscious and aware. As a matter of fact, I know a lot of people who eat right and don't do any work on looking at their demon, don't do any work on improving and developing and cultivating release. They're holding back the inevitable. Diet is going to give you the fuel to do that, now you have to take the step to move forward.

VIKTORAS KULVINSKAS

Yes it is essential. It's the sattvic diet in Bhagavad Gita that states very clearly: in order to be a spiritual aspirant, you need to be on a raw food diet. With it, you are increased into extension and moving into what is coming into our domain. It's called the one mind—we will be one mind. As a result, our bio computers link up and we will have the true humanity, the new frontiers of human evolution. We'll be one essence and we will function as one organism.

GABRIEL COUSENS

This cuisine will create potential for greater consciousness and spiritual connection. I did a study on one group of spiritual people, and I found that as they got involved spiritually, 95% naturally gravitated toward a live food cuisine.

I also find that given the right direction, people on a live food cuisine are more likely to find a greater enhancement of their spiritual life. My book, *Spiritual Nutrition*, specifically discusses this from every single angle.

Jesus, all of His disciples, and His brother James, were all at least vegetarians. James, the brother of Jesus, only drank water and ate vegetables and bread. The ancient Rishis were 100% live foodists and the Taoist sages were as well. Genesis 1:29 prescribed a live food vegan cuisine as the optimal cuisine for spiritual life 5,774 years ago. There's no question that this is the optimal diet to support spiritual life. The only question is, why aren't people choosing to follow it?

FRED BISCI

Yes, no doubt about it. You have to experience it to believe it. If you're doing it halfway, bouncing back and forth in your diet, eating a raw food diet while cheating a lot, it's not going to happen. I do recommend that you believe the people who are telling you that this is true, and take the steps you need to take to experiencing this for yourself.

81. DO YOU BELIEVE IN TELEPATHY, PREMONITIONS, AND OR TELEKINESIS? HAVE YOU SEEN EVIDENCE OF THIS IN YOUR MANY YEARS OF HELPING PEOPLE HEAL? CAN A HEALTHY DIET AND MIND OPEN UP SOME OF THESE HIDDEN POWERS?

GABRIEL COUSENS

Over time, on a live food diet, we increase our biophoton energy. That biophoton energy connects us to the biophoton field, and we become more connected to all there is.

In that process, there is acceleration in opening up telepathically and psychically. These things really do happen. When people eat a live food cuisine there is an increase in these abilities.

FRED BISCI

I'm not an expert when it comes to that, so I'm not going to make any outlandish statements, but I have seen that a healthy diet and mind can lead people to have unusually heightened insights into things. As far as telekinesis and telepathy, it's certainly possible but I don't have any experience with this sort of thing. Beyond a shadow of a doubt, by cleansing your chemistry you will develop an enlightened consciousness, with a better understanding of our role in nature, and be able to see the truth. I have also noticed that a negative attitude is a detriment to most kinds of change, including lifestyle. Those with a positive attitude will do much better and go much better in all lifestyle changes. We have to learn and experience what we don't know. Attitude helps.

BRIAN CLEMENT

The answer is yes. All of us instinctually have what we call ESP and we know what to do. I always say, just shut off the brain and think from the heart. The Chinese say it so well, they have two ways to think about the mind, the mind of the brain and the mind of the heart. The one they cherish is the mind of the heart. Your instinct always gives you the right answer. Now, when I go with my instinct, which I try to do all of the time, I don't make mistakes. When I go with my mind, I make mistakes quite often.

The way I like to describe this is, if you were on a beautiful sailboat and you were going across the Pacific Ocean from San Diego to Hawaii and in the middle of that trip, 50% there, the wind stopped and the sails went down and you heard the voice of God from Heaven and God said, "Now, we're going to give you an opportunity to see who you really are. We're going to make the rudder on this boat the mind and we're going to make the rest of the sailboat the heart. Now, if you think the mind is so important, take the rudder off the boat, jump into the Pacific Ocean and swim to Hawaii. If you think the heart is more important, throw the rudder over the side, stay in the sailboat and allow the tides to take you." The way I differentiate the mind from the heart is quite simple. We're not going to grab the rudder and try to swim 2,000 or 3,000 miles in the middle of an ocean. The rudder helps to gently and slowly move the heart, the instinct, the awareness in the right direction. But, you could actually live with just the instinct.

Ann Wigmore was wildly instinctual, thank God, and she instinctually understood how to spark the beginning of the raw and living food movement here in North America. Every great person I've ever met spoke from their heart, and those women and men have actually helped us all expand our understanding of our potential. So we all have that which we call telepathic or instinctual ESP. It's cultivated, but don't get mystical or new age about it. Any of you that has to create fantasy, you feel yourself lacking something. Your life is magnificent and magical to begin with, you don't have to create something—it already is beautiful.

VIKTORAS KULVINSKAS

All animals on their natural diet have intuition, a sense of premonition. During the last Tsunami in the Pacific Rim, over a quarter of a million people lost their lives, whereas animals were leaving the seashore days before the event happened. Raw foodism, alkalinity, certainly helps optimize the neurological functioning. Keeping stillness and quietness while fasting are the ultimate ways to increase premonition, psychic telekinesis.

I practiced telekinesis many years ago, and just by focusing my concentration, I could move objects at a distance. This is not at all an uncommon phenomenon, especially among many of the raw food people who still are also involved in the process of serious deep meditation and experimentation with projecting their consciousness. Of course, it has to do with genetic predisposition and with your astrology and the reasons for your incarnation. It's not an option that is readily available to everybody. Certain individuals are more predisposed than others through exploration of this kind of phenomena, but we all have unlimited powers accessible.

During fasting and practicing meditation, I was able to download all my study material that I never studied and scoring top grades without ever looking at the books, by practicing days at a time mindlessness and stillness.

82. WHAT KEEPS YOU MOTIVATED AND PATIENT ENOUGH TO KEEP HELPING PEOPLE?

BRIAN CLEMENT

If in life you learn this one thing, and nothing else I say today matters to you, this should matter to you. All human beings are universes unto ourselves, connected with the other universe, and all we have to do is find our mission, find our purpose and, on a daily basis, 24 hours a day seven days a week, fulfill that mission. Any of you who look at people who are devoted to what they do as heroic, you're wrong. We're not heroic.

"If you find your passion, it will help others around you, your family, your friends, humanity on a whole—the ripple effect, the domino effect is inevitable." – Brian Clement

What we're doing is what every human being should do, contributing, and why we contribute and why we do what we do I'm sure I'm speaking for all of the Elders and all of the people in the world who are contributing today is fulfillment. It's because we're fulfilling our own reality and, yes, in this case, we're working with lifestyle that helps to bring back people and prolong life. We are mono-focused inherently.

So, why we do what we do? Every one of us, the truthful ones of us, will tell you that we do it to perpetuate our own passion. If you find your passion, it will help others around you, your family, your friends, humanity on a whole—the ripple effect, the domino effect is inevitable.

VIKTORAS KULVINSKAS

Unlimited, unconditional LOVE for LIFE.

FRED BISCI

It is frustrating sometimes, especially with the confusion and the nonsense that's being promoted on the Internet. It is difficult to stay with it at times when I see people who fail because they don't stay on track, or people who come to see me when it's actually too late. But I stay motivated because I see a lot of wonderful results and miraculous changes. People often tell me how well they're doing and how their doctor can't believe what a wonderful recovery they made; or I hear from people who could hardly walk before who are now running. I've seen some great recoveries. First and foremost, I believe in God, and this has been my purpose. I believe that I am an ordinary person that God has given a small gift to, which was meant to be shared by helping others.

GABRIEL COUSENS

This is my dharma. When I was four years old, I knew I wanted to be a doctor. When I was eight or nine, I began having spiritual visions and seeing what I now know were the Essene elders, as well as the other healers in the Eastern and Native American traditions.

I was fortunate to open up to my healing interest. Healing was not part of my recent family tradition. I am from a Levite priesthood lineage in Bialystok, Russian (now Poland), but my immediate family were bakers, and they even helped created the Bialy. I have become more in alignment with the original Levite tradition started 3,200 years ago.

I am motivated because I enjoy it. I love to see the play of God in people. I love to see the joy, the spiritual unfolding in people as they get holistic insight into their healing process, and I love to see the joy of their healing and the whole activation of the spiritual enlightenment process.

But the truth is, my motivation doesn't depend primarily on that. My motivation is that it is truly my dharma, my life work, and it's the inner joy. My non-causal inner peace and inner love is actually what drives me. It's certainly enhanced by seeing so many people come back to life, which is part of my mission in helping people wake up to their purpose of life and to activate their spiritual energy with shaktipat/haniha. To see and experience a person light up from within is great joy. Spiritual nutrition supports this.

WATER/HYDRATION

"In the Western world, 60% of the population is dehydrated. 40% of the people in the West and probably worldwide, that I don't know, are lacking the mechanism in the brain that tells you to drink."
- Brian Clement

"Inadequate hydration means that there is not enough liquid through your system to excrete the waste products and you accumulate waste products due to lack of hydration."
- Viktoras Kulvinskas

"By the age of 60 and older, our level of hydration can get as little as 55 or 60%." - Gabriel Cousens

"Many people are sub-clinically dehydrated especially the elderly." - Fred Bisci

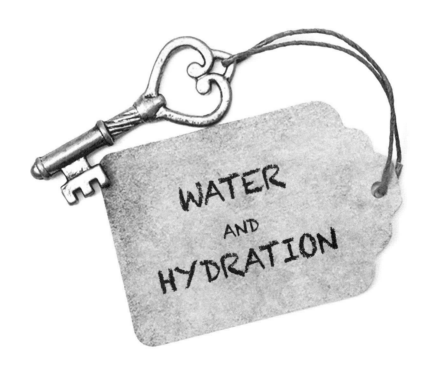

83. WHY IS WATER IMPORTANT AND WHICH IS BEST?

VIKTORAS KULVINSKAS

Our body is composed, at the start of our life cycle, from about 80% water. Inadequate hydration means that there is not enough liquid through your system to excrete the waste products and you accumulate waste products due to lack of hydration.

Any kind of water is better than no water, but our water systems are becoming more and more contaminated especially with plastics, medicines, etc. Over 60 of these pollutants have been identified coming out of all major city faucets, and none of the filters are able to eliminate it. There's only one effective system and that is distillation. You can get the least expensive water distillers, stainless steel, from about $100, from a water distiller company.

BRIAN CLEMENT

Hydration is the most important nutrient other than oxygen. The number one nutrient is oxygen, number two is water. Most of the oxygen your body gains every day comes from water and hopefully raw juices. So, water is hydrogen and oxygen, it needs to be pure, it needs to hydrate the cell and allow the brain to work with the greatest conduction of electricity. The neurons in the brain require water, 80% of the brain is made of it. You'll die if you're dehydrated and so, please don't avoid this one—go back to the facts I gave earlier. In the Western world, 60% of the population is dehydrated. 40% of the people in the West and probably worldwide— don't know they are lacking the mechanism in the brain that tells them to drink. You have to really, mechanically figure out how to drink and drink adequate amounts if you have this concern.

Everyone needs to drink a minimum of ½ of an ounce of pure water or raw organic juice, for every 1 lb. of body weight. For example, a 150 lb. person requires a minimum of 75 ounces of pure fluid a day. If they are in an arid climate, more, if they are in an arid climate and they're exercising, more, and exercising in a humid climate, even more.

GABRIEL COUSENS

Water is one of the most important factors for life. In fact, for life it's the most important factor besides air. There are basically three stages of how we relate to water. The first stage is as a fetus. In the uterus, the baby is floating at a very high level of water, close to 75% hydration. Stage two is growth. Until we reach full height and weight, somewhere between ages 18 and 25, we are not fully matured. Our cells are functioning at a pretty high level, and we move out of the kapha phase, which is really the highest amount of water. This occurs until pre-puberty, where we maintain a high level of hydration more naturally.

After that, around the age of 40, we enter another phase where we actually begin to diminish our degree of hydration. By the age of 60 and older, our level of hydration can get as little as 55 or 60%. Aside from this general process, dehydration is made worse by drinking coffee, soft drinks, and alcohol, and inadequate hydration.

Our hydration levels and needs change as we enter the different phases of life. The kapha stage (pre-puberty) is when we're the most hydrated. Pitta (post-puberty to approximately 45-60 years old) will sustain maximum hydration. Finally, there is a slow dehydration as we enter the vatta stage (age 60 onward), and one begins to more actively dehydrate. We must increase our efforts to stay hydrated with increasing age. A simple sign that we are adequately hydrated, given our kidneys are fine and we have no bladder infections, is if we urinate every two hours during the day.

The two simple ways to do this are: 1) drink more fluids and 2) add a little bit of high quality, living salt to the fluids we drink.

Adequate hydration is something that affects every organ of one's body. For example, drinking one or two glasses of water 15 minutes before eating creates a well-hydrated and cleansed stomach mucus barrier, which will then retain bicarbonate and neutralize acid as it passes through the mucus. Hydration will provide a much superior hydrochloric acid barrier and allow us to be much better protected from any sort of excess acidity.

We need water to adequately hydrate our lungs. The lungs control evaporative water loss through breathing. When that function isn't optimal, the bronchial can constrict, activating asthma.

Water is necessary for proper gastrointestinal tract function, so that we don't have our blood so concentrated that we're able to pull the digestive solid foods through the stomach and intestines and get them past the liver for further biochemical unfolding. It is important that we have adequate water to create blood that's able to absorb nutrients.

As an athlete, I'm aware that poor hydration can lead to inflamed joints. The reason for that is that water is a lubricant in our joints. When people do not have proper lubrication, it's easier to have joint inflammation and arthritis. I have suffered injuries to almost every joint, but I'm not having the usual arthritis. In fact, I have zero arthritis. I believe that's partly because I am well hydrated, and, as a result, the water protects my joints. With age we tend to dry out, and, of course, then our joints dry out, and we may have joint inflammation.

> *"Hydration will provide a much superior hydrochloric acid barrier and allow us to be much better protected from any sort of excess acidity." – Gabriel Cousens*

A dehydrated brain contracts and disrupts the function of the neurons, because they become contracted and the neurotransmitter flow is interrupted. In regards to hypertension, contrary to common belief, in dehydration, the vascular system will adapt and bring blood flow to critical areas, but in so doing, it may actually raise the blood pressure.

Perhaps the most obvious place where dehydration plays a role is on the intervertebral spinal discs. Seventy-five percent of our spinal column is water. The fibrous material in the discs supports only 25% of the spinal column. The point being that, when we're dehydrated, the space between our discs shrinks in size, and therefore our height diminishes. Therefore, we may have a general intervertebral contraction, putting pressure on the vertebral nerve and lymphatic fluid passing through the vertebrae.

When we are adequately hydrated, the spaces between the discs expand, allowing proper lymphatic circulation and proper nerve flow to our body. Proper hydration protects against sciatica and other problems that happen when the spine is compressed. Proper hydration also helps maintain our healthy height. By the age of 60, many people lose up to two inches off their height. At 70, with proper hydration and spinal hygiene, I may even be ¼ inch taller than when I was 20 years old.

Water plays an important role in many aspects of our life. A well-hydrated person lives longer and their mind thinks well. Some suggest that even 2% dehydration can negatively affect cognition.

The best water is spring water taken from within the first 10 feet of the head of the spring. Short of that, there are other waters available. One of the best is matured, distilled water. It is the cleanest water, which is important in this highly polluted world. Distilled water is valuable because radioactivity, pesticides, and herbicides are leaking into wells and into springs. We don't have any control over the water besides our ability to monitor it. The advantage of distilled water is that it is 100% free from of the pesticides, herbicides, heavy metals, toxins, and radioactivity. However, from my perspective, distilled water is still immature water and may not yield the most energy.

Once the water is distilled, I like to mature it, reactivate it, and restructure it. I do this through a particular process. Per gallon, I add 12 drops of ionic minerals, or it could be a pinch of a high-quality living salt. This brings the water to its optimal 50 parts per million. Next, I structure the water. This can be done through a variety of mechanisms. Once the water has been restructured, it can lose its structure under heat or exposure to sunlight. But if its structure is intact, water may hold considerably more energy. Life force energy is a whole science, part of which addresses how to build the life force energy of water.

Then, I create an implosive vortex in the water by stirring it with a wooden spoon and creating vortexes of energy. People have machines to do that too, but I prefer to do this manually. These vortexes of energy pull energy into the system. This technique reflects research that was done in the 1930s, so it's not a new idea. I vortex the water in both directions, bless it, and then put it out under the moonlight. Moonlight resonates very strongly with the quality of the water and further increases the energy.

If one is not able to put it out under the moonlight, one could also put on a Tachyon disc, which further energizes the water. Now we have fully energized water.

The next issue is the pH of the water. Based on all the research I've seen, and based on the way that nature gifts us, except for some rare circumstances, the pH of pure spring water is between 6.5 and 7. Slightly acid water seems to be the more optimal water. Of course, distilled water and rainwater are all slightly acidic or neutral.

In the short term, alkaline water has helped people get a temporary alkalization. However, some of the Japanese research suggests the long-term use of alkaline water may be detrimental because the highly alkalized water acts like light acid, in a sense, and may melt the cell. This is a controversial point, but it is certainly a point worthy of careful consideration. I do not recommend alkalized water on a long-term basis.

FRED BISCI

Water is a solvent and a transport medium. A large portion of your body is water. It is extremely important that you stay hydrated. Many people are sub-clinically dehydrated especially the elderly. In order to detoxify your body, you have to make sure your water is clean. Your water must be pure; you want to drink clean water that doesn't have any additives and has a low Total Dissolved Solids (TDS) factor so you know it doesn't have a lot of chemicals in it. You can get your water tested to make sure it's clean. Vitamin waters and all these waters with additives are completely unnecessary, as far as I'm concerned. You're wasting money. I am not a big fan of bottled water. Some of the bottled waters that were tested had too many dissolved solids and chemicals I myself have a very good filtration system on the main source of water entering my house, and a reverse osmosis system that comes from the main filter to our showers and kitchen water.

SUPPLEMENTS

"The one that everyone requires, period, without any more consultation, is a bacterial form, a living form of B12."
- Brian Clement

"Ninety-nine percent of the people are enzyme deficient, and enzymes rule not only the digestive function, but also the immune function and metabolic activity." - Viktoras Kulvinskas

"Take food concentrate supplements containing the real essence of the food." - Gabriel Cousens

"I believe that taking supplemental enzymes is a big help—they can prevent disease and slow down the aging process " - Fred Bisci

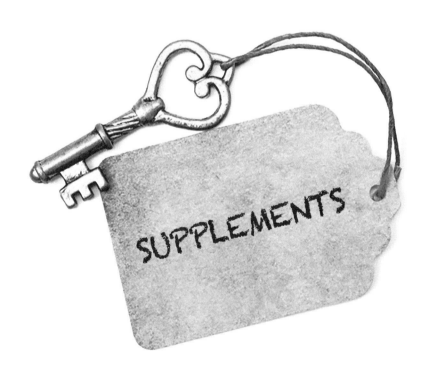

84. IS SUPPLEMENTATION NECESSARY? WHAT IS THE MOST IMPORTANT REASON TO TAKE SUPPLEMENTS? A HEALTHY IMMUNE SYSTEM?

BRIAN CLEMENT

Yes, start with that. It's all about the immunity. Now, when I began my work in the mid-70s at Hippocrates Health Institute, we did not suggest or utilize supplementation. The excuse could have been that we didn't have many available at that point, which was true. We also have a mantra, which was incorrect, that if you eat enough healthful, nutritious food, you do not require supplements. When I accepted the position as the Director, there were a few stipulations, and one of the stipulations was, we had to start to employ science appropriately. We began this with seriously ill people and then the emerging healthy people that came to Hippocrates. I had to evaluate for them where they were and where they needed to go. We needed a guidepost. We needed light that showed us the progress, or lack of. When we started to test, we were stunned, even people who lived impeccably good lives were lacking nutrients, in many cases.

"Supplementation is a requirement." – Brian Clement

Supplementation is a requirement. Only 9% of supplements are proper supplements today worldwide. The effective ones are whole-food based supplements. In my book, *Supplements Exposed,* which I put together over the course of a decade, I scientifically validate that more than 90% of supplements are oil-based, chemical-based, and not natural in any way and very dangerous for you. But I'll still say to you, after four decades of work, and being on the frontlines of disease and health, that people require whole food supplementation. The one that everyone requires, period, without any more consultation, is a bacterial form of B12. Beyond that, there are many others, but we personalize and tailor via bio-frequency testing, bioelectric frequency testing.

VIKTORAS KULVINSKAS

Yes. Ninety nine percent of the people are enzyme deficient, and enzymes rule not only the digestive function, but also the immune function and metabolic activity. It's extremely important for everybody to take enzyme supplementation, as well as to reach for optimization of your genetic makeup. Every new cellular system that is produced is going to have optimum genetic material, and that means consumption of a full mineral spectrum of nutrition coming from sea salt and from sea vegetables.

More targeted evaluations can give you more details and indications of deficiencies. Though, overall,

"It's extremely important for everybody to take enzyme supplementation." - Viktoras Kulvinskas

if you're going to take enzymes, consume all forms of living foods in conjunction with sea vegetables and fermented foods, I wouldn't be concerned about it. In the long term, your body will get everything straightened out without additional supplementation, but supplementation is going to accelerate the whole healing process, and of course, it has to be from whole organic foods. Anything else is contraindicated to health.

GABRIEL COUSENS

If one eats a variety of different whole, raw foods and does not limit oneself to excessive amounts of any specific food, one can derive a modest level of nutrition. However, because of soil depletion, most people thrive with supplementation. To discover if one is sufficientaly nourished by their diet, one should be evaluated by a healthcare professional and/or get blood tests. But blood tests use statistical averages and may not reflect one's true state of health.

FRED BISCI

In most cases, supplementation is not necessary, but it can complement a healthy diet and give you a better chance to make sure you're covering all the bases nutritionally. You have to realize that a lot of supplements are not only unnecessary, they could be detrimental. Be very careful, because tremendous claims are being made about a lot of supplements that are not valid. Some people claim their supplements are raw and I have found out that this is not always true.

If a person is on a raw diet, they should be aware of the potential of B12 deficiency, and if they're starting to see problems with their short-term memory, they might have a B12 deficiency. Of course, have your vitamin B12 checked if you suspect that you are having a problem. The normal range in B12 is 200 to 1100 milligrams per Pico liter. Anything under 450 picograms is a gray area. Many people are already into a serious B12 deficiency in this gray area. Many B12 deficiencies are misdiagnosed because the normal ranges are too low. This is becoming very evident in the last 5 years. This is nothing that should be taken lightly by any raw food eater or a vegan. Many people that eat animal protein are also suffering from B12 deficiencies. There are a number of different reasons why our diet alone might not solve our B12 issues. You are still better off being a vegan, but make sure that if you need some supplementation, that you become aware of it and that you do it.

Now, living in the north, in the winter I recommend taking vitamin D. I also take my own blend of super green foods, which is for sale on my web site. I take blue-green algae almost every day, but that's about all. Again, it's an individual thing that you should really discuss with a professional. I also recommend probiotics and enzymes.

85. WHAT ARE THE TOP 3 SUPPLEMENTS EVERYONE SHOULD BE TAKING?

BRIAN CLEMENT

Number one, B12, number two, algae like AFA and chlorella which is a green algae, number three, I would probably say, a mineral supplement, since it's one thing I see lacking. The top minerals lacking that I see in people are magnesium, zinc and selenium. It doesn't mean that people do not miss others, but when I discover they are missing—they are very important minerals—this is what I'm seeing. Number 4 is vitamin D Manganese is number five. So, an ionic form of mineral supplementation, with the inclusion of sea vegetable supplementation, is really important for you.

VIKTORAS KULVINSKAS

Enzymes, with their meals, to support the digestion, as well as, rebuilding up their enzymatic reserves, at least once a week for a few days, enzymes between meals to clean out the blood stream and for surplus build up.

Number two: mild herbal laxative on an as-needed basis. Most people need this until they get to three bowel movement evacuations per day. For monitoring the function of the bowels, as well as regenerating the bowel activity, take some form of probiotics or fermented foods.

Number three: as long as it's available, blue-green algae is the ultimate superfood for consciousness, regeneration of the immunological system, maximizing our intellectual powers, as well as athletic performance.

GABRIEL COUSENS

Humans do not make vitamin C and do not make B12. Therefore, these are the top two supplements to take, because people are generally deficient in them. Additionally, deficiencies commonly occur in antioxidants, long chain omega-3s, and nascent iodine.

FRED BISCI

The top three supplements, as far as I'm concerned are probiotics, enzymes and vitamin B12. I'm not saying everybody should be taking these supplements, however. I always say consult with a professional because, again, I don't want to give a blanket answer and I don't want to turn this into an infomercial. In some cases, one might have to consider additional supplements based on symptoms. If there's any doubt, consult a professional.

86. WHAT ARE THE BEST SUPPLEMENTS FOR BOOSTING ENERGY?

VIKTORAS KULVINSKAS

There is no free lunch—neither is there free energy, unless you work your divine. Besides the three supplements mentioned for increased energy, energy is increased by oxygenation practicing Pranayama. Exercise will increase your energy. Perhaps some ginseng or many of the medicinal mushrooms will work for some people. Of course, also green juices and wheatgrass.

BRIAN CLEMENT

Bee pollen and algae, these are the two we found to be great. There are some herbal medicines out of the Chinese medicine cabinet that give you exceptional amounts of energy, just make sure they're plant-based botanicals.

GABRIEL COUSENS

In the Traditional Chinese medical model, the Three Treasures provide a good way to view energy. Jing represents both pre-natal and post-natal primordial essence. Jing is what we come in the world with. It is our energetic primordial reserve. Chi is one's general daily energy. Shen is one's brightness or spiritual energy. Different approaches and supplements support these three deep energies.

This requires a full discussion of Jing, Chi, and Shen, which is beyond the scope of this book. Think about all levels of energy, and not simply about chi, which is daily everyday energy.

FRED BISCI

You really don't need any. I mean they will help you if you're really training hard, but the best way to increase energy is to detox, clean out your system, eat a nourishing diet, get enough calories, get plenty of rest, and drink enough water. Then add in some E3Live, wheatgrass or super green foods. D-Ribose increases your ATP production, which gives you more energy; you can get it from meat and certain fruit. Consult a professional to find the right protocol for you. Drink adequate amounts of fruit and vegetable juices.

87. WILL I GET ENOUGH NOURISHMENT IF I ELIMINATE UNHEALTHY FOODS FROM MY DIET, OR DO I NEED TO ADD SUPPLEMENTS AND CLEANSE?

BRIAN CLEMENT

When I was pondering in the early days supplementation use, I started to ask questions to my Elders. They pointed out that what made the difference between our great grandparents and grandparent's generation and ours, is stress. That stress burns nutrients out of the body quicker, and more effectively than anything else. I said, "Well, some of us are not stressed," and they laughed and said, "Remember, a hundred years ago and before, people were agrarian, and before that, nomadic and they didn't have outside influence. They knew what was going on in their family, their community and beyond that, they didn't know what was going on, because they didn't have radio, television, media, they didn't read." They were colloquial, a very calm existence at that point.

"...stress burns nutrients out of the body quicker, better and more effectively than anything else." – Brian Clement

As we became universal, as the information age took over and we're on computers, cell phones, and have 900 channels to pick on our televisions worldwide, we are constantly being influenced and stressed 24 hours a day, 7 days a week. You have a secondary stress, the invisible stresses of what we call wireless. These are the things that didn't exist decades ago, and all of these stress the body. We burn out nutrients at a much higher level—this is one reason why we require nutrients today versus not long ago.

VIKTORAS KULVINSKAS

Everyone is toxic and everyone needs to cleanse. No matter how good your diet is, a unique meal would be enzymes and sea vegetables and fermented foods or probiotics. You can grow your enzymes in a high concentrated form and then incorporate with probiotics. Watch me talk about this on *youtube.com/ ViktoraskKulvinskas*. For most people, this is most convenient through supplementation. The Hippocrates diet is the one that is going to get you everything that your body needs.

GABRIEL COUSENS

First, eliminating unhealthy foods plays a big positive role in increasing energy and life force. Second, eating live food will increase your vital life force. Third, supplementing with herbs that particularly build Jing, Chi, and Shen, can contribute to the overall long-term building of your deep vital life force. Finally, cleansing optimizes the flow of energy in one's system, as toxins detract from energetic flow and production because so much energy is used to neutralize toxins.

FRED BISCI

You have to cleanse so you can utilize all the nourishment in the healthy foods you're eating. Remember, eating unhealthy foods is the reason why you won't get enough nourishment. You can usually get everything you need from a raw living food diet. If you can't get enough B12, add a good probiotic. Consult with a professional, go to a health retreat or start reading some good books by people who have long time clinical experience.

88. SHOULD I TAKE SPECIFIC VITAMIN AND MINERAL SUPPLEMENTS, OR A SUPERFOOD THAT HAS EVERYTHING IN IT?

VIKTORAS KULVINSKAS

Unless it's prescribed by someone who has done clear cut evaluation, then you should get all this from organic whole foods.

GABRIEL COUSENS

Take food concentrate supplements containing the real essence of the food. This is in contrast to synthetic supplements. Superfoods are natural foods containing concentrated nutrition. These are highly energetic natural foods. Superfoods are preferable, because they are the most alive and the most natural.

BRIAN CLEMENT

Well, no food has everything in it. Go to the Hippocrates website, *hippocratesinst.org*, and you will see our magazine archives and there we talk about multi-vitamins as an example. One of the alumni of Hippocrates, Dr. Lily Link, who reversed a stage four cancer, writes about how most of that is a misnomer and an embellishment. What you have to do is specialize or specify supplementation rather than taking one fits all.

FRED BISCI

You really don't need a lot of supplements. There are raw food vitamins that you can take and some of the super foods are fine—you just have to find out which one works best for you. The first thing to do is find out if you have a deficiency. It's a good idea to go for a blood test to learn what's really going on. Then detox, clean up your diet. Make sure you're moving your bowels regularly, sleeping consistently, and drinking clean water. Once you're doing all that, see how you feel and add supplements as needed. Try superfoods first before you use supplements. Everyone is a unique individual and their need for supplements varies. Some people need a few, some people might need more and some people do not need any. Those who eat 100% raw, in my experience and observation over a period of 20-30 years, are going to need a B12 supplement and possibly something else.

89. IF I CAN GET SOMEONE I CARE FOR TO TAKE ONLY ONE WHOLE FOOD SUPPLEMENT WHAT WOULD YOU SUGGEST?

GABRIEL COUSENS

I have been working with the blue-green algae from Klamath Lake since 1982. Blue-green algae is the single best superfood in general and for brain function in particular. Because brain function is, in a sense, the most important function, I favor it. I've used E3Live on a daily basis for years, and I am happy with it.

When I look at the product as a whole, when I look at the minerals, and when I look at the fact that the E3Live actually is one of the only vegan foods that has the long-chain omega-3, the DHA, and the EPA, I see that E3Live provides total nutrition. But, more than that, E3Live provides a total green mentally elevated energy, unique in the plant and the algae kingdoms.

BRIAN CLEMENT

Let's preclude, as an example B12 (as everyone requires B12), then what should the supplement be? I would say, no-question, hands-down, that would be the algaes. Things like Life Give LIVE, E3Live, the same exact supplement I tell people to take this worldwide. You can find E3Live inside the frozen cooler section. BrainOn is another excellent E3Live product. We also suggest things like chlorella and marine phytoplankton.

VIKTORAS KULVINSKAS

There's only one choice, everybody is deficient in enzymes and if you can get them to take the most potent enzymes, with meals and between meals, it will make a radical difference in their life. If you could get them to take an additional supplement, then I would recommend a mild herbal laxative. Between those two, you will see miraculous results. If you want the third miraculous component, then it would be adding blue-green algae—this will create miracles in anybody's life.

FRED BISCI

They're all good. I take E3Live and the bio superfoods. I have my own super green food, which is really fabulous. So I use that in juices or coconut water or smoothies. That works well for me and I don't have to eat a lot of food.

You should make sure they're clean by looking at the certificate of analysis because some of these things have a lot of heavy metals. Some of the chorella I checked had lead in it. I'm very wary about anything that comes from outside the country, particularly from China, because the supervision might not be there. Chlorella from Japan can be problematic because it is grown in outdoor ponds near Fukushima, so that has to be a consideration. A lot of the new chorella is being grown in 480KM of glass tubing and it's actually much better because there's no contamination.

90. WHAT ARE ENZYMES AND WHY DO I NEED THEM?

BRIAN CLEMENT

In medical school biology classes, you're taught that enzymes are proteins. Let me try to describe this for you. To call an enzyme a protein is like me looking at your skin and saying, "All you are is your skin." Now, yes, part of you is your skin, just as the outer shell of an enzyme is the skin, it's a protein, but what is the purpose of an enzyme? Well, your body is first and foremost electric. You're a bioelectric person, and

"For premature aging prevention, use enzymes."- Brian Clement

even the most conservative of mainstream physicians and researchers know this. This is why when they do testing on you, they test with an MRI or a high speed CAT scan or an ultrasound. You're an electromagnetic field. We know you're electric, everyone knows you're electric. If you pass out and fall to the ground, I don't give you a vitamin supplement. I take two large electric probes and stick them on your chest to start your electric body up. With that clear understanding now, that you are a biofrequency body, your first question should be, "Where do I get electricity from naturally?" You get it from an enzyme, although an enzyme's outer shell is a protein that carries electricity to your bioelectric body, keeping your body alive is the enzyme's job. Literally, when a sperm and an egg come together and create a baby, a fetus, it's an enzyme activity that does that.

When we die and our body begins to decompose and becomes soil again, it's an enzyme activity that does that. How I picture enzymes is as a continuum of electrical frequencies that govern the universe that we live in. In the dietary form, we call it an enzyme that's in the living fresh, raw plant-based food. In my upcoming book, *Quantum Human Biology*, we're actually going to talk about studies that were conducted by my colleague, Dr. Valerie Hunt, all the way back in the 1970s and 1980s.

In a current worldwide lecture series I'm doing and presenting at the Elders Conference, I'm going to show bioelectric frequency photographs of people when they're dying of disease and what happens when they stay on a living diet. We're at a very clear scientific threshold now of really validating, on a bio frequency level. Correction of disorder is the core contribution from nature, this is raw plant-based food, because it again corrects the wrong frequency and enhances the right frequency. This is why enzymes are important.

Now, there are those who say, that an enzyme doesn't get into the body and do anything because it's wiped out by stomach acids. Sadly, they're only reading the literature, they're not doing the work that we've done with enzymes for 60 years. Watch what happens, both microscopically and biologically, on the person. Enzymes supersede, and do not have to go through the enzymatic. It goes into the body instantaneously and it enhances the bio-frequency and life of the cell.

One of the experiments we have conducted is taking students and showing them microscopically the coagulation or coordination of cells called, *Rouleaux*. We then administered enzymes, and within three to five minutes, in 100% of the cases, we actually see that the cells no longer were stuck to other cells, they move independently and start to glow and flow. We did this testing about 500 times—this is what enzymes do. This is why, in my household, Dr. Anna Maria and my children and I choose to take supplemental enzymes.

For premature aging prevention, use enzymes. Consuming appropriate digestive enzymes in the early stages of adapting a raw food diet is essential. Our bodies were meant to consume raw food, since in nature, 100% of every other species do so. We are the only ones who choose to consume denatured, cooked food.

With this established fact, we must also acknowledge that our bodies have lost their potential to break down this high-roughage and enzyme-rich fare, so the use of enzymes will help reignite the anatomy's ability to accept and flourish on its original fuel.

There are two reasons one would adopt a raw living diet. Either, you're frightened because you're sick and you instinctually understand raw food can help, or you're enlightened and say, "My God, I want to have more energy so I can feel better, happier, etc." When you adopt a raw diet and your body's muscular structure in your digestive and elimination canal is not prepared to do the work, enzymes are extremely helpful in breaking down those foods. I take these for an anti-aging effect. I take 20 enzyme supplements every evening before I eat my meal, and boy, they're one of the great anti-aging supplements you can have this at the top.

VIKTORAS KULVINSKAS

I have written about using enzymes for health and longevity in my book, Survival in the 21st Century. I did pioneering work with Dr. Edward Howell, who is considered the father of immunology. Enzymes should be on the recommended daily allowance. They are, first of all, an assurance that the digestion of food is going to be complete.

At one time in history, we lived on totally enzyme rich diet, which were laden with all kinds of friendly bacteria and the bacteria ate the foods within your gastrointestinal tract and made a lot of enzymes. We also consumed a lot of fermented food in a normal fashion. As a result, our elements levels of enzymes were pretty strong.

Enzymes are needed for supporting digestion, so that its protein is converted to amino acids and enzymes. Starches and carbs are converted into sugars that your body can utilize. Crude fats are converted into essential fats that your body can utilize. The whole thing is, what can your body use? It cannot use the food, it needs to have the food broken down to its essential components, and enzymes do the job.

"Without enzymes, there is no life." – Viktoras Kulvinskas

Enzymes drive the immune system function, which is the police force against pathogenic microbes and industrial waste radiation and also rejuvenation of your body. And of course, in every form of reactions in the body, the metabolic activities are driven by enzymes. There are over 4000 enzyme systems presently identified or more being discovered on a weekly basis.

The enzymes are your blue-collar workers. They do all the physical work. All other nutrients don't do any kind of work—it's the enzymes that do it. They are associated in your healing and recovery, and without enzymes, there is no life. Most people are living on an enzyme-less diet; the only reason they stay alive is that there are certain amounts of friendly bacteria that are on your skin and in your gastrointestinal tract, that make some enzymes for the individual.

When should enzymes be taken? With meals, and in between meals. Dr. Leskovar showed in published studies that enzyme use helped to reverse 79% of the cancers. Dr. Max Wolf of Fordham University showed up to 95% recovery of all forms of cardiovascular diseases with the administration of adequate volumes of enzymes. One of the key components of accelerated recovery, in terms of influence, is adding enzymes.

GABRIEL COUSENS

Enzymes are biologically active proteins that catalyze all levels of human biological function. We need enzymes for proper brain function, for proper digestion, for proper metabolic function, and for repair. Every function of the human organism requires enzymes.

Dr. Howell suggests that our vital life force runs out when our enzymes run out, and then we die. It is important to take enzyme supplements, particularly for digestion, because they aid digestion and help the enzyme reserve maintain itself.

Enzymes are life force energy. Taking enzyme supplements supports the enzyme life force energy. Under chronic disease, the enzyme reserves diminish significantly.

I believe that we are able not only to stop enzyme loss with age, but by taking the proper herbs and eating in a way that preserves enzymes (eating 80% to 100% live foods), we are able to minimize the loss, and essentially, begin to build and regenerate new enzymes and turn on the DNA programs that continue to build enzymes. In other words, we can, as we lengthen our telomeres, reactivate enzyme production through our genes.

This is a change from the view that we have a limited amount of enzymes. I believe that it is possible, with the proper use of diet and herbs, to actually increase enzyme production to avoid enzyme depletion with age.

FRED BISCI

Enzymes are catalytic proteins and there are different kinds of enzymes. They're required for every function of your body. Your body produces about 3,000 metabolic enzymes. Digestive enzymes are produced from the metabolic enzymes. Vitamins are a co-enzyme. There are enzymes in a plant-based diet. Your body produces digestive enzymes to break down your food so the nutrients can be absorbed.

In our society, where we are under significant stress, I believe that taking supplemental enzymes is a big help—they can help prevent disease and slow down the aging process. I've been using them diligently since I was in my sixties. I definitely noticed a difference, and I believe that, if it wasn't for the enzymes, I probably would have some pain from my injuries. They reduce inflammation and slow down deterioration from aging. I've seen fantastic things happen when people start supplementing their diet with enzymes. It's not absolutely necessary, but they do have a lot to offer. Digestive enzymes help with digestion and systemic enzymes help to reduce inflammation and reduce blood viscosity. A plant-based diet keeps your blood viscous.

91. ARE THERE DIFFERENT KINDS OF ENZYMES FOR DIGESTION AND DETOXIFICATION?

GABRIEL COUSENS

There are specific enzymes necessary for digestion, such as amylase for carbohydrates, lipase for fats, and a variety of proteases for protein. Enzymes for detoxification are primary proteolytic. If one is taking enzymes for that purpose, one shouldn't take them with food, because those enzymes would then contribute to a secondary function, namely, digestion. Enzymes for detoxification should be taken without food.

VIKTORAS KULVINSKAS

Not really, but primarily, for digestion, you need all the full spectrum of enzymes—protease, amylase, lipase. You want at least 50,000 HUT of protease; you want at least 6000 units of amylase or comparable digesting abilities. You want at least 500, but preferably 1000 and higher, of lipase activity. You want at least 100 units of cellulose activities.

The higher the potency, the more active, you will get more bang for your buck. For immune function, it's primarily protease, that's why you have different components of the protease complex protein digesting enzymes, and you take them between meals. For cleansing and detoxification, take the digestive enzymes between meals, because what you're trying to do is cleanse and detoxify yourself of all the incompletely metabolized foods that are stored within your blood vessel, within cancer cells, within your lymphatic system. By taking enzymes in between meals, you can absorb up to 90% of the enzymes.

For immune enhancement, take the ones that have at least 150 units of protease.

FRED BISCI

Yes. Digestive enzymes support our digestive system, especially as we age. Many older people don't secrete enough hydrochloric acid, and taking digestive enzymes is a simple way for them to enhance their digestion and absorption. A lot of people, as they get older, are actually in an early stage of starvation because they're not absorbing a lot of the nutrients from their food. So, digestive enzymes play a very important role.

Systemic enzymes have a dramatic effect. They're taken on an empty stomach with plenty of water, so they go directly into the small intestines. Some people who have pain or discomfort see a difference right away, even after taking their first two. It's almost amazing—and it's not working like a drug. It's a natural way to help with your digestion and get relief from pain. You might want to try and replace aspirin with enzymes.

BRIAN CLEMENT

The answer is, absolutely, yes. We have two other forms of enzymes—a fat eating or fat digesting enzyme that's been incredibly effective in helping people with obesity and overweight problems. People who encounter gallbladder concerns would flourish on a lipase enzyme that we call MELT AWAY.

The second one we have comes from mainstream medicine in Northern Europe, which is commonly used in mutagenic diseases like cancers, tumors, fibroids, as well as microbial, bacterial and viral diseases. It's what we call a systemic enzyme, and it's plant-based. That one is called "Life Give Systemic Enzymes."

These enzymes are spectacular and we know that in this century, even in mainstream medicine, enzymes are becoming great agents for health recovery. We've been showing that for all these decades now at Hippocrates.

92. WHAT NUTRIENTS ARE BETTER FOUND IN SUPPLEMENTS BUT HARD TO FIND IN WHOLE FOODS?

FRED BISCI

If you're eating a variety of whole foods, you can get just about everything you need. To make sure, you can have yourself evaluated by a healthcare professional and get a blood test. Remember, though, the bottom line is how you feel. I've seen people get a blood test and the doctor says something doesn't seem right, but meanwhile the person is not symptomatic. Remember, the normal range is really just a rough average; you could be slightly out of the normal range and there'd be nothing wrong with you. A lot of people on raw food come out below the normal range, and it doesn't mean there's anything wrong; in many cases it actually means they're healthier. On a whole food diet, we must eat a variety of different fruits, vegetables, nuts, seed, sprouts, avocados, and with enough calories. Periodically, we should check to see that we are thriving and absorbing what we eat by getting tested. I have seen people who refused to do this and later found out that they were suffering from deficiencies over a long period of time, especially vitamin B12. I'm talking about long-term raw food eaters or vegans.

BRIAN CLEMENT

B12 is one example. Vitamin D is another. We make our "Sun D" out of Shiitake mushrooms. Of course, the best way to get "Sun D" is to go out into the sun itself wearing natural fiber clothes year-round. Minerals, again even though you get minerals, we burn them out. There are certain forms of elements that you'll get in the green and blue-green algae that you don't find in other food at all because they're unique to aquatic life.

VIKTORAS KULVINSKAS

Enzymes—that's the only thing.

GABRIEL COUSENS

This is a relative question. Clearly B12 is very difficult to find in vegan, whole foods.

Adequate amounts of omega-3 may be difficult for everyone to find (in meat-eaters, vegetarians, and vegans alike) in adequate amounts in whole foods; however, it is certainly available in whole food concentrates, such as yellow algae, and to some extent, in blue-green algae.

Vitamin D is not in the whole foods we eat.

Vegans need to consider concentrations of vitamin A and even vitamin E in therapeutic doses. We may also consider therapeutic doses such as what I may use in orthomolecular psychology. These remain unavailable in supplements in the sizes that I wish to prescribe. For example, something like tryptophan, as a precursor for serotonin and a major aid for helping women with hot flashes, as well as women and men with insomnia.

At least 80% of people in the U.S. are deficient in magnesium. I personally do a certain amount of supplementation to boost my magnesium. There is a great variation in what people need for magnesium.

Zinc is another supplement that is hard to get in high enough concentrations.

Neither meat eaters nor vegans get enough carnosine. Meat eaters do get a certain amount of carnosine. It is, in fact, possible to get 1,000 mg of carnosine by eating three steaks a day, but this is unhealthy. Carnosine is an anti-glycation supplement and is a supplemental protein that protects against aging and excess sugar combining with protein, i.e. glycation. Carnosine may also lengthen the telomeres. These are not readily available to vegans and vegetarians.

Certainly, there are necessary supplements. Selenium and nascent iodine are very important for protection against cancer and against developing fibrocystic breasts.

LIFESTYLE

"...the chemicals in the home and the environmental toxicity of the home is about five times higher than it is of the outside world" - Viktoras Kulvinskas

"Everyone, at minimum, also requires approximately an hour and a half or more of weightlifting, strength bearing, muscle building, bone developing, resistance exercise three days a week."
- Brian Clement

"I think in the long run, the price in our quality of life, health, and life span far outweighs the lesser short-term expense that one saves with synthetics." - Gabriel Cousens

"The fact remains that those who eat a plant-based diet, juice, blend whole foods, in general, are far healthier and get less opportunistic infections than those who are not following this lifestyle." - Fred Bisci

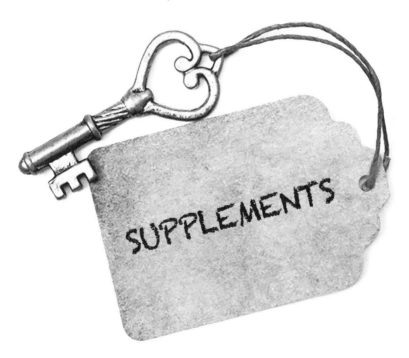

93. SHOULD I VACCINATE MY KIDS OR PETS?

VIKTORAS KULVINSKAS

Definitely, no. Go to www.mercola.com and search vaccinations. That should convince you with all the studies. The best way to strengthen your immune function is through the consumption of fermented foods and taking enzymes with meals and in between meals. It will protect you against everything. Also, at the same time, stop eating poisonous food, start eating real food, which is plant-based and uncooked, undestroyed by our social culinary arts as well also our technology.

Work with some of your local church groups or have your holistic alternative healthcare doctor provide the needed documentation for you to get your children into school.

Honestly, you're better off to do Internet-based education, home schooling. You'll get a much better educated child and without being contaminated by the insanity and the indoctrination that exist in our school system.

GABRIEL COUSENS

There are a lot of recent studies that show that vaccinations aren't healthy.

Neil Miller writes (and this is in a journal article) that the U.S. child immunization schedule asks for 26 vaccine doses for children less than one year old. Yet 33 nations have lower infant mortality rates in the first year. We're 34 out of 34. There is a direct correlation between the amount of vaccinations and infant mortality rates in the first year of life.

Other research shows that there is an increased hospitalization and mortality rate among infants, directly correlative to the number of vaccinations they receive. The more vaccinations received, the higher the mortality rates.

There are many reasons to not vaccinate children. One of the primary reasons is that vaccines don't work very well, and so their risk/benefit ratio is poor. Neither the herd concept nor the herd protection concept has been shown to work. These theories have proven to be inaccurate. In highly vaccinated areas, the populations still have very high rates of the diseases they are vaccinated against, even if 95% of the population is vaccinated.

A third point is the serious side effects of vaccines. One of them is brain inflammation and swelling. There is a theory that Sudden Infant Death

"There are many reasons to not vaccinate children." - Gabriel Cousens

Syndrome is correlative within four days to three weeks after vaccination, related to the fact that the infant's brain swells, and it pushes against the actual skull, suppressing the respiration center. The potential devastating and permanent side effects of that far outweigh the potential advantage.

Looking at the controversial research, it is my opinion that there exists a correlation between vaccinations and autism. There are no cases of autism in certain communities where they do not vaccinate—such as the Amish. These communities do not have any vaccinations. That's the kind of thing that we're talking about. In a study done in Oregon, 900 unvaccinated children were compared with 900 vaccinated children. There were significantly lower amounts of autism, hyperactivity, and dyslexia amongst the unvaccinated children.

As far as I can tell, children really do suffer from vaccinations. Their immune systems are weakened; their neurological systems may become disorganized; and the risk/benefit ratio doesn't merit vaccinating.

Back in the '70s, when I was working as a general practitioner, there was an outbreak of whooping cough. I gave all my patients homeopathic pertussis vaccinations, and 100% of my patients did not get whooping cough/pertussis. Those who were vaccinated and those who were not vaccinated indeed contracted whooping cough. The results of research done in Buenos Aires also support the superiority of homeopathic vaccinations over allopathic ones. There was a plague of diphtheria, and those people who received homeopathic vaccinations had far less diphtheria and no side effects as compared to those who actually received the allopathic vaccination.

One of the most effective protections, and the best thing to do, is to build a very healthy immune system and use vitamin D as a very potent protector of the immune system. With vitamin A and vitamin D, we have a great deal of protection against illnesses like measles, which can be a serious problem. I also grew up in the '40s without particular vaccinations, and I had chickenpox and measles and whatever else. Basically, in the long run, my immune system is stronger from those exposures than that of children who have been vaccinated.

One of the things we're looking at with mumps, measles, and other communicable illnesses is that vaccination can postpone their onset, but when one gets mumps as a teenager, it can affect sexual function and create sterility. By this measure, the downside of vaccinations far outweighs the upside.

There are many other issues, such as the adjuvants they are putting in the vaccines. Mercury and other additives cause brain and immune system damage. Other adjuvants may cause devastating whole body autoimmune attacks on the neurological system, causing life-threatening reactions like multiple sclerosis and various whole-body demyelinating diseases.

The research does not show a significant advantage with flu vaccinations. In fact, for the swine flu in Canada, they found that those who got the swine flu vaccination had 250% more swine flu than those who did not receive the vaccine.

The bottom line is that it is best and safest in the risk/benefit analysis to avoid vaccinations and avoid whatever is put in the vaccinations. Many things that shouldn't be put in are affecting the consciousness and long-term health of the human population.

If it's not broken, don't fix it. Vaccines are maybe good money for the vaccine companies, but when we look at the overall statistics, a veritable volume of information, the risk/benefit ratio doesn't justify their use.

FRED BISCI

I am not a medical doctor and this should not be misconstrued as medical advice. My personal opinion is that the problems far outweigh the benefits. Children who are taught to follow a healthy lifestyle very rarely get any common diseases. Children who are vaccinated get the diseases in many cases. I believe that people should do their own extensive research and come to their own conclusions. We must remember that we are programmed, through fear and intimidation, to believe that which is profitable for other people who have a vested interest in our poor health. I have never had a vaccination as a child and was very healthy and had no problems. I was never vaccinated until I entered the military during the Korean War. At that time, I got very sick and ran a high fever for 3 or 4 days. I do not encourage people to vaccinate their children. Of course, this is a personal decision. Do your own research and the truth will be obvious.

The same applies to pets. If you believe in God and the sanctity of the human body, it is your Constitutional right not to vaccinate because of your religious beliefs.

BRIAN CLEMENT

Well, all you have to do is read the archives of evidence against vaccines and you'll see that putting a little disease in your body permanently reduces your immune function. It will make 100% of the people more susceptible to other diseases. With that said, have vaccines saved billions of people's lives? Absolutely. Vaccine's intent was a really good one.

Today, sadly, the pharmaceutical cartel has a plan not only to give the 18 prerequisite of vaccines to infants, but every five years throughout the human life, they're going to propose you take new vaccines they have invented and fabricated vaccines since the U.S. Supreme Court has removed liability from the companies that make them . This is something one must think a lot about—do I want to contaminate my body? Yes, it may protect me from certain diseases if I live in a fully vaccinated culture. It's an easier decision to make because those sorts of diseases are not prevalent. If you live in parts of the world where the diseases are prevalent, that's something you have to think long and hard about.

One of the remedies is homeopathic medicine—the good effect without the side effect, that's one way to do it. I chose not to vaccinate my children; they're grown adults and I have grandchildren now. In most places in the West, almost all that I know of, it is not required by law that you vaccinate your children to get into school. So, don't get railroaded into this, make decisions based upon knowledge, not fear. Today, there is a major move by the vaccine manufacturers to force vaccinations.

94. WHAT ARE THE BEST EXERCISES FOR OUR HEALTH?

VIKTORAS KULVINSKAS

All forms of exercise essentially should be done minimally six days a week, seven days a week would be best. As far as exercise, my cardio and lymphatic workout is on a rebounder. You can also do certain Qigong exercises that will get your cardio ripped up as well as also your rebounder type of a workout. I think that we all need a certain amount of resistance training on a daily basis in order to have a higher bone density and prevent bone degeneration and osteoporosis. It's the only thing that seems to work. Flexibility—by way of all kinds of stretching exercises that are found in yoga. Yoga is, as far as I'm concerned, the ultimate science. That's something you can do for the rest of your life and it can give you stretching, toning, increased flexibility, adjustment of your spine, the squeezing and cleaning out your hormone system, as well as lymphatic and cardio, depending on the rate you're doing it. It can also provide resistance training by using your own body weight as the resistance. It's the ultimate. That's something that you'll be able to do at the age of 90, a hundred, two hundred years of age.

BRIAN CLEMENT

What we do know is that everyone requires a minimum of 35 minutes of aerobic exercise five days a week. That's just for maintaining your health. Everyone, at minimum, also requires approximately an hour and a half or more of weightlifting, strength bearing, muscle building, bone developing, resistance exercise three days a week. Everyone, especially as we get older, should be doing stretching exercises. Now, that's normal stretching and you can get books and look at videos and also look at the Internet. Yogic exercises do that, Pilates exercises do that. When I'm doing weight lifting exercises, I use body bearing exercises, dips, pull-ups etc.—all of those are also stretching exercises. These are more important as we age because our body starts to pull together and elasticity and flexibility will be lost if we don't continue these movements.

FRED BISCI

All forms of exercise, done correctly in the correct amounts are beneficial. Walking, jogging, resistance exercise, body wight exercises such as chinning and dipping, yoga, palates, Tai Chi and Qigong. Biking, roller blading, swimming and even dancing are all good forms of exercise. My favorites are Qigong, walking, jogging and biking. Proper breathing is life-changing, like the breathing that is done in Qigong. Exercise with oxygen therapy, or EWOT, is therapeutic. Extreme endurance and resistance exercises, when overdone can be counter-productive.

GABRIEL COUSENS

There is a wide range of beneficial exercises. There are stretching exercises, and I particularly like yoga, which I've done for 40 years. I do yoga at least six or seven days a week and find it immensely beneficial. There is core strengthening, that you also get with yoga, such as Pilates. Then you also have heavy aerobic exercises, and you have exercises to support the lymphatic system.

Exercise is immensely good for you. Moderate exercise is all we really need. Exercise physiologists suggest we may not need more than 16 to 22 minutes of aerobic exercise three or four times a week to actually maintain healthy function. This level of aerobic exercise improves all levels of brain function and growth.

95. DO YOU HAVE ANY ADVICE ON KEEPING A HEALTHY HOME BESIDES FOOD & DIET?

FRED BISCI

Use non-toxic cleansers that are void of chemicals. Use natural, non-toxic shampoos that are food based and flouride and chemical-free toothpaste. I do not have carpets in my house, only wood floors. It is best to use non-toxic paints if you have a choice, because they off-gas. Also, be aware of molds and funguses in your house. I found out first-hand what black mold can do. If you are living in a polluted environment, it might be a good idea to have an air filtration system in your house. We are living in a highly toxic environment in most areas of big cities. You can't walk around with a mask on. That is why I recommend that you detoxify 3 or 4 times a year. I don't get paranoid about what I cannot control. I only change what I can control. I believe many people are walking around in fear over things they have no control of. When dry-cleaning your clothes, use a dry cleaner that uses organic and safe chemicals or better yet, use only washable clothing instead of dry clean only. Your house water is extremely important. If possible, put a high quality filtration system on the main line coming into your house and an extra, reverse osmosis preferably, filtration system for your drinking water. The totally disolved solids should be zero. This water will be safe for drinking and taking showers.

BRIAN CLEMENT

First, let's imagine the worst. Let's imagine that you're living in a toxic nightmare at this point, which I did for a good part of my life in the area of the United States that was super toxic compared to the rest, it is a factory laden area of the Northeast. Well, at least begin today as you listen to us, or as you read this, to crack your windows open when you drive a car and, when you are sleeping at night.

Second, the things that you are most connected to—your bed linens, the bed itself—try to make those organic varieties. Again, if money is the concern, which with most of us reading or listening, it is, this has to be done systematically, slowly and over a period of time. Carpets, other than 100% wool or natural fiber, are dangerous—so slowly but surely remove those. You replace them with the environmentally safe bamboos, or at least, wooden floors. I like bamboos, they're sustainable resources. A lot of the new building I do at Hippocrates, I either use tile or I use bamboo flooring. Use those available green coverings

Obviously the things to use for washing your clothing, the inside of your house, cleaning the windows, etc., all of these are available at your local health food store, or on the Internet now and, if you get on the Hippocrates website, www.hippocratesinst.org, look back at our magazine archives. I've done a feature magazine on different solutions you can make with vinegar and water, lemon and water, these are very inexpensive and you can use them to clean your house in a more effective and helpful way protecting your family, your pets, yourself.

Healthy Home, a great book that was written on this topic, and many other books, you can get on Amazon. Look up Environmental Homes, when you're building a home, certain materials should be used. All of these things need to be contemplated today because you could live right and be positive and healthy and eat raw living food and still be sick if you have your body surrounded by these toxins.

Your most important surrounding is your clothing. Everyone immediately needs to purchase and to wear organic undergarments and then from that point forward, ideally, organic clothing. But that's not always available, so wear at least natural fiber clothing. When you're buying clothes that are suspect of being chemically treated, even if they are 100% linen, 100% cotton, soak them in inexpensive vinegar, mixed of course with lots and lots of water in your bath tub and let them drip dry themselves. Search out dry cleaners that are organic or soy-based. All of these are important and easy to find on the Internet or in that book or in magazines like the one Hippocrates speaks about.

GABRIEL COUSENS

I tend to be a little bit more on the fastidious side. I do whatever I can to minimize anything toxic. I'm willing to make the extra expense to get the highest quality and go with everything organic, from organic sheets and so-forth. I think in the long run, the price in our quality of life, health, and life span far outweighs the lesser short-term expense that one saves with synthetics.

At the Tree of Life Center US, as well as in our own home, we absolutely use nothing but the highest quality organic shampoos, cleansers. Toothpastes with fluoride are an absolute disaster. Fluoride is an absolute disaster, and it should be avoided at all costs. Air purifiers are a good idea. Living in the country, we don't really need much of that, but certainly in city life, I would consider air purifiers a must. Even though you can control the fabric in your house and toothpaste and wall paint and so forth, you can't really control the air quality without an air purifier. It is important to put that fastidious effort in, as we genuinely are overwhelmed with toxins in our environment.

VIKTORAS KULVINSKAS

As they say, the chemicals in the home and the environmental toxicity of the home is about five times higher than it is of the outside world. As a starter, I would suggest, unless you're living next to a very toxic environment, keep your windows open so as to minimize the amount of retention of the chemicals that are in your home. For moldiness, get rid of the damp spots, clear up the condition. At the same time, introduce air filtration systems such as Alpine, or others. It will help get rid of molds, mildew and all kind of microbial and chemical elements that are part of whatever housing structure.

The biggest helper would be getting a good air filtration system into your home. There are many choices and you can find them online and do an Internet comparison of the different air filtration system. Decide on the one that will fit best for your home needs. If you continue living in a major city with all kind of harmful chemicals, it's definitely very essential to give consideration to adding this component, especially at your bedside.

96. THERE HAS BEEN PUBLICITY ABOUT FOOD-BORNE ILLNESSES LINKED TO RAW PLANT FOODS. WHAT CAN WE DO TO PREVENT THEM?

GABRIEL COUSENS

I question just how true that is. Given that possibility and having lived in India for seven years without anyone in my family, my two kids or my wife, getting sick, I would say that the best thing you can do is not only wash everything with hydrogen peroxide, but use potassium permanganate. Those two things will take care of any food borne illnesses that we face. The solutions are simple, if that's a concern. We do wash all of our food in hydrogen peroxide at the Tree of Life Center US. In India, those people who didn't use the potassium permanganate actually didn't do so well. In a possibly pathogenic environment, I use both.

BRIAN CLEMENT

What's really interesting to me is how, in the mainstream media, which is controlled by the corporate interest, nobody ever mentions that hundreds of people daily die from food-borne diseases coming out of meat and dairy food. That is a non-existent discussion in mainstream media globally. Interestingly enough, every time one of these food-borne diseases hurts somebody, the usual suspect isn't looked at. They always pick an organic grower of some kind, when in fact, here in the United States, wild boar feces got onto plants and this E-coli they said was caused by people eating plants. Number one—E-coli always has to come from animal feces, either another creature or human, E-coli does not grow on plants. So, there was an animal involved or an animal food involved in this. Very few people have ever died from eating a plant. If animal feces or an animal food was implicated in this, they died at an alarming rate.

You protect yourself quite simply by getting a natural organic germicide, and there are many companies that sell these, get on the Internet and look for them. Even companies like Shaklee, have a germicide. Add little bits of that in water and then put your plants in, if you're overly concerned about this, then soak them for a minute or so, rinse them off and then that's when you eat them. I'm not concerned with this, for more than four decades I've eaten this way, fed my family and fed hundreds of thousands of people this food via Hippocrates, and not one person has ever gotten sick from a food borne illness, where I can show you on a daily basis people who've gotten sick from eating meat and dairy food and fish.

FRED BISCI

Some professionals tell people not to drink fresh juices because they haven't been pasteurized and not to eat uncooked vegetables because of the pathogens. They are worried about E-coli and salmonella. Many juice bars are high-pressure pasteurizing their juices because of this kind of advice. With whole foods, people are concerned about some types of food poisoning. When food is handled correctly and is fresh, I do not see any of this to be a problem. The fact remains that those who eat a plant-based diet, juice, blend whole foods, in general, are far healthier and get less opportunistic infections than those who are not following this lifestyle. If there was a special hospital for raw foodists and juicers, it would be loaded with empty beds. When all processed food is cut out of the diet and the lymphatic system and GI tract are cleansed, and you stick to this lifestyle, you are not a good host internally for bacteria proliferation.

VIKTORAS KULVINSKAS

Try to emphasize utilizing organic produce, for one. Minimize the purchase of anything that comes in plastic bags. Check for dates of expiration. Learn to do kinesiology or muscle test and determine if the food is good for you, for your own wellness. At home, wash the produce in water. Always carefully examine your food so that it's not spoiling. It is a problem that has been with us forever and as soon as we don't pay attention to our food, the microbial or the pathogenic microbes help to break down the foods for recycling. They are already old, they are not worthy of being consumed by humans, and humans consume such foods because they haven't paid attention to the food.

"Always carefully examine your food so it is not spoiling." - Viktoras Kulvinskas

There is food that is contaminated. Often, it's found by poorly sprouts, as well as old vegetables, as well as introduction of contamination at the farms that are using poor sanitation, especially runoff water from animal husbandry, which is so contaminated with pathogenic microbes. Try to do, as much as possible, your own indoor gardening and sprouting. Also, be very careful, paying attention to the freshness of your food. That includes what you keep in a refrigerator. If food has been in your refrigerator for two, three days, it's always a good idea to wash it carefully and examine each piece before using it. I've been eating vegan and a raw foodist for over 45 years—I've had not a single bout of poisoning.

97. WHAT ABOUT THE CLOTHES I WEAR—DO THEY HAVE AN EFFECT ON MY HEALTH?

BRIAN CLEMENT

I'm not trying to sell you a book, I'm just trying to inform you and give you greater knowledge. Please read Dr. Anna Maria's and my book called *Killer Clothes*. This is a definitive publication on clothing and the toxic effect of wearing bad clothing. I petition you to do this because you could be doing everything else right and wear the wrong clothing and end up sick. The part I want you to be acutely interested in and if you're a parent or thinking about being a parent, is what they do to children's clothing and infant clothing. I am absolutely, scientifically and personally convinced that much of the brain cancers that you see today come from fire retardants that are mandated worldwide to be placed on children's clothing and children's products as well as infant products. Please spend time and do this.

VIKTORAS KULVINSKAS

Yes, they do, especially if you take your clothing to dry cleaners. Use only soy-based cleaners. Use minimal detergents in washing, ones that are approved by dermatologists and have no chemicals or fragrance and no enzymes to irritate your skin. Get natural material such as cotton, hemp and bamboo. Try to get as much of it organic, especially the clothing that you wear directly on your skin, your undergarments. Read the book by Dr. Brian Clement, *Killer Clothing*, for further guidelines.

GABRIEL COUSENS

Absolutely. Synthetic clothing blocks the flow of energy and blocks the flow of oxygen. One should select clothing that can breathe and that doesn't block one's energy. I wear all organic clothes and generally recommend that for everybody's optimal health.

FRED BISCI

Yes. Of course natural fibers such as cotton and wool are preferable. Dry cleaning fluids are highly toxic, unless you can find a dry cleaner who does not use toxic chemicals. There is plenty of information; do your own research and make your own choices. I, myself, wear natural products and keep it simple.

PROTEIN

"The top protein foods on the planet are blue-green and green algae, sea vegetables, and sprouts and grasses, by far the best, most complete and highest levels of protein." - Brian Clement

"The fastest animals with the highest endurance are the green-eaters." - Viktoras Kulvinskas

"Animal protein, by and large, builds up toxicity in the muscles. The research on athletes, as the measure, is that non-athletic vegetarians had two to three times the endurance as meat eating athletes." - Gabriel Cousens

"A truly healthy person does not need as much protein as they have been led to believe. You can get more than enough from a raw plant-based vegan diet, with some cooked food." - Fred Bisci

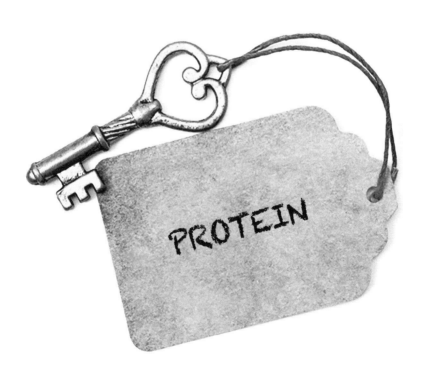

98. ANY TRUTH TO THE IDEA THAT ANIMAL PROTEN MAKES A PERSON STRONGER? MANY PEOPLE I KNOW WHO WERE ONCE VEGETARIAN REPORT GAINING STRENGTH AND FEELING HEALTHIER AFTER GOING BACK TO MEAT. IS THIS A TEMPORARY FEELING?

VIKTORAS KULVINSKAS

One of the major reasons why they might have felt stronger and healthier after getting off a vegan program is the fact that they were not digesting the proteins. Many of them were on heavily starch-oriented vegan diets, thus when they got the stimulation of the animal protein, and that is the stimulation, from the uric acid structure of trioxopurine, which is latent in the flesh and the skin of the animal, and it gives you the booster, so you have a temporary influence just like you would from coffee. The results will be short-lived. They're going to move into more and more acidity and degenerative diseases. Even if they stick to a raw meat diet, the results will be disastrous because you're consuming the fear of the animal slaughterhouse, and also you're consuming very acid-forming foods.

Temporary results is ignorance on their part. If they only consumed a diet more like Hippocrates' program, nobody would ever want to go back to any form of consumption of meat.

BRIAN CLEMENT

Many people I know who were once vegetarian report gaining strength and feeling healthy after going back to meat—this is a temporary feeling. Well, it's an illusion to begin with. If you spend the next minute with me you're going to learn everything you ever need to know about protein. All life in this planet comes from the sun, it's captured on the green leafy plant and that's called photosynthesis. All of the protein in the world comes from UVA and UVB rays from the sun, through photosynthesis on the plant, so where protein comes from is a plant. For one to say that you gain strength by eating a secondary protein is not only absurd but also fantasy and illusion. If you think not eating a plant, but allowing an animal to eat it, then slaughtering the animal, and in most cases, cooking it and eating it, is making you stronger, you are way off track.

What you have to know is that the strongest people in the world are plant-based eaters. In an upcoming book, I'm going to show you a plant-based eater, the only one that has ever been shown to do this in history—lift over 7,000 lbs. with one arm. Nobody in history, even the top, strongest Olympic athletes, has ever lifted anything more than 7 hundreds of pounds over their head. It's, of course, mind over body, but on the other hand, it's a plant-based diet that does this. I'm a body builder, have been for 35 years. I'm stronger today in my 60s than I've ever been in my life. My muscles are bigger than they were when I was in my 20, 30s, 40s and 50s. It's totally a state of mind to think that you need meat. Now, I know it's very difficult for people when they're out there and they're the one person who's a plant-based eater, and the entire culture and the entire society and the entire educational system that's manipulated by the meat and dairy industry, and the entire medical profession is pushing the misinformation that meat protein is complete and makes you strong.

I know it's easy to fall right back into your old patterns, but let me tell you, you're in fantasy land. The truth of the matter is, we train Olympic athletes. We have Olympic athletes that came to us on meat-based diets and now have created greater endurance, reversed diseases, prevented the premature aging process, etc. Look at the work of my colleague, Dr. Neal Barnard who successfully sued the dairy industry when they put a fraudulent ad out internationally saying that you lose weight on dairy. The opposite is true. I mean, look at the work at Hippocrates Health Institute, that for 60 years on the frontlines doing clinical research on humans, and validating positive change. Do not listen to the vested interest of the meat and dairy industry, or the cheerleaders who are not emotionally capable and spiritually capable of maintaining a plant-based diet. Have the integrity to not only heal your body, but heal the very planet earth that we live on?

It takes integrity. It takes strength. It takes viability. It takes absolutely commitment to self. If you find that avenue in life, you don't have to slaughter animals and eat their flesh to think you're manly and strong and healthy, you just want to be normal, but unfathomally normal is totally abnormal. Just remember that. My first mentor, this wonderful little lady, Lilian Gulfin, said to me "Whatever everyone thinks is right, look at the opposite and that's the truth." Boy, was she correct on that. The older I get, the more I know that to be true.

GABRIEL COUSENS

Animal protein, by and large, builds up toxicity in the muscles. The research on athletes, as they measure, is that non-athletic vegetarians had two to three times the endurance as meat eating athletes. There are about 10 research studies that show that vegetarians have more strength and endurance.

Many of these people who enthusiastically discover meat are fast oxidizers who were previously trying to do a high-complex vegetarian cuisine for theoretical and ideological reasons, rather than eating according to their constitution. Likely, they failed to thrive because they needed more protein, as does about 70% of the population. Flesh food has been shown to be both addictive and a stimulant. It's not whether or not it's flesh food, but, rather, on the vegetarian/vegan diet, the outdated tendency is for most people not to work out their individual needs, but instead follow a low-protein, low-fat, high-carb diet, which, at best, works for 25% of the population.

"The highest-quality proteins in the world are spirulina, chlorella, and blue-green algae." – Gabriel Cousens

The highest-quality proteins in the world are spirulina, chlorella, and blue-green algae. They are 90-95% absorbable, which is considerably more than even eggs, which have a 44% assimilation rate. Truly one can get the very highest quality proteins from plant-source foods. One's strength is determined by whether one is eating the best combination cuisine for their particular constitutional type. After 30 years on a 99-100% live food cuisine, and with the proper macronutrient ratios necessary for my constitution and metabolic type, I did 601 push-ups at 60 years old and 29 pull-ups at 70 years old. Both these feats far surpassed what I could do as a 22 year-old, meat-eating athlete.

FRED BISCI

In order to answer this question I would like to tell you a little bit about my own history. I was a competitive, olympic-style weightlifter—not a bodybuilder—at a state level and was a Navy champion. When I gave up animal protein, I lost a lot of weight. It took a lot of detox and quite some time before I got enough strength to start working out with weights. I did get quite strong for my new body weight. I could not be as strong at 145-150 lbs. as I was at 195-200 lbs. With that said, pound for pound, I was very strong, and I was not stimulated as I was from the animal protein. Of course, I was a much healthier person and I believe I slowed down my aging process dramatically.

"I believe they are better off by using the super greens such as E3Live, spirulina, etc." - Fred Bisci

I also believe that I would not be here today if I had stayed with that same lifestyle. I was in my sixties and was able to do 3 sets of 10 repititions in a squat with 300 pounds. There are those who eat high protein diets consisting of 5 meals a day with hundreds of grams of protein and added protein shakes who are extremely stimulated by the excess animal protein, which is not a true indication of real health or healthy strength.

As far as answering the question, many people go back and forth to their old eating habits after trying a raw plant-based diet and feel what they consider to be better. In all honesty, there could be a number of different reasons why they are having this experience, and there are many variables to this answer. They might not have ever gone through the cleanse and also could have been doing many things within the concept of the raw vegan diet that were holding them back. This can happen when you get up in all the confusion and abstract science available on the Internet. Some people are not getting enough calories to sustain their lifestyle.

I personally find that I have to eat enough fruit to sustain my activity level and my body weight.

Sometimes, a person is not eating a large enough variety of fruits and vegetables to get all of their nutrients, especially minerals. I have seen raw fooders who did not exercise enough, or at all, and because of this, they did not feel strong and healthy. By exercising, you will increase your metabolism, digest your food better, absorb more and feel stronger and healthier. There are those who eat a raw plant-based diet and supplement with vegan protein powders and claim that they feel stronger. I believe they are much better off by using the super greens such as E3Live, spirulina, etc. With that said, there are those who eat a moderate amount of animal protein in the context of a plant-based diet and feel well and strong. I believe that sometimes it could be a B12 deficiency that causes people not to be successful. You must make sure that you are connecting all of the dots and getting all of your nutrients, which can be done without animal protein.

I am not a dogmatic person. I do not lump everyone into the same category. I do not believe one size fits all. I try to meet people where they are and help them achieve their goals. I believe everybody should leave out all of the processed foods and chemicals. I have seen those who said they tried a raw vegan diet and it did not work for them. After looking at their circumstances, in many cases, I can see why. People have to walk their own journey and become as well informed as they possibly can. They should want to have their own experience. I would be careful about following the advice from a person who has the same answer for everybody. To summarize the answer to this question, I have a varied background in all athletics, including weightlifting, long distance running and Qigong. I live on 100% raw vegan diet. I'm still doing this at 85 years of age, but that is my choice. You must choose for yourself.

99. IS THE HUMAN DIGESTIVE SYSTEM DESIGNED TO HANDLE ANIMAL PRODUCTS?

BRIAN CLEMENT

Absolutely not. In a book I wrote 20 years ago called *Living Food for Optimum Health*, which is still being published and an international bestseller, I show you exactly what a carnivore, an animal-based intestinal tract is like, with the high acid in there that you could put hand in and have it eaten by the hydrochloric acid. My dog has that. I feed my dog animals. The best animals to feed a dog are raw.

They're built to eat raw and best, raw organ meat.

The human digestive tract, like that of all plant-based eating creatures, is an elongated sophisticated tract, that requires the length and the villi in the small instestines, to systematically pull nutrients out of plants. The majority of the world's population today, well over half, are basically plant-based eaters. The sickest people in the world, in general, are meat eaters and dairy eaters. The healthiest people in the world, generally, are plant-based eaters. Now, these are statistical facts. This is what every clinician speaking to you in this book is going to tell you. This is what our emprical

"The healthiest people in the world, generally, are plant-based eaters." - Brian Clement

evidence from clinical research on humans show us. Then you have people who are weak emotionally and spiritually, without experience, without evidential science, without empirical research, that are going to tell you something different. Either become independent and responsible and understand truth, or stay back in the old paradigm and go down with the old paradigm.

VIKTORAS KULVINSKAS

Yes, temporarily. We can even handle eating garbage. We can digest maggots. We can digest grasshoppers and many insects, but it's the least efficient form of food. The strongest animals are the ones that are green-eaters. We have a digestive system, an anatomy, like the anthropoid apes, and the majority of their diet is from succulent greens. The fastest animals with the highest endurance are the green-eaters.

So, we would do best to take lessons from nature and our comparative anatomy and physiology, and choose foods that are appropriate to our structure. We can live on poor quality fuel temporarily, but eventually, we start sputtering and break down, and the more we move from one generation to the next, eventually old age diseases start appearing in childhood.

GABRIEL COUSENS

This is of course an endless debate, but I do believe we are omnivores. I choose to be just a fruit and vegetable person, and my system is really good for that, but I do believe our systems are somewhat in-between and can handle both, again, depending on our constitution.

FRED BISCI

I believe the answer to that question should be obvious. From an optimal standpoint the answer is, no. Of course, if you look at our dental structure, our enzyme system, the length of our digestive system, the answer is obviously, no. There are many, many other factors here, so if somebody is eating a small amount of animal protein added into a heavily plant-based diet that enables everything to move through just as quickly as if the animal protein was not there, it's possible for this person to be healthy.

This is a complicated question that many pages could be written about. It is obvious, looking at the world epidemialogically, that there are many cultures that eat some animal protein and are thriving. But, they live in a pristine environment and none of their food is processed. This does not mean that this is optimal. In fact, everybody I knew that lived beyond 100 years of age, ate only a small amount of animal protein. The bottom line with me is results. I know 5 or 6 people personally that lived up to 105. All of them ate a small amount of animal protein. I still believe that these people could possibly have done even better. My mother was one of them. She died at 101. She ate a Mediterranean diet, with very small portions. I believe the raw vegan diet and lifestyle, taking into consideration all of the other factors, is still the best way to go. Of course, anyone who has serious disease, including cancer, should focus on a raw plant-based vegan diet.

100. DO PEOPLE'S CONSTITUTIONS REALLY VARY THAT MUCH? IS THERE ANY TRUTH TO THE CLAIM THAT WE ARE DESIGNED DIFFERENTLY AND THEREFORE NEED TO EAT DIFFERENT TYPES OF FOODS? FOR EXAMPLE, DO SOME PEOPLE HAVE TO EAT MEAT TO THRIVE?

BRIAN CLEMENT

Nobody ever has to eat meat. Where the problem came in is when people started to settle and not be nomadic. Now, to make this a very simple conversation, for most of the time that we've been on this earth, we were moving from place to place. In the winter climates, when it became cold, we would not be there at those times. We would be in the southern climates. We didn't move from place to place to have holidays and to travel. We moved to follow the food. You would be in Africa in the wintertime, you would be in Lapland, in Norway or Sweden in the summertime. Again, this constant move to temperate climates, to tropical climates, back and forth, picking the food available and eating it was the way our bodies evolved.

The human body still renders the evidence of that by the fact there are certain nutrients you only require every 9 or 10 months. What you would maybe get in the north in the deep green leafy vegetable or a berry in the middle of summer, you wouldn't require until the next time you came up to that area, tropical food in the middle of winter time. This is how we were. All at once, we became insecure as soon as we started to depend upon the intellect and relinquish the instinct, the heart, and we started to create boundaries, borders, limits, countries, states and protect those lands. Many of us settled in unlivable surroundings, and in those unlivable surroundings, we started to do abominable things like slaughter animals. Now, if you're in the middle of winter and the only thing you see running around is an animal, you go and eat the creature for survival.

That's how I think is the common sense way to think about this all began, but it doesn't mean we should be doing that, because the evidential science is clear. People who eat animal-based foods are sicker and live less time in general than people who eat plant-based diets, or in great part plant-based diets. Constitutions do not matter. Life matters.

GABRIEL COUSENS

They've actually discovered the genes that determine the constitutional variations. They found that 75% of the population needs a higher protein diet, and that 25% needed a lower protein diet and a higher complex carbohydrate diet.

My observation, clinically, was closer to 65% and 35% respectively, but generally the trend still says that there are more people that need a higher protein diet than a lower protein diet. I basically eat about 10% of my calories from protein, and I tend to go to the very highest quality proteins anyway, which are blue-green algae, spirulina, chlorella, and nuts and seeds. People needing more protein in their diets need to do the same thing, but with more intensity.

The superiority of a high protein concentrate of foods such as blue-green Klamath Lake algae, spirulina, and chlorella work directly, and there are now many kinds of combinations of vegan protein powders out there. Extracted proteins, pumpkin seed, nut protein concentrates and so forth. The best protein source in the animal world is eggs—they are 44% assimilable. Meat, fish, and chicken are 16%, 17%, and 18% assimilable, respectively. No one needs meat. Flesh food also does decrease insulin sensitivity.

In my 40 years of clinical work, I've only found one person who was born and raised near the Arctic Circle, who wanted to be successful on live foods, but they had to eat fish once a week. Otherwise, there's no one that needs to eat meat to thrive, except under those extreme conditions I just mentioned. The highest quality proteins are in blue-green algae, and really give you the highest amount of protein for the concentration. In this context, flesh food, compared to plant-source protein, is more of a bloodlust comfort food.

The people who eat according to their constitutions are going to be the most successful with live food cuisine. If a person needs higher protein (somewhere between 10% and 25% of the calories from protein, averaging 15%), they will not thrive on a fruitarian diet. It's amazing to hear people proclaim that they have found the miracle of meat eating after having spent a few years wasting away on a fruitarian diet. Clearly, they don't comprehend the fact that they simply have constitutions that require a higher protein macronutrient ratio. A plant-source cuisine would be adequate for them if only they were eating more protein.

In the same way, a person eating a high protein cuisine (who's in that 25% of people who genetically require lower protein) will not thrive on a higher protein diet. They may find the miracle of a sprout-based, plant-source cuisine perfect for themselves. Eating according to one's constitution is the key to all cuisines.

In the revised edition of *There Is a Cure for Diabetes*, I report that people eating according to their constitutions did well with 10 to 25% protein, 25 to 45% fat, and, initially, on phase one, 25 to 35% carbohydrate, which are sprouts, leafy greens, and green vegetables. They had amazing success in curing their diabetes. When they go to phase 1.5, when their fasting blood sugar is less than 100 for more than three consecutive months, then I may recommend that they move up to approximately 40% of calories from carbohydrates in their diet.

Again, constitution plays an important role. A spectrum of our work is to find the optimal combination of macronutrients that best energize the TCA cycle, operating inside the cells in the mitochondria. It's all about how to supply them with the right mix to create optimal ATP (Adenosine Triphosphate Phosphate) production, which is the primary source of biological energy.

VIKTORAS KULVINSKAS

Everything that is cooked, you lose up to 85-90% of the protein, it becomes disorganized and not recognized by your own protease (protein digesting enzyme) to be able to digest it successfully. It has been totally denatured and creates the conditions for degeneration and mental disorders and premature aging. According to the Institute of Traumatology, there's an inverse relationship between longevity and the consumption of heat-treated protein. Raw protein is the only choice. You want to have your protein in predominantly predigested form. That's why you soak your seeds and nuts and grains, thus allowing the hydrolytic enzymes that are in the seeds to predigest the protein, starch and fat, creating a very easy to digest type of food. We need at most 35 grams of protein per day. I've shown that you can get more than 30 grams of protein in a healthy gastrointestinal tract from just one fixation of nitrogen by the friendly bacteria. It's impossible to have a protein deficiency.

I get my protein from raw plant sources. Secondly, from soaked seeds, nuts and grains, which are very high in protein, up to 20%. I get it also from blue-green algae, which is up to 65% protein in a bioactive form. Also, I get protein from all my greens, just like all the wild animals and domesticated animals, mammalians.

FRED BISCI

I think I answered much of this question in the previous answer. I believe the answer to this question is somewhat complicated. I believe that we are not designed differently. We have 1 heart, 1 brain, 2 lungs, 2 kidneys and all the same organs along with 2 legs, 2 arms, etc. So obviously, we are designed the same. What else is obvious to me is that we have different chemical predispositions. I believe that most everything about the human body is chemical and is action and reaction. If you came from an area of the world and your family in that culture was eating the same way for thousands of years, your chemical predisposition is going to be different from someone coming from another culture in another area of the world and has been eating a different diet for thousand of years. For instance there are people from the Mediterranean that do not have a problem with aged cheese, but if you take some Asian people and give them dairy products, they could get very sick. With that said, I do not recommend dairy products for people. This is just an analogy. Your chemistry adapts its genetic expression to what has been passed down from generation to generation over a long period of time. This is different than your genetic blueprint, like the color of your eyes or the shape of your nose. This adaptation is called epigenetic.

If you come from the orient like Dr. Hiromi Shinya, who is probably one of the best Doctors in the world, inventor of the Shinya technique for colonoscopy surgery and author of a book called The Enzyme Factor, where rice is probably their main staple, it could be considered an optimal food, as Dr. Shinya states. They have been eating the rice for thousands of years, and under his hypothesis, he is probably correct. He states in his book that he has treated thousands of people, after they had cancer and were in remission and followed the diet that he recommends in his book and they never had a reoccurring cancer. I have a great deal of respect for Dr. Shinya and he is a brilliant medical doctor. Again, I state that his diet recommends no processed food, which I think is the main key. There are no simple answers to all of these questions. I believe there are certain foods that people are consuming that are not processed and are not optimal, and yet these people seem to be doing ok. Again, I will repeat, what you leave out is the key. Processed food is the killer.

101. WHERE DO YOU GET YOUR PROTEIN?

BRIAN CLEMENT

The top protein foods on the planet is blue-green and green algae, sea vegetables, and sprouts and grasses, by far the best, most complete and highest levels of protein. Again, this is what we train Olympic athletes on. This is what I've raised four children and our grandchildren on. This is what we've placed hundreds and hundreds of thousands of people on, collectively millions of people. And people not only get better, they flourish on these types of proteins.

GABRIEL COUSENS

Personally, 10% of my calories come from protein. My main protein sources are nuts and seeds and, specifically, one tablespoon of E3Live concentrate daily.

VIKTORAS KULVINSKAS

Where does the cooked food meat eater get their protein? When animal protein is cooked, up to 85% of the protein is destroyed by fire. All the research can be found in my book Survival. The better question would be to ask the meat eaters how they manage to get their protein when they lost most of the protein in the cooking process. In the raw food program, you will have predigested protein in the form of amino acids and peptides found in soaked seeds and nuts and grains, as well as in sprouted form at values as high as 30% protein levels.

Furthermore, many of the superfoods consumed, such as grass powders, are up to 45% protein, the algae family is up to 65% protein and then lastly, see research in my book *Survival in the 21st Century* where Dr. Oolong and Dr. Huxley researched a vegan tribe in Papua, New Guinea that exhibited exceptional health on 5 grams of protein per day. Extensive investigation by the two doctors showed that because these vegan individuals were on a high complex carbohydrate diet with a huge volume of probiotic activity, the friendly bacteria fixated nitrogen from the air, creating over 30 grams of protein per day. All the most progressive research indicates that 30 grams of protein per day is more than adequate. Hence, a very important dietary intake for vegans is a high-fiber diet and probiotics to be assured of optimal levels of essential amino acids and overall protein.

FRED BISCI

The information that is available I believe is inaccurate and mythological. The more you use, especially animal protein, the more you are going to think you need. A truly healthy person does not need as much protein as they have been led to believe. You can get more than enough from a raw plant-based vegan diet.. I get more than enough protein from eating a variety of fresh fruits, vegetables, a moderate amount of nuts, seeds, avocados, sprouts and green smoothies, super foods such as E3Live, spirulina, etc. I particularly like chia seeds, sesame seeds, pistachio nuts and almonds. I do not believe in protein powders of any kind.

My meal on a consistent basis is fruit, the quantity of the fruit I eat is based on the extent of my exercises. If I am training hard, I eat more fruit. I find that the fruit that are fructose-based, like berries, cherries, peaches plums, pears and apples, rather than glucose-based, like bananas and other starchy fruits, work better for me because fructose-based fruit does not require insulin. Glucose-based fruits and vegetables require insulin. I never consume any form of animal protein. I do not like it and over the years, have found it to become repulsive and have no desire to eat it. It is a big part of my spiritual and moral standards. I am against it and it is not for me and I would never go back to it no matter what my circumstances. My beliefs have been severely tested a few times in my life. It is not for me and I would not go back. I am an animal lover and have always loved my dogs. I would not eat my dogs, no matter what the circumstances. When I feed my dog some raw meat, there is a certain amount of moral and spiritual discomfort. There are people who would not choose to live this way. This is the way I choose to live no matter what happens. I am glad I made this choice. It was the right choice for me.

102. IS IT OK TO EAT RAW MEAT—AND DO YOU GET NUTRITION OUT OF IT?

GABRIEL COUSENS

The issue of raw meat is a moral and spiritual one, as well as a physiological question. As a person who's a committed vegan live foodist, it's not okay to eat raw meat for moral, ethical, and spiritual reasons. It's certainly not okay to eat raw meat because it clogs the subtle energetic spiritual channels called the nadis and fills the nadis and chakras with energies of death. Also, from a vegan perspective, it creates pain and cruelty. From a health perspective, whether it's wild game or not, you're still eating higher on the food chain, and that means it will have more concentrated radiation. Meat has 15 to 30 times more concentration of pesticides, herbicides, more depleted uranium, I-131, and radiation in general.

Whether you're killing animals in the wild or going hunting in the supermarket, where most of the "raw meat" people ultimately end up eating, you're still going to get food that will be more toxic. The newer research from Harvard School of Public Health clearly shows that there's a 20% decrease in life span by eating more junk meat and an 18% decrease in life span eating the highest quality of grass-fed meat. In any case, meat eating decreases life span. An excellent meta-analysis of 12 studies shows that the incidence of diabetes is increased 35% to 50% from eating meat.

Is this okay? If moral, ethical, spiritual, and health concerns are not an issue for a person, then by definition, it's acceptable. Eating raw meat is better than cooked, because when one cooks meat, 50% of the protein, according to the Max Planck Institute, is lost.

Eating raw meat also carries the risk of parasites. I remember in Hawaii some raw meat, live-food people ate a fish while it was still alive, which is against the Noahide principles. One died from the parasites and one became very ill. There are a lot of problems in eating raw meat and cooked meat, but these issues are non-existent if one eats a plant-source only cuisine.

FRED BISCI

Based on my experience and the people I have counseled, I do not recommend it. With that said, there are people in the world that eat insects, like the Aborigines in Australia who eat grubs. There are cultures in the world where people eat raw fish, such as raw ceviche and sushi. I do not believe that you have to eat these foods. Weston Price, in his book, *Nutrition and Physical Degeneration*, recommends these types of foods based on his travels and studies with pristine cultures. We must remember, these people ate no processed foods and were under very little stress and had no problems from all of the things we encounter in modern-day society. They were leaving out all of the processed food. This does not mean that what they were doing was optimal. We can thrive and excel in many cases, if you so choose, without the animal protein. Whatever you choose to eat should be clean, without chemicals, antibiotics, pesticides, etc.

BRIAN CLEMENT

I think anyone who would propose eating raw fish or meat should take a microscope, even if it's a $30 child's microscope and look at it. It would cure you immediately of wanting to eat anything uncooked from the animal kingdom.

Number two, the same thing applies to raw flesh as would apply to cooked flesh. Please, don't be absurd.

VIKTORAS KULVINSKAS

A well-chosen, meat-oriented diet, organic, eating the whole animal, has been the case with Eskimos and Laplanders. You can find all the documentation in my book coauthored with Dr. Edwin Howell called Good Enzymes for Health and Longevity. These individuals lived right into their 90s, as long as they ate it in a raw state. But they ate every part of the animal, even the head. By the time they were in their mid-90s, they all were dying off from acidosis, even though they ate the sweet meat.

The typical raw meat eaters eat predominantly the muscle tissue, which is the most acid-filled with urea and urine. These individuals smell bad. They are very vulgar to any humane considerations. They are involved in the act of killing. There is nothing ethical about them. They will reap the karma of killing. No human has the claws that are needed to kill an animal, to tear it apart and to consume and delight in it. No healthy child would ever want to conceive of choosing meat over a bowl of salad greens, sprouts or fruit.

Such individuals, as a rule, why they made such great progress on the raw meat is the stimulating effect of meat, and, they weren't cooking the protein and they were getting the stimulation and the protein in an easily assumable form. As a background, most of them were probably hygienists. They were not consuming the sprouted high source of predigested amino acids and proteins.

Such a dietary approach is also mentally unsound. It's unsustainable. The seven billion people on planet earth could not in any way thrive and live healthy or well by consuming raw meat. It is also more contaminated than fresh vegetables by the environmental contaminants. These animal fare consumers are poisoning themselves.

103. WHAT ARE YOUR THOUGHTS ON CONSUMING FISH AND SEAFOOD?

BRIAN CLEMENT

My book, *Killer Fish*, will absolutely frame why one would never consider fish a food, much less a healthy food. It is not only the contaminants, it's the unacceptability for the human body to consume the saturated fats, the discombobulated essential fats in it and the absurdity of the fact that now we're fishing out the ocean so much that the top oceanographic scientists at this point in history say that by the mid-21st century, three decades from now, there will not be fish as we know it in the ocean. Please, wake up. Fish is not a health food. It's a destructive food to you and the planet earth. Do no eat fish.

FRED BISCI

Fish and seafood are animal proteins. They are aquatic animals. To me, it is pretty much the same and I don't eat fish. I don't eat shrimp and I don't eat lobster. New studies have shown that people who eat animal protein on a regular basis have a 28% better chance of having a stroke. People who eat fish, which is an aquatic animal, have a 6% chance of having a stroke. All shell fish and scavengers are high stress foods. The body has to work harder to metabolize shell fish and it is best avoided. Those that ate a plant-based vegan diet had a 52% less chance of having a stroke. People have to make their own choice. If a person wants to eat animal protein, fish would probably be their best choice. I try to meet people where they are and try to put together a healthy lifestyle for them, which I have been able to do. Most people who come to see me do not want to eat a 100% raw plant-based vegan diet.

VIKTORAS KULVINSKAS

Just read the Hippocrates' magazine article issue on fish, as well as the book by Brian Clement, Killer Fish. Even when raw, it is infested with all kinds of pathogenic microbes. It rots. It smells bad. You could go past the fish market—it's the most stinking place. It's worse than meat in terms of stink. That's what you become. That smell, that rot.

The oceans have been contaminated by all form of heavy metals, including mercury. Fish concentrate the poisons of the ocean many times over what you would find if you were consuming sea vegetables.

GABRIEL COUSENS

At this point, with the amount of radiation pollution in the Pacific and, ultimately, the world over, fish, whether this year or in next year, will be far more radioactively contaminated than any other animal source. The fish concentrates the toxins in the water 9 million times. Oysters and clams concentrate their toxins 70,000 times. The problem with fish is they don't urinate, so they're literally building up toxins in their bodies. From this perspective, I wouldn't recommend eating fish.

104. I LOVE THE TASTE OF MEAT—BACON, BURGERS. MY DIET REVOLVES AROUND TASTE AND CONVENIENCE. HOW CAN I OVERCOME THIS AND BECOME AND STAY HEALTHY WHILE STILL SATISFYING MY TASTE BUDS?

FRED BISCI

This is an unusual question. To me it's like saying "I like to smoke crack and do cocaine, how can I get around this and become a healthy person and still satisfy my cravings for drugs?" That's pretty much impossible. What I can tell you is that you are heavily intoxicated and have been poisoned. In order to change, you have to cleanse your lymphatic system, your GI tract and your cells. Your taste buds have been perverted. If you do this, your chemistry will change. Remember, everything is chemical and every action has a reaction. If you change your actions and your lifestyle, the reactions in your cells, your lymph system and GI tract will change. Your tastebuds will desire clean, whole, raw, fresh foods. When I go to social events such as weddings and parties, I watch people eat the Standard American Diet, see their obesity, hear about all of their illnesses, hear about the medications they are on and the surgeries that they had, and my answer to this question is to change what you are eating and your perception of how food should taste. I hear this story every day, and many of these people now have life threatening illnesses. We must remember, the human body is a miracle in progress. Cleanse and detox, change your lifestyle and claim your miracle.

BRIAN CLEMENT

Well, this was me. I wasn't a conscious kid. I loved meat and I loved the worst meat and I used to fry the worst meat in butter. You have to make a decision based not upon your addiction, but upon your will. If your will is centered, if you say to yourself, "I know this is making me sick. I know it's contributing to disease and shortening my lifespan. I have enough knowledge and understanding of why that's bad for me." Once you have that knowledge and understanding, it gives you the ability to have the will to say no.

Now, the first year I had given meat up, I was climbing walls. I wanted to eat meat again, but my will prevented me from doing that. I assure you, by the beginning of the second year, you're going to say, "I actually used to eat meat?" The things that used to attract you when you've been putting them into your body repel you and make you sick and nauseous by even considering it. The hardest one for me to give up wasn't meat, as much as I loved it, it was dairy food because dairy food wasn't as offensive. I wasn't killing animals. That was my easy way to stop eating meat. I wanted to stop killing animals. The fact was, dairy food wasn't that easy because I was justifying it and in so many areas it's mixed into foods, it's prepared into foods. It's ice cream that was my biggest crutch. I mean, ice cream was one-stop shopping; it was high fat and high sugar. My God, I didn't have to go anywhere else to get that. I used to eat it literally by the gallon, liters and liters at a time.

What you have to understand is that you've got to make a conscious decision based upon an emotional and spiritual truth and then maintain that. Make it almost your dogma for a while. Then, after that, your body's going to be singing hallelujah, thank God, this person's stopped contaminating me! We're the only creatures that I've observed, other than the poor domestic animals, that actually crap where we live. We just do it by destroying our bodies and destroying the earth by consuming animals. That's one of the sad ways we do it.

VIKTORAS KULVINSKAS

This sounds like an alcoholic who says, "How can I continue to not be consuming alcohol and satisfy my taste for alcohol?" You cannot. You've got to make a choice between poison and non-poison. The taste that you find in the animal protein can be satisfied by the veggie burgers. You can try out all the delicious vegetarian restaurants, vegan restaurants and raw food restaurants around the world. You'll find that there will be many dishes that you will totally enjoy far more than you will enjoy the consumption of flesh food. Learn how to spice up your meals. It's in the spices that create the taste that you delight in. By experimenting in these directions, you'll be able to overcome.

There's also the idea that you might need to go to a detox center, one of the raw food spas, resorts, and go on a juice program. Eat fresh produce. Get some colonics. Entertain some new way of living. Get reeducated. Right now, you are conditioned by the social matrix that has inculcated and indoctrinated you, and force-fed you toxic food, and as a result what you are made of is what you crave. In order to get over this addiction, you need to go to a place that will support you breaking the addiction. Then go to potlucks on a daily basis if you need to, where you can enjoy a variety of good, healthy foods, as well as vegan restaurants, until you lose that craving. You will. We all had it. You're not alone. So you can do it.

GABRIEL COUSENS

Meat is indeed addictive, not only to humans but also to vegetarian animals. This was something noted by some of the seafaring voyagers from Denmark and the Vikings. They found that when they fed fish to the animals like the cows and the sheep on their ships, the animals became addicted over time. Meat has an addictive quality because it stimulates endorphins.

For people who are really serious about breaking that addiction, a one-week green juice fast is extremely helpful. It clears the cellular memory of the addiction. This is why, during my 21-Day Transformation Program, we have the seven-day green juice fast followed by a Zero Point course, a psycho-spiritual course that teaches one how to psychologically let go of addictions. In the first week, participants address the physiological aspect through juice fasting. During the second week, participants deal with the psychological aspects. During the third week, we have the Conscious Eating course, where we teach people how to develop all kinds of delicious foods that are plant-source only. In that process, people also understand their constitutions, so that they can make delicious food suited to supporting their individual constitutions.

MEN'S HEALTH

"The less one eats, the longer one lives. Never eat such a big meal that you aren't fully energized and ready to go within a few minutes after eating." - Gabriel Cousens

"The idea here is to slow down our aging process, which we definitely can do by changing lifestyle to a raw vegan or close to it lifestyle with minimum or no animal protein." - Fred Bisci

"The answer lies in the high electro voltage charged alkaline foods of the raw vegan program, which is predominantly oriented in the green food, which leads to maximizing the red blood cell and hemoglobin levels within the blood, thus maximizing oxygen delivery, which leads to maximal metabolic activities—thus creating power and endurance." - Viktoras Kulvinskas

"The two nutrients that help prevent premature graying and baldness are zinc and copper." - Brian Clement

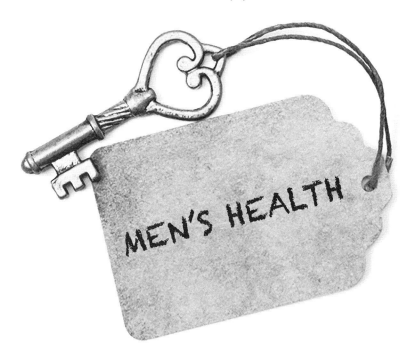

105. IT TAKES FOREVER TO BUILD STRENGTH—AND EVEN AFTER TAKING LOADS OF SUPPLEMENTS, PROTEIN AND CREATINE, I STILL STRUGGLE TO MAINTAIN IT. HOW CAN ONE GET AND MAINTAIN STRENGTH?

GABRIEL COUSENS

There is no simple way. One has to eat according to their constitution. One has to exercise and also stretch and do a variety of exercises throughout the week. One common mistake is that people do heavy weight training more than once or twice a week. Some of the newer research is suggesting that once or twice a week of heavy weight training can actually give you more sustaining strength more quickly than lifting heavy every single day.

FRED BISCI

Let's start from the beginning. First and foremost, supplements, in most cases, are not the answer. In this case I'm talking about protein powders and creatine. If you want to be super strong, it is best to cleanse and detoxify your GI tract, your lymphatic system and at a cellular level, as I have stated in many of the previous questions. Then you must free yourself of processed food. Get all the nutrients that you need and connect all the dots. In order to be strong and maintain your strength, you have to do resistance exercises and employ stretching. The human body, when it is healthy and clean, responds very well to strenuous exercises. By increasing the resistance and making the right changes in your diet and getting adequate rest, you can become super strong. In my sixties, at 140 lbs. body weight, I was able to do repetition knee bends with 300 pounds. With the right diet, adequate rest and the right mental attitude and discipline, the sky is the limit. You don't have to have tremendous size to be super strong and healthy. You do not want to end up being the best built guy in the cemetery, like some people I have known. Some of these questions you could write a whole book on.

BRIAN CLEMENT

Most importantly, you have to be consistent with weightlifting. I'll give you my story. I don't want to become over-focused on me, but I went through a lot of these struggles. When I read this question, it was really resonating with me because this is the question I had. I hated exercise. When I was a kid, I was very cerebral and I was very musical. I had a mantra along with my fellow musicians, we don't exercise and we don't dance. With that said, when I began to eat a proper diet, I lost an enormous amount of weight. I lost 120 lbs. and became very thin, and I started to realize that healthy raw plant-based foods are not going to put weight on my body because they shouldn't put weight on your body. Foods should nourish you and give you energy and build the cells and build the anatomy. They shouldn't be making you fat. Was I going to go back to eating fattening, bad foods, unhealthy foods—or was I going to build true weight, namely muscle? The first two months I went into a gym, I thought I was going to die. I mean, I had never done anything like that in my life. By the fourth month, I never looked back and now I can't live without weightlifting exercise. I gained 55, 60 lbs. 40 years ago, and have maintained that, even in spite of the fact that I eat very little. I drink a lot of juices. I take whole food supplementation and I eat very little solid food. Not to say that that's what you should aspire to do today, that's where I am at this point this many years later.

All of us need to go and be where we are at the time. This is what you have to know. Every one of you will gain strength. Keep your youth, keep your vitality, but you have to do it properly. You have to eat the right foods. You have to eat adequate amounts of those foods. In the early days, I had to eat to get from thin to strong, enormous amounts of food, rather than high-caloric, sugary foods like fructose-rich fruit, which have 30 times more sugar than the original fruit. I was eating sprouted grains, which were slowing down my metabolism, sprouted beans, some nuts and seeds, but proteins do not build muscle unless you rip your muscle. Even these protein powders you're taking, if you take a pound a day, a half a kilo a day, you will not build muscle if you don't rip your muscle through weightlifting. Weightlifting is the way you maintain strength and weight.

VIKTORAS KULVINSKAS

First of all, it's no wonder you have difficulties in maintaining strength. Creatines and protein powders are not a way to maintain it. You want predigested protein that comes from soaked seeds and nuts. The creatine is totally unnecessary. It's a fake food. It's the green super foods you need. Make it from soaked seeds and nuts, spirulina, add some fresh fruit if you need to, or Stevia. Add enzymes and probiotics to such smoothies, and you're going to get all the essential necessary food for building strength, and that means providing the essential amino acids for creating a physique that you want on a raw food based type of a diet, just like any bodybuilder or strength builder.

During the building phase, you would be consuming small meals, 16-20 ounces per meal, with high protein, high carbs, that center around well-combined soaked seeds and nuts, as well as blue-green algae, grass powders, enzymes, probiotics. They'll be digested in two to three hours. You'll be consuming it about every three hours. You can put on one to two pounds of lean muscle mass per week on such a program. You don't need anything more than that.

To maintain it, then you can do it on two meals a day. Initially, to jump start it, you'll have to do more. Smaller meals are better. But eventually, as you cleanse and detoxify, you need less and less food in order to obtain the maximum results.

106. IF I UNDERTAKE STRENOUS PHYSICAL ACTIVITY AT WORK (LOGGING, POURING ASPHALT, ETC.) ON A DAILY BASIS, HOW CAN I GET ENOUGH ENERGY TO MAKE IT THROUGH THE DAY? I'VE ALWAYS BEEN TOLD TO EAT A BIG BREAKFAST—LOTS OF CALORIES— FOR ENERGY. IS THERE A HEALTHY ALTERNATIVE?

GABRIEL COUSENS

The first rule is to eat according to your constitution, because eating according to your constitution will support the mitochondria, where you make the optimum amount of ATP. This will allow you to maximize our strength.

At least 10 research projects since 1917 have also shown that vegetarians and vegetarian non-athletes have two to three times the endurance needed in athletics. By going vegan and, even better, going live food, one is more likely to have the energy to go all day. Generally speaking, according to Ayurveda, the biggest meal should be between 10 am and 2 pm, when our digestive power, or the fire element, is highest. That's the time to eat your biggest meal. However, one could have a moderate meal at breakfast and the smallest meal at dinner.

The less one eats, the longer one lives. Never eat such a big meal that you aren't fully energized and ready to go within a few minutes after eating. When one eats live food, one can get twice the quality of nutrients than when it's cooked. When cooked, food loses 50% of the protein, 60 to 70% of vitamins and minerals, and up to 95 to 100% of the vital nutrients.

Clearly, if eating cooked food, one must eat at least twice as much, or even more, calories to get the same nutrition. If one is eating live food, one needn't eat as much, and therefore, there's less digestive stress, and therefore, one definitely has more energy all day long. Personally, I find that the less one eats, the more energy one has over time. My goal, as I stated earlier, is to have full-on energy all day long. My goal is to have no drops in energy for my full working day, which is often 12 hours.

VIKTORAS KULVINSKAS

I have easy to digest eco foods for breakfast. For one, sprouted grain cereal with soaked overnight sunflower blended to a cream with one carrot. Add a little sea salt to taste. Have as a side dish flax crackers, maybe dulse, and that will keep you going right up to noon. Have a cream made out of soaked sunflower or almonds, which can also be served in a form of cheese or in a form of cream. Serve it with banana and some other fruit. You'll have a very high calorie, high protein breakfast that will keep you going right up to noon.

For a noon meal, take along in a thermos bottle green juice and a protein green smoothie. Have a cup of green juice. Thirty minutes later, have the green protein drink. You will have all the energy you need to work through the day. Toward the mid, end of the day, have some more green protein smoothie, and that will cover you with excellent power with no slowdown.

I had a very good friend, she was in her 60s and still working on weekends as a dancer. At the same time she did that, she got paid to exercise in public. During the week, she had a full-time job. When she was trying to earn money for graduate work in school, she worked in construction. On her raw food program, yet being in her 60s, she outdid men who were one-third her age, whether it was climbing to the top of a tree or logging or doing any of the heavy labor-intensive work. Whatever was difficult, they would send her, because they knew she could do it.

In the evening, you can serve a more comprehensive meal made out of sprouts, avocados, sea vegetables and fermented foods. Take your time in chewing all the salad greens and other high fiber foods. You will have a very delightful, non-stressed, long evening for yourself, instead of being totally wasted like the rest of the public.

Remember, in the studies that have been done on endurance—and this is what we're talking about—the vegans outdid the meat eaters. And that's true in the field. It is the ox that outdoes the lion who might be a short sprinter, but cannot keep up with that, whether it is an antelope or a hardworking elephant or a hardworking mule or a hardworking donkey. The answer lies in the high electro voltage charged alkaline foods of the raw vegan program, which is predominantly oriented to the green food, which leads to maximizing the red blood cell and hemoglobin levels within the blood, thus maximizing oxygen delivery, which leads to maximal metabolic activities—thus creating power and endurance.

FRED BISCI

The answer to that question is no for the first part, and yes for the second part. If you mean, "Do I have to eat eggs and pancakes with a protein shake for breakfast to give me the strength and energy to carry me thru the day?" the answer as stated before is, no. I've known many vegans who ate plenty of raw foods, myself included, and had plenty of strength and all-day energy. The key is, leave out all the processed food. Make sure you're getting enough calories to sustain your physical activity, with a 10% increase of your normal amount of protein. If you are a vegan raw foodist and are advanced eat plenty of fruit, chia seeds, sesame seeds, pistachio nuts, E3Live, spirulina and combination supergreen foods in your green smoothies. In place of a heavy protein breakfast, a supergreen smoothie with plenty of calories from fruit, coconut water, chia seeds, hemp seeds, nuts, raw spirulina and a small amount of coconut butter is good. A person could go all day on a drink like this. There is much more I can add to this question. This is a good and important question. Many people on raw diets are healthy but feeble because they are living in the past and are being confused by the mixed bag of information that is on the Internet by people who never had to work hard or were strength or endurance athletes. You might want to try a consultation from a professional that has this kind of experience. Doing hard labor all day is a lot different than working out in a gym or running in a race.

BRIAN CLEMENT

I don't eat breakfast. I haven't eaten breakfast in four decades. One day's supply of juices and supplementation are probably the same nourishment I used to get in one month before I began eating a healthy way.

I did an experiment. Before I went to Europe for Hippocrates back in the 1970s, I took a two-month sabbatical and went essentially to get an extremely strenuous job. I was working with a demolition crew disassembling the Apollo launch pads at Cape Kennedy. I experimented on myself during that nine-week period where literally I was doing my one-day-a-week fast and then by the fourth week added a second day and by the seventh week added a third day. I was just on raw juices. I made sure that my body was exposed to as much sunlight as possible, so that I got as much direct nutrient loads and energy and immune boosting as I could. This wasn't hard to do in sunny Florida, out in the middle of a peninsula that was a wildlife refuge. Other than the Apollo launch pads, I've never done work nor have I ever seen anyone do work any more strenuous than this. I mean the lightest things we were doing was picking up 200 pounds with another guy, using heavy equipment where I had to throw my entire body on top of it to turn the wheel of the machine. This was again from 6 in the morning till 1:30 or 2 o'clock in the afternoon.

They made me the foreman by the fourth week because I was the only guy with energy after the 10:30 in the morning when we had lunch. They finally learned, by about the fifth week, that I was a wild, non-meat eating creature and their manhood was challenged at that point. They liked me—they saw that I was a great worker. They saw I was building muscle and strength and they saw I had more energy than them, but they thought I was some kind of a deranged character because I chose not to eat meat. They called me all kinds of names, but I just laughed about it and went on.

The saddest day I had was when I had to tell them I was leaving and going to Europe. I felt almost a little bit dishonest, but I can tell you anyone who would like to have that conversation, I intentionally went out of my way and did this work to prove that you can do the most strenuous, the most intense heavy work and flourish on it by getting nutrients. It's a lot of heavy solid stuff like a heavy big breakfast that weighs you down, that your poor body has to use all of its energy to discard, but it's light, easy to digest nutrients, high protein nutrients like you get from the sprouts and the algae and the juices, that literally are going to make you flourish and strong as an ox. It's amazing what you can do with this. Again, when we train Olympic athletes, they get stronger and healthier and make better time.

107. IS THERE A NATURAL WAY TO SLOW DOWN OR PREVENT BALDNESS?

FRED BISCI

If you look around today and are observant, you will notice that more young men are going bald than ever before. I also have noticed a lot of professional athletes are bald. I am a big baseball fan and watch the New York Yankees every chance I get. It's amazing to me how many of these young guys in their 20s and early 30s are bald. I also remember watching the Giants, the Yankees and the Brooklyn Dodgers when I was a kid. Very few of the athletes were bald. In fact I don't remember any. There is a direct connection between

"There is a direct connection between male pattern baldness and elevated testosterone and diets that are high in animal protein, not to mention growth promoting hormones." – Fred Bisci

male pattern baldness and elevated testosterone and diets that are high in animal protein, not to mention growth promoting hormones. Many of the massively built bodybuilders today are bald or going bald. If you are eating a vegan diet with plenty of raw foods and reducing or eliminating animal protein and getting an adequate amount of protein from a vegetarian source and lowering your testosterone, you will slow down your hair loss. Genetic predisposition, of course is a big factor. There are some men who lose their hair in their early 20s and their father and uncles had the same thing happen to them. There are many men who are losing their hair because of their lifestyle and accelerated aging. The idea here is to slow down our aging process, which we definitely can do by changing lifestyle to a raw vegan or close to it lifestyle with minimum or no animal protein.

BRIAN CLEMENT

Yes, there is. The two nutrients that help prevent premature graying and baldness are zinc and copper. I would get an ionic form of zinc, a liquid ionic form of zinc, take double the amount of that as copper in the mornings, zinc and then copper at night. I would use a brush, like a Fuller Shampoo Brush, to scrape your scalp on a daily basis when you're in the shower to get blood flow up to that area. Biotin, silica and then magnesium, better taken in the oil form topically on the body—all of these contribute to hair growth. Of course, why so many young people are having baldness today, especially the young men, is because of the incredibly high incidence of animal food consumption. The University of Buffalo reported in a study a number of years ago where they actually showed the follicles were clogged with cholesterol, smothering the hair. That's one of the big reasons you see so many young bald people. It was an anomaly when I was boy. Now, it's a common-place event.

VIKTORAS KULVINSKAS

Absolutely! I was moving toward baldness at the age of 29. Some youngsters are nowadays already bald by that time because they're suffering from old age diseases, as I was at 29. I used to count up to 400 hairs lost on some days, as I was brushing my hair out of my scalp. I had quite a high density when I was a teenager. It was very clearly indicated that I had an acid soil, that is the scalp, within which the grasses, which we call hair, grows. When it's acidic, you have lots of dandruff and an itchy scalp, which I did. This means that the pH of the soil was totally inappropriate. It should be slightly on the alkaline side, or at least, mildly acidic. Due to a mucus-forming diet, the soil became claylike in the scalp extremities, thus poor circulation of nutrition. Of course, the minerals and the quality proteins feed the hair rootlets. I had an acidic, enzyme-depleted internal environment, lacking in proper hydration. I never drank water; instead, choosing Coca-Cola and other sweet beverages, such as an extremely toxic milk. I had many other health challenges, of course, but upon joining Ann Wigmores' Rising Sun Christianity, I started changing my lifestyle habits. Hair loss stopped. Though the re-growth was sparse, as I increased my mineral resources and also the enzyme intake with improved quality of amino acid profile due to my ability to digest the plant-based proteins, I saw quite a great deal of re-growth of my hair.

In my late 60s, I had an embarrassing receding hairline. I was introduced to a well-researched nutritional algae stem cell accelerator, which doubled the daily production. Within a matter of a few months, the receding hairline disappeared. Now, in my mid-70s, I have a full head of hair.

Cold laser is being researched with excellent results. At Hippocrates Health Institute salon, they showed me many photos of individuals with extremely thinned out hairline. Within a period of a year of ongoing treatments, many again had a full head of hair. Call Hippocrates and ask for the organic beauty salon.

Things you can do on your own, independent of any other assistance: number one—hydrate, especially with alkaline green juices. You need to increase the water content of your scalp and stop having itchiness and dandruff. Clean up the compromised cardiovascular system to increase circulation, with not only live and raw food, but also with the use of enzymes with meals and systemic enzymes between meals, as found at Hippocrates Health Institute. Daily, massage your scalp. Rinse your hair daily with diluted lemon. Wash out the lemon, and then rub into your scalp wheatgrass juice—not only for your scalp, but also for your facial toning. You want to rejuvenate the whole head. Keep the wheatgrass on your head for twenty minutes, and then shower again. Avoid the desert winds that come from hair blowers. They're one of the deadliest things for destroying your hair rootlets. It's cooking your hair. Use only organic quality shampoos and conditioners on your hair once a week, or less frequently.

You can purchase an inverse slant board and lie on it at continually increasing angles, until, eventually, you're hanging by your feet. Do this very gradually, because it'll place a lot of pressure on your head area in terms of blood circulation, which will provide nutrition. Until your cardiovascular system is cleaned up, only marginal, gentle slant board uses are suggested. In yoga, you can be doing the shoulder stand, as well as utilizing inverse hanging by an Iyengar-style rope system.

Daily indulgence in cayenne, unless you are allergic to it, in all your liquids, whatever you can tolerate, will make a difference in terms of circulation. Consuming sea vegetables for the full mineral effect is also recommended.

Nutritional guidelines. One of the key driving factors for the start of baldness is consumption of heat-treated animal protein, especially pasteurized dairy products. In that category are also sugar products, as well as white flour products and processed grains of all sorts. That includes organic pasta, organic spaghetti, even though it's made from whole grains. It is a processed food. Products such as vinegar.

GABRIEL COUSENS

I don't have as much experience in this area, but increasing circulation to the scalp is good. Inversions that bring the blood to the scalp would be a general suggestion.

WOMEN'S HEALTH

"Exercise has a great influence on the duration and the severity and discomforts associated with menstruation." - Viktoras Kulvinskas

"I know many women who follow this type of a lifestyle and have no symptoms from menopause." - Fred Bisci

"...some of the research is suggesting that adequate iodine supplementation can decrease rates of breast cancer." - Gabriel Cousens

"You shouldn't have pain, or be suffering from PMS—which 6 out of 10 women do today." - Brian Clement

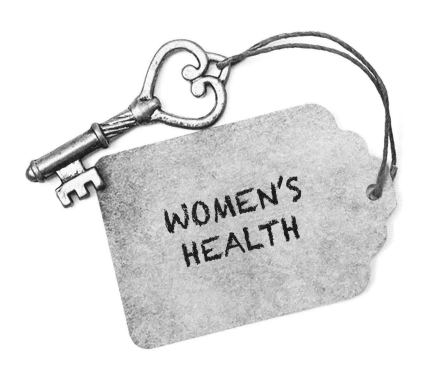

108. THERE SEEMS TO BE A HIGH RATE OF WOMEN WITH ESTROGEN AND OTHER HORMONAL PROBLEMS. WHAT IS THE BEST AND MOST NATURAL WAY TO BALANCE YOUR HORMONES?

BRIAN CLEMENT

Estrogen is pervasive because the body looks at chemicals, heavy metals, etc., as estrogen. If you look at men becoming more feminine, and women becoming more masculine, it is because when these chemicals get into the bloodstream, they mimic estrogen. When you have more estrogen as a woman, your body creates testosterone, masculinizing you, more estrogen in a man is feminizing. For the first time in human history we now know that that there are 2% fewer boys being born than girls, it used to be 50% female, 50% males. Now, for the first time, they predict that by the year 2025, it may be up to 5% disparity in birth rates, fewer boys, more effeminate men, and this is because of estrogens. We have to avoid all of the things I just mentioned, starting with food, air, water, clothing, certainly those polyester, nylon undergarments which are deadly. I can't invent a better word to give you about this then "chemical toxiema."

There are certain foods, cruciferous vegetables, the cabbage family, that help to knock it back. We have a product called Life Give Est-Toll that acts as an estrogen lowering agent, it's phenomenal. It's an Ayurvedic formula made from the plant that all cabbage came from. We've seen it to be quite effective over the years we've used it. Hormonal problems should be tested by a great bio-identical hormone doctor. That woman or man should tell you what's going on. In some cases, with the concern of disorders, you have disease that has to be part of the discussion. You may want to temporarily take bio-identical hormones.

VIKTORAS KULVINSKAS

Hormones are your platinum elixirs that are involved in monitoring and creating appropriate responses to the environment, internal and external, as well as to the emotional states. Consumption of animal protein, especially processed foods, has led to the appearance, earlier and earlier in the life of a woman, of her first menses. The duration of the bleeding has also increased. During the menstrual flow, a tremendous amount of hormones are lost and the aging process accelerated.

The first phase of recovery would be to get on a plant-based vegan diet. Second, start consuming bioflavonoid-rich vegetables and taking some bioflavonoid-source, organic quality vitamin C complex supplementation, as found at Hippocrates Health Institute. Bioflavonoids have a structure almost identical to estrogens and other female hormones, thus rejuvenating one's own hormonal levels, while also increasing the strength of capillaries and arteries.

Women are subject to a tremendous amount of impossible stress to meet standards that are found in the fashion world, as 18-year-old girls are held up as the expression of the ideal form for a woman at 30, 40, 50. Women are continuously under stress about their breasts, about their overall appearance. They never feel good enough. One should read *Biological Superiority, A Woman in Survival in the Twenty-First Century*. Find out who a woman is. Read Dr. Anna Maria's *The Power of a Woman*.

Meditation, yoga and all other forms of exercise are necessary to get yourself out of that depressive condition. Get on a vegan diet. Start having self-respect and worth. Do not accept degrading commentaries from males or competitive females. You are perfect and beautiful as you are. You can create whatever form you wish through exercise and nutritional modifications.

Some of the most healthful foods, besides the bioflavonoid-rich greens, are sprouted grains. They can be made into delicious cereals that I describe. They're a source of the hormones for the regeneration of the reproductive cycle. Cleansing and detoxification regenerate these and other ductless glands, which absorb nutrients through the skin and excrete the hormones through the skin. If it's coated with mucus and phlegm from pasteurized dairy products, the consumption of corpses of animals, raw or cooked, as well as the mucus-laden processed foods, yoga postures will allow you to activate all your hormones and exercise the ductless glands, thus increasing the production and regenerating and renewing and youthing yourself.

The only other superfood, besides the herbal female formulas, that I've seen extremely helpful from the nutritional point of view is blue-green algae. The results we have seen are phenomenal in terms of not only assisting males, but also females, in regenerating the hormonal system.

GABRIEL COUSENS

When women eat a healthy live food plant-source-only cuisine, their hormonal balance is significantly improved. Also, when they cut out all white flour, white sugar, high fructose, high sucrose, high glucose foods, the hormonal balance improves.

PMS symptoms increase up to 246% when people are taking a high sugar diet. Living on a live food plant-source only cuisine, having a relatively low sugar diet, eating according to one's constitution, and moderate exercise, all can significantly, in my experience, help rebalance your hormones. These are my first recommendations, before I would consider adding herbs or homeopathics that can further refine the rebalancing of the hormones. Let the body do it first.

FRED BISCI

Give up all processed food, go through a cleanse and detox the right way, follow a good diet that connects all the dots, and see how you do. Most likely, the hot flashes and all of the other symptoms will disappear. Get into the outdoors, where there is plenty of fresh air—walk, jog, swim, ride your bike, do yoga and Pilates, use some whole food supplements if you need them and you will do fine. The right kind of herbs, superfoods such as E3Live, spirulina, wheatgrass can specifically be of help to women. Wheatgrass is very good in this kind of a concern.

109. HOW CAN I PREVENT HOT FLASHES?

VIKTORAS KULVINSKAS

Due to the dead food aging process, one has a limited amount of enzymes, which are needed for the activity of the immune function. One way to make enzymes work harder takes into account that, for every degree rise in temperature, there's a 35% increase in enzyme activity. Thus, by increasing the temperature by one, two, three degrees, all of a sudden, you're doubling and tripling the enzymes, thus enabling the immune system to clean up the bloodstream of toxins that would have been normally eliminated through the excretion of the menstrual flow, which right now is not taking place.

Take enzyme supplements. Why? There is toxemia for excretion, due to the fact that you're consuming animal protein and processed foods and pasteurized dairy products. Stop it! Go on a vegan diet, go on mostly raw, and you will see the hot flashes disappear. Also, increase the consumption of liquids, especially in the form of green vegetable juices.

GABRIEL COUSENS

The heat system is controlled by the hypothalamic function, and I've had very good success with patients working with tryptophan. Tryptophan has been very successful in treating hot flashes, because tryptophan works on the temperature control areas. It seems to be the single easiest remedy. Tryptophan is an amino acid. In addition to a holistic lifestyle with live-food nutrition, tryptophan will minimize hot flashes.

BRIAN CLEMENT

By having balanced hormones. What I just suggested is by far the most intelligent and prudent way to do that—eating properly, not taking hormonally-rich foods like animal-based food, etc.

FRED BISCI

It goes without saying that stimulants such as coffee, alcohol and certain medications are detrimental to anybody's well-being, including women who suffer from hot flashes. A woman that has been following a healthy lifestyle, omitting all the processed foods, will find that meopause can actually be a rewarding part of her life. When a woman goes into menopause, she does not stop all of her hormone production. She reaches the point where she is just not reproductive. I know many women who follow this type of a lifestyle and have no symptoms from menopause. They just stop menstruating. Of course, there are vitamin supplements, nutraceuticals and herbal formulas and homeopathic formulas that can help. The real answer is to cleanse your GI tract and lymph system, and follow a plant-based diet devoid of all processed food, and your meopause symptoms should be minimal to none.

> "A woman that has been following a healthy lifestyle, omitting all the processed foods, will find that menopause can actually be a rewarding part of her life." – Fred Bisci

110. WILL CHANGING MY DIET AFFECT MY MENSTRUAL CYCLE?

GABRIEL COUSENS

Yes. My experience with women on the live food cuisine is that there is a decrease in the time spent menstruating. I recommend that women menstruate at least a day in their cycle as it denotes a normal physiological function. Women who stop having periods are often those who don't eat enough fat, women who are very athletic, or women who are more fruitarian in their approach. In nature, infertility is a sign that one is not healthy enough to reproduce.

My overall observation is that when women go onto a live food diet, their length and intensity of flow is significantly decreased. It is important, however, not to go to an extreme in thinking, by idealizing not having any period. Nature has a way of protecting the survival of the species. Not having any period can definitely happen on a low fat, low protein, live food cuisine.

If one is not having one's period, it can be interpreted as nature's way of protecting the survival of the species, because one does not have enough nutrients and hormonal base to actually carry the baby or, in a sense, create a healthy baby.

I recommend, for health, to maintain a certain amount of body fat and be very happy when the period comes because it still has its function. I would definitely be concerned if one's period disappears, as that is a potential sign of infertility and general nutrient weakness.

BRIAN CLEMENT

The answer is, yes. Women experiencing menstrual cycles in indigenous tribes I visited don't wear pads or tampons and they don't bleed profusely. At least, I never saw one in the several times I've been in these tribal areas over weeks in my life. What we find is that an odorless gel comes out about 10 or 11 months a year, and only a little bit of blood comes out with these women.

In our culture, because we're collecting debris, problems, chemicals, God knows what is absorbed into our bodies, animal fats, things that ought not to be there, female bodies start to purge all of that through the menstrual cycle. You're used to profuse bleeding via all of these chemicals coming out and that, in some part, is why women have historically lived longer than men. Men don't have that outlet. The debris we collect stays within the tissue mass of the body. When you change and get rid of all of that, you don't have this profuse menstruation occurring. You're not having the fats in your body that actually propel hormonal imbalance and you regulate. Now, there's an unhealthy level of this. If somebody becomes too skinny and doesn't lift weights and doesn't build muscle, then you have an abnormal menstrual cycle. You shouldn't have pain, or be suffering from PMS—which 6 out of 10 women do today—you shouldn't be bleeding profusely. It should be odorless and it shouldn't be problematic, the way it seems to be.

VIKTORAS KULVINSKAS

It certainly will. It obviously has affected you by changing your diet from the natural Genesis 1:29 diet to the modern diet of our society. It has brought on where the menstrual cycle begins at the age of 8 or 10, and the breast development starts by the time girls are 12, and earlier. That's called accelerated aging due to the consumption in high volumes of the processed, genetically modified, and/or heat-treated animal protein that abound for breakfast, lunch and dinner.

The influence of natural components, such as vitamin C and bioflavonoids, has been studied by Dr. Dobson at Methodist Hospital in Brooklyn, New York, which I document in my book, *Life in the Twenty-First Century*, where the research was done on 100 nurses. By introducing merely a vitamin C complex, the consequence was the number of menstrual pads used was reduced by over 66%. That's how dramatic it can be, because it strengthens the capillaries and arteries.

"The real answer is to improve your dietary habits." - Viktoras Kulvinskas

During the normal cycle of menstruation, the body is being prepared for conception and fertilization by a male sperm. In the event that that does not occur, the lining, the endometrium, gets reabsorbed. The percentage of re-absorption is a function of how good the circulation is in the endometrium. Dr. Bieler, a medical doctor, in his book, *Food is Your Best Medicine*, made strong commentaries that the processed starches, as well as the consumption of heat-treated animal protein, creates a severe impact on the arteries. If the arterioles in the endometrium go to varicosity stage, during the change in blood pressure that occurs during the reabsorption of the endometrium, they end up hemorrhaging. Breakage and seepage of blood, of toxic waste products, and the tissues that have been destroyed by the toxicity of the blood itself, are parts of the menstrual flow.

In my book, *Survival in the Twenty-First Century*, I document everything I state and much more, on the whole subject of menstruation. I've done a study with 90 women, 60 of them stayed on the program for a whole year. These were raw food eating women, mostly on living food. None of them had a menstrual period. All they had was a slight mucal discharge and a change in basal temperature during the time of ovulation. All ovulated normally. Thus, they were capable of conception.

Exercise has a great influence on the duration and the severity and discomforts associated with menstruation. Generally, exercising women are also on a better nutritional program. Menstruation is very short in comparison to the average American girl, when you look at the menstrual cycles associated with competitive athletes.

By improving your nutritional intake just for a duration of four days before the onset of menses, that is by staying on vegetable soups, away from animal protein, away from pasteurized dairy products, eat only whole vegan foods, you'll find that the menstrual flow will be quite comfortable and it will be shorter in duration.

Blue-green algae is one singular product that has made a radical difference during the many years that I have been involved in the blue-green algae related research—in the influence on female hormones, as well as on the menstrual cycle. One classic example was a woman who was in her early 30s. Her menstrual would be at least 15 days, during which time she would be disabled. By consuming blue-green algae and enzymes, within a duration of four months, she didn't even know she was going through the cycle. That's how radical of an influence it could have.

The real answer is to improve your dietary habits to where you're consuming predominantly, or altogether, not only vegan but mostly raw, and you will find that the menstrual cycle will be reduced to a comfortable level.

A very close relative of mine, as an example, came to work at Hippocrates Health Institute when I was running it in Boston. Within a period of six months during her stay there, her cycle was reduced to only a few hours, like six, seven hours, when before that, it was eight days in duration, even though she consumed a little bit of cooked food outside of our environment, as well as smoked occasionally, as well as drank a cup of coffee.

Radical influence of dietary habits on the menstrual cycle is very clearly observed.

FRED BISCI

Changing your diet and lifestyle to a plant-based diet, with reduction or elimination of animal protein, will have a beneficial effect on your menstrual cycle. Everything is chemical and action and reaction. By making these changes, your body should, in most cases, normalize the menstrual cycle. There are some cases where raw food females get too thin, do not have enough fat on their body and could stop menstruating, or just stain and still be ovulating. In many of these cases, they need more calories. I do not like to recommend intervention with supplements unless it is absolutely necessary. In most cases, when the lifestyle and diet is correct, supplements are not necessary.

111. WHAT IS THE BEST WAY FOR ME TO PREVENT BREAST CANCER?

VIKTORAS KULVINSKAS

The worst culprits are always pasteurized dairy products, and then the contribution from animal protein is extremely significant. There are many studies to confirm that. Even if you do have breast cancer, do not be dismayed. Fourth stage breast cancer, with radical lifestyle alterations, the cancer potentially can be reversed within a matter of five months. It involves radical dietary changes. The whole subject of cancer in its full details can be found in *Survival in the Twenty-First Century*, with documentation.

Some of the lesser-known causes for the development of breast cancer, or contributing factors in the cancer, are the kind of bras that women wear where it leads to reduced circulation in that region, thus predisposing to low oxidative states. Read *Killer Clothes* by Brian Clement.

Further, is the emotional state. Louise Hayes does it great justice in her exploration of the relationship between emotionality and all forms of cancer. Anger issues—in a relationship to the male partner who is abusive, non-appreciative and non-communicative—lead to a lot of

"...the kind of bras that women wear where it leads to reduced circulation..." - Viktoras Kulvinskas

emotional stress, which shows up with poor self-worth, leading to comfort foods and the appearance of either breast cancer or ovarian or uterine cancer and tumors. Use her DVDs, as well as her book, to start changing your attitude by forgiving, self-loving, unconditional love toward yourself and others. And if necessary, if there is no chance of resolution, leave your partner. You are much better off to be alone and with God and develop quality friendships, especially with women. Don't rush into another nonproductive relationship until you raise your standards.

GABRIEL COUSENS

The best way to prevent breast cancer is a live food plant-source-only diet. Also, some of the research is suggesting that adequate iodine supplementation can decrease rates of breast cancer. The research also shows that high amounts of omega-3 fat in the diet decreases the incidence of breast cancer by 50%.

FRED BISCI

A diet, mostly raw and vegan, devoid of all processed food, along with cleansing the GI tract, the lymphatic system and at a cellular level, is best. This will optimize your immune system. We must remember, we are living in a very toxic environment, and some of these elements we do not have control over. It is best to try to detoxify and cleanse your system 3 or 4 times a year.

BRIAN CLEMENT

Number one—exercise, exercise, exercise.

Number two—manipulate or massage the breast area to keep the lymphatic fluid flowing. Certainly, living properly is the way we do it. Also, infrared saunas are amazingly good to help you heal yourself. If you have high estrogens because you've been tested for that, you want to be taking an estrogen blocker that is natural, like a cruciferous vegetable, or a product like Est-Toll—that could be very, very helpful for you. Do not wear synthetic undergarments or clothes.

VIBRANT HEALTH

"Fall in love with life. Find out who you are, what makes you happy, what turns you on, and do it." - Brian Clement

"Realize that life is a series of changes. Don't expect everything to be a constant sameness. Make use of every opportunity to express your highest creative potential." - Viktoras Kulvinskas

"My definition of success is to be a super conductor for the Divine, with a cuisine that supports every aspect of my physical, emotional, mental, and spiritual life." - Gabriel Cousens

"Unconditional love, kindness, generosity and an attitude of gratitude goes a long way in keeping us healthy and happy."
- Fred Bisci

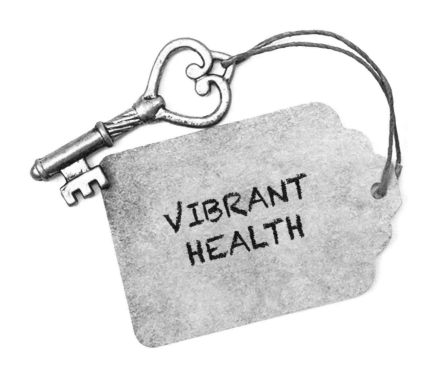

112. IF YOU COULD GIVE ME ONE PIECE OF ADVICE, WHAT WOULD IT BE?

BRIAN CLEMENT

Fall in love with life. Find out who you are, what makes you happy, what turns you on, and do it. In spite of what anyone else says, what anyone else is telling you to do, whatever the economics look like if you do what you love, you're going to be a healthy person. We won't have to be guiding you and telling you how to eat and how to exercise, etc. This is going to naturally and inherently occur for you. This has happened in thousands, in tens of thousands of people's lives I've worked with. It's really about that. It's about finding out who you are. You came to this world with that and slowly but surely, through parental training, so-called education, religious dogma, pieces of your beautiful marble were chipped off you. Now, it's time to pick those up, glue them back on and become whole again. You are a person who has something to offer. You may just not know that at this point. Find out what that is and start giving it out, because the greatest joy in the world is to give yourself, in an authentic, unadulterated form, to all other life.

VIKTORAS KULVINSKAS

In my book, *Love Your Body*, I created a quote: "It is better to do nothing than to waste time." Most people do time in this incarnation, but waste time by not discovering who they are and becoming who they are, namely becoming self-realized human beings. You can do that through self-love, forgiveness and non-judgment.

I cannot over emphasize how important it is to develop a sense of happiness. Happiness with your life and who you are, that is, entering the state of unconditional love for yourself and for others, enjoying your chosen profession, your chosen work and, whatever you do, do it with the highest intention and caliber of service. Realize that life is a series of changes. Don't expect everything to be a constant sameness. Make use of every opportunity to express your highest creative potential.

Step out of the myth of the insanity that has been propagated by our materialistic oriented, greedy society and step into the domain of freedom, liberation, and be free forever of all disease, to be happy until you die and to die in a youthful body, without any pain and suffering - that is, you're finished, you've had enough of planet earth. You're ready to go to your next level of cosmic evolution, so going back to doing nothing. That means totally nothing. That means no physical activity. That means going into savasana.

That is nothingness. Stop eating. Stop drinking. Stop all activities. That includes your brain activity and what happens all of a sudden, you reach for the divine. You are in a state of self-realization and bliss. It's the hardest thing that you could ever achieve or accomplish.

Set those kinds of goals if you wish, if it's for you. Each one of us has a totally different numerological destination or configuration of the zodiac, so it's maybe not for you, but it is for you to be healthy, happy and holy. God Bless You.

GABRIEL COUSENS

The most important thing to understand is that eating is not rocket science. There's an amazing amount of physical, mental, emotional, spiritual, ethical, and moral benefit from eating at least an 80% live food plant-source-only cuisine. Everyone (99.99% of the population) can be successful if they pay attention to all the aspects of what it means to be healthy—including eating according to your constitution, getting enough water, eating a moderate-low glycemic high mineral diet, eating live organic plant-source-only food prepared with love and not overeating.

None of this is complicated. Adjusting one's dietary requirements to age and the seasons also reaps benefits. The other piece of advice is to move one step at a time, according to how you feel you can succeed.

Then, define what you mean by success.

My definition of success is to be a super conductor for the Divine, with a cuisine that supports every aspect of my physical, emotional, mental, and spiritual life.

FRED BISCI

To keep it simple change your lifestyle. Stop eating all processed food. This is a modern day curse. I do see people in my practice and the best I can get them to do is to eliminate all processed food. The results from that alone speaks for itself. In 90% of the cases, their blood profile normalizes. Their energy goes way up. By leaving out processed food, the body goes through a major detox. Try to work towards an 80/20% plant-based raw, as much live food as possible, vegan diet.

Of course, when I talk about a lifestyle change, we are also talking about being spiritually grounded and having a personal relationship with our Creator, developing a sound, emotional and psychological attitude in our life. Unconditional love, kindness, generosity and an attitude of gratitude goes a long way in keeping us healthy and happy.

REFERENCES

Anderson, M. (2009). *Healing Cancer From Inside Out*. RaveDiet.com.

Bisci, F. (2009). *Your Healthy Journey*. Bisci Lifestyle Books.

Carrel, A. (1938). *Man of the Unknown*. Halycon House.

Clement, A. M. (2014). *The Power of a Woman*. Hippocrates Publications.

Clement, B. (2012). *7 Keys to Lifelong Sexual Vitality*. New World Library.

Clement, B. (2014). *Food IS Medicine, Foods that Undermine your Health, Volume Three*. Hippocrates Publications.

Clement, B. (2013). *Food Is Medicine: Edible Plant Foods, Fruits, and Spices from A to Z, Evidence for Their Healing Properties*, Vol. 2. Hippocrates Publications.

Clement, B. (2012). *Food Is Medicine: The Scientific Evidence - Volume One*. Hippocrates Publications.

Clement, B. (2007). *Hippocrates Lifeforce: Superior Health and Longevity*. Healthy Living Publications.

Clement, B. (2011). *Killer Clothes: How Seemingly Innocent Clothing Choices Endanger Your Health...and how to protect yourself!* Hippocrates Publications.

Clement, B. (2012). *Killer Fish: How Eating Aquatic Life Endangers Your Health*. Hippocrates Publications.

Clement, B. (1998). *Living Foods for Optimum Health : Staying Healthy in an Unhealthy World*. Harmony.

Clement, B. (1998). *Living Foods for Optimum Health*. Harmony.

Clement, B. (2006). *Longevity: Enjoying Long Life Without Limits*. Jouvence.

Clement, B. (2009). *Supplements Exposed: The Truth They Don't Want You to Know About Vitamins, Minerals, and Their Effects on Your Health*. New Page Books.

Cousens, G. (2000). *Conscious Eating*. North Atlantic Books.

Cousens, G. (2001). *Depression-free for Life: A Physician's All-Natural, 5-Step Plan*. William Morrow Paperbacks.

Cousens, G. (2005). *Spiritual Nutrition*. North Atlantic Books.

Cousens, G. *Spiritual Nutrition and the Rainbow Diet*. Cassandra.

Cousens, G. (2013). *There is a Cure for Diabetes*. North Atlantic Books.

D'Adamo, P. J. (1996). *Eat Right 4 Your Type: The Individualized Diet Solution to Staying Healthy, Living Longer & Achieving Your Ideal Weight*. G.P. Putnam's Sons.

Ehret, A. (2011). *Mucusless Diet Healing System*. Ehret Literature Publications.

Epstein, S. S. (2009). *Toxic Beauty: How Cosmetics and Personal-Care Products Endanger Your Health... and What You Can Do About It*. BenBella Books.

Fitzgerald, R. (2007). *The Hundred Year Lie: How to Protect yourself from the Chemicals That Are Destroying Your Health*. Plume.

Hawkins, D. R. (2014). *Power vs. Force*. Hay House, Inc.

Hunsberger, E. M. (1992). *How I Conquered Cancer Naturally*. Avery.

Kulvinskas, V. (2010). *Survival in the 21st Century*. Book Publishing Company.

Mini, J. (2012). *Marijuana Syndromes: How to Balance and Optimize the Effects of Cannabis with Traditional Chinese Medicine*. CreateSpace Independent Publishing Platform.

Pacholok, S. M. (2011). *Could It Be B12?: An Epidemic of Misdiagnoses*. Quill Driver Books.

Pilzer, P. Z. (2007). *Wellness Revolution, The Next Trillion*. Wiley.

Ratey, J. J. (2013). *Spark: The Revolutionary New Science of Exercise and the Brain*. Little, Brown and Company.

Robbins, J. (2010). The Food Revolution: How Your Diet Can Help Save Your Life and Our World. Conari Press.

Romieu, e. a. (2012). *Dietary glycemic index and glycemic load and breast cancer risk in the European Prospective Investigation into Cancer and Nutrition (EPIC)*. American Journal of Clinical Nutrition.

Shinya, H. (2010). *The Enzyme Factor*. Millichap Books.

Szekely, E. (1981). *The Essene Gospel of Peace*. International Biogenic Society.

Wentz, D. (2012). *The Healthy Home: Simple Truths to Protect Your Family from Hidden Household Dangers*. Vanguard Press.

INDEX

T

U

V

W

X

Y

WITH APPRECIATION

Thank you for reading Our Elders Speak! Although the 4 authors have slight variations in their opinions, they all lead to the same conclusion: a tried and true formula to keep your body and mind healthy and prevent dis-ease. It is clear that you must remain alkalized, mineralized, hydrated, and keep your body, mind and spirit sound and strong. Incorporating more living foods, juices, fermented foods, in other words— trying to eat an 80% living foods diet—will help you thrive. But also, it's important to know that your diet may require additional superfood supplementation—including algaes, B12 and more. Your body is self-healing and self-preserving. It just needs proper nutrition, guidance and self-love to flourish.

Our Elders have given you the key to unlock the door to vibrant health, longevity and happiness.

May your life journey be filled with blessings!

For continuing education, and ongoing dialogue with
Our Elders please visit

OurEldersSpeak.com